# MYOFASCIAL TRIGGER POINTS

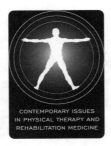

Jones and Bartlett's
*Contemporary Issues in Physical Therapy and Rehabilitation Medicine* **Series**

**Series Editor**
Peter A. Huijbregts, PT, MSc, MHSc, DPT, OCS,
FAAOMPT, FCAMT

**Other Books in the Series**

*Now Available*

*Tension-Type and Cervicogenic Headache:*
*Pathophysiology, Diagnosis, and Management*
César Fernández-de-las-Peñas, PT, DO, PhD
Lars Arendt-Nielsen, DMSci, PhD
Robert D. Gerwin, MD, FAAN

*Orthopaedic Manual Therapy Diagnosis:*
*Spine and Temporomandibular Joints*
Aad van der El, BPE, BSc, PT, Dip. MT, Dip. Acupuncture

*Wellness and Physical Therapy*
Sharon Elayne Fair, PT, MS, PhD

**Coming Soon**

*Clinical Prediction Rules:*
*A Physical Therapy Reference Manual*
Paul E. Glynn, PT, DPT, OCS, FAAOMPT
P. Cody Weisbach, PT, DPT

*Post-Surgical Rehabilitation After Artificial Disc Replacement:*
*An Evidence-Based Guide to Comprehensive Patient Care*
John N. Flood, DO, FACOS, FAOAO
Roy Bechtel, PT, PhD
Scott Benjamin, PT, DScPT

# MYOFASCIAL TRIGGER POINTS
## Pathophysiology and Evidence-Informed Diagnosis and Management

Edited by
**Jan Dommerholt, PT, DPT, MPS, DAAPM**
President
Bethesda Physiocare/Myopain Seminars

**Peter Huijbregts, PT, MSc, MHSc, DPT, OCS, FAAOMPT, FCAMT**
Assistant Professor
University of St. Augustine for Health Sciences

**JONES AND BARTLETT PUBLISHERS**
*Sudbury, Massachusetts*
BOSTON    TORONTO    LONDON    SINGAPORE

*World Headquarters*
Jones and Bartlett Publishers
40 Tall Pine Drive
Sudbury, MA 01776
978-443-5000
info@jbpub.com
www.jbpub.com

Jones and Bartlett Publishers
Canada
6339 Ormindale Way
Mississauga, Ontario L5V 1J2
Canada

Jones and Bartlett Publishers
International
Barb House, Barb Mews
London W6 7PA
United Kingdom

Jones and Bartlett's books and products are available through most bookstores and online booksellers. To contact Jones and Bartlett Publishers directly, call 800-832-0034, fax 978-443-8000, or visit our website, www.jbpub.com.

Substantial discounts on bulk quantities of Jones and Bartlett's publications are available to corporations, professional associations, and other qualified organizations. For details and specific discount information, contact the special sales department at Jones and Bartlett via the above contact information or send an email to specialsales@jbpub.com.

The authors, editors, and publisher have made every effort to provide accurate information. However, they are not responsible for errors, omissions, or for any outcomes related to the use of the contents of this book and take no responsibility for the use of the products and procedures described. Treatments and side effects described in this book may not be applicable to all people; likewise, some people may require a dose or experience a side effect that is not described herein. Drugs and medical devices are discussed that may have limited availability controlled by the Food and Drug Administration (FDA) for use only in a research study or clinical trial. Research, clinical practice, and government regulations often change the accepted standard in this field. When consideration is being given to use of any drug in the clinical setting, the health care provider or reader is responsible for determining FDA status of the drug, reading the package insert, and reviewing prescribing information for the most up-to-date recommendations on dose, precautions, and contraindications, and determining the appropriate usage for the product. This is especially important in the case of drugs that are new or seldom used.

**Production Credits**
Publisher: David Cella
Associate Editor: Maro Gartside
Editorial Assistant: Teresa Reilly
Production Manager: Julie Bolduc
Marketing Manager: Grace Richards
Manufacturing and Inventory Control
  Supervisor: Amy Bacus

Composition: Glyph International
Cover Design: Scott Moden
Cover Image: © Sofia Santos/ShutterStock, Inc.
Printing and Binding: Malloy, Inc.
Cover Printing: Malloy, Inc.

**Library of Congress Cataloging-in-Publication Data**
Myofascial trigger points : pathophysiology and evidence-informed diagnosis and management / [edited by] Jan Dommerholt, Peter Huijbregts.
    p. ; cm.
Includes bibliographical references and index.
ISBN 978-0-7637-7974-0 (alk. paper)
1. Myofascial pain syndromes.  I. Dommerholt, Jan. II. Huijbregts, Peter.
[DNLM: 1.  Myofascial Pain Syndromes—physiopathology. 2.  Myofascial Pain Syndromes—diagnosis.
3.  Myofascial Pain Syndromes—therapy.  WE 550 M9975 2010]
RC927.3.M965 2010
616.7'4—dc22
    6048                                    2009041284
Printed in the United States of America
13  12  11  10  09    10 9 8 7 6 5 4 3 2 1

# DEDICATION

Jan Dommerholt would like to dedicate this book to Mona, Taliah, and Aram.

Peter Huijbregts would like to dedicate this book to his parents, who taught him to work hard, and to Rap, Arun, and Annika, who gave him a reason to work less.

# CONTENTS

**Chapter 5**  Interrater Reliability of Palpation of Myofascial Trigger Points in
Three Shoulder Muscles

**Carel Bron, PT, MT**

**Jo Franssen, PT**

**Michel J. P. Wensing, PhD**

**Rob A. B. Oostendorp, PT, MT, PhD**

**Chapter 6**  Contributions of Myofascial Trigger Points to Chronic Tension-Type
Headache

**César Fernández-de-las-Peñas, PT, DO, PhD**

**Lars Arendt-Nielsen, DMSci, PhD**

**David G. Simons, BSc, MD, DSc (Hon), DSc (Hon)**

| Part 4 | **Future Research Directions** |

# INTRODUCTION BY THE SERIES EDITOR

Peter A. Huijbregts, PT, MSc, MHSc, DPT, OCS, FAAOMPT, FCAMT
Series Editor, *Contemporary Issues in Physical Therapy and Rehabilitation Medicine*
Victoria, British Columbia, Canada

Other than a summary mention of myogelosis as a possible palpatory finding that might be relevant when choosing from among massage techniques, I remember no discussion of pain of myofascial origin as part of my entry-level degree in physical therapy in The Netherlands. And although at least one of the required texts for the postgraduate degree in manual therapy that I completed in Belgium discussed the topic in depth,[1] clinical diagnosis and management of myofascial trigger points similarly was not dealt with in class during this degree program. During further postgraduate study in orthopaedic manual therapy in the United States, myofascial trigger points were either not discussed or were summarily dismissed as a nonexistent condition.[2] When I served as a physical therapy clinical instructor while working in the United States, I insisted that my interns provide some convincing evidence or otherwise stop wasting their time (and, more importantly, their patients' time) on unproven concepts and instead concentrate on the tried-and-true articular dysfunction as the main cause for most patients' complaints. I considered any myofascial abnormality I found in my patients to be secondary to the primary articular dysfunction and was quite convinced that such minor issues would disappear once I had adequately dealt with the dysfunctional joint.

Of course, I could deny some of the responsibility for my past joint-centered convictions by stating that the account above is just reflective of earlier and simpler times. However, to some (certainly not minor) extent this primacy of the articular dysfunction remains at the core of many educational programs in orthopaedic manual therapy available to physical therapists today. For me personally, myofascial trigger points only entered into my clinical reasoning process as a relevant construct after completing a course in dry needling. It was not that I agreed with the hypothesis of a radiculopathic etiology for all chronic myofascial pain presented there.[3] Rather it was the admittedly anecdotal evidence of clinical effects I observed in my patients once I incorporated dry needling into my existing approach of education, manual therapy, and specific exercise interventions. Perhaps even more important was the fact that I started considering myofascial trigger points as a possible primary or at least contributory dysfunction rather than solely as an almost irrelevant secondary problem. Based both on the literature and on my own clinical experience, I started considering myofascial trigger points in the differential diagnosis for a great variety of patients, including those with radiculopathy, intervertebral disk dysfunction, joint dysfunction, tendinopathy, craniomandibular dysfunction, headaches (including migraine, tension-type, and cluster headache), whiplash-associated disorder, pelvic pain and other urologic syndromes, postherpetic neuralgia, fibromyalgia, and complex regional pain syndrome.[4-6]

However, even as I eagerly incorporated myofascial trigger points into my everyday clinical practice, I realized that there were a lot of questions that remained to be answered. The expanded integrated trigger point hypothesis has been proposed to explain trigger point pathophysiology. Centering on endplate dysfunction and a cascade of associated biochemical changes, this elegant hypothesis has the potential to guide both clinical management and ongoing research.[7] In fact, recent microdialysis studies of the local chemical milieu of active myofascial trigger points seem to support the hypothesis.[8] A multitude of genetic abnormalities have been described that can lead to the endplate dysfunction that is central to this hypothesis.[9] The integrated hypothesis also allows us to almost seamlessly integrate emerging knowledge in the area of pain neurobiology on the role of central and peripheral sensitization, as have been shown to occur in chronic myofascial pain states. But how does this hypothesis relate to suggestions seemingly plausible in some of my patients that neuropathic changes of the nerve root or peripheral nerves might be responsible for the clinical signs and symptoms that we commonly associate with myofascial trigger points?[3,10]

Questions also remain with regard to diagnosis and management. With equivocal opinions on the relevance of the electrodiagnostic findings of endplate noise proposed to be specific to trigger points,[8,11] recent research into magnetic resonance elastography[12,13] is promising from a research perspective, but it hardly has the potential to provide us with a readily accessible clinical gold standard test. Many interventions have been described for myofascial trigger points, but research support often barely exceeds the anecdotal level. Dry needling can serve as an example. Although preliminary evidence exists for its use in patients with chronic low back pain,[14] a recent meta-analysis[15] could not support that it is superior to other interventions or even to placebo. However, this might be due less to actual effect size of this intervention and more to lack of study homogeneity which, considering the multitude of treatment and interaction-related variables, may not come as a surprise.[16] Similar problems occur when studying other proposed interventions.

This book does not purport to answer all of the questions surrounding myofascial pain and myofascial trigger points; admittedly, there are many. In fact, on many occasions it will provide the reflective clinician with new and unexpected questions. It is also not meant as a comprehensive or uncritical resource on all things myofascial. Rather, with its combination of research, clinical experience and expertise, suggestions relevant to everyday clinical practice, critical analysis, and the presentation of hypotheses, it intends to serve solely as an introduction for those clinicians willing to look beyond the joint-centered paradigm that is still so central in many schools of thought within orthopaedic manual therapy and thereby perhaps provide some suggestions for managing patient problems not adequately addressed under that paradigm.

# References

1. Van der El A. *Orthopaedic Manual Therapy Diagnosis: Spine and Temporomandibular Joints*. Sudbury, MA: Jones & Bartlett; 2010.

2. Paris SV, Loubert PV. *Foundations of Clinical Orthopaedics*. 3rd ed. St. Augustine, FL: Institute Press; 1999.

3. Gunn CC. *The Gunn Approach to the Treatment of Chronic Pain: Intramuscular Stimulation for Myofascial Pain of Radiculopathic Origin*. New York, NY: Churchill Livingstone; 1996.

4. Borg-Stein J, Simons DG. Focused review: Myofascial pain. *Arch Phys Med Rehabil* 2002;83(suppl):S40–S49.

5. Fernández-de-las-Peñas C. Interactions between trigger points and joint hypomobility: A clinical perspective. *J Manual Manipulative Ther* 2009;17:74–77.

6. Calandre EP, Hidalgo J, Gracia-Leiva JM, Rico-Villademoros F, Delgado-Rodriguez A. Myofascial trigger points in cluster headache patients: A case series. *Head and Face Medicine* 2008;4:32.

7. Gerwin RD, Dommerholt J, Shah JP. An expansion of Simons' integrated hypothesis of trigger point formation. *Curr Pain Headache Rep* 2004;8:468–475.

8. Shah JP, Gilliams EA. Uncovering the biochemical milieu of myofascial trigger points using in vivo microdialysis: An application of muscle pain concepts to myofascial pain syndrome. *J Bodywork Movement Ther* 2008;12:371–384.

9. McPartland JM. Travell trigger points: Molecular and osteopathic perspectives. *J Am Osteopath Assoc* 2004;104:244–249.

10. Butler DS. *The Sensitive Nervous System*. Adelaide, Australia: Noigroup Publications; 2000.

11. Huguenin LK. Myofascial trigger points: The current evidence. *Phys Ther Sport* 2004;5:2–12.

12. Chen Q, Bensamoun S, Basford JR, Thompson JM, An KN. Identification and quantification of myofascial taut bands with magnetic resonance elastography. *Arch Phys Med Rehabil* 2007;88:1658–1661.

13. Chen Q, Basford J, An KN. Ability of magnetic resonance elastography to assess taut bands. *Clin Biomech* 2008;23:623–629.

14. Furlan AD, Van Tulder MW, Cherkin DC, Tsukayama H, Lao L, Koes BW, Berman BM. Acupuncture and dry needling for low back pain. *Cochrane Database of Systematic Reviews* 2005; Issue 1. Art. No.: CD 001351. DOI: 10.1002/14651858.CD001351.pub2.

15. Tough EA, White AR, Cummings TM, Richards SH, Campbell JL. Acupuncture and dry needling in the management of myofascial trigger point pain: A systematic review and meta-analysis of randomised controlled trials. *Eur J Pain* 2009;13:3–10.

16. Rickards LD. Therapeutic needling in osteopathic practice: An evidence-informed perspective. *Int J Osteopath Med* 2009;12:2–13.

# INTRODUCTION

Myofascial pain is arguably one of the more common clinical findings in patients presenting with musculoskeletal pain. However, only a very limited number of academic programs in physical therapy, medicine, osteopathy, and chiropractic include specific courses on the identification and management of myofascial trigger points. Despite the impressive surge over the last decade in the number of high-quality research articles, literature reviews, and case studies providing a solid basis for integrating myofascial pain concepts into clinical practice and academic preparation, there seemingly remains a noted degree of resistance among health-care providers, academicians, and legislators. Some state boards of physical therapy, associations, charters, and societies continue to be reluctant when it comes to acknowledging and incorporating trigger point therapies. For example, as recent as October of 2008 the Nevada Board of Physical Therapy Examiners concluded unanimously that trigger point dry needling would not be within the scope of physical therapy practice.

Interestingly, although skeletal muscle constitutes nearly half of our body weight, it is the only organ that is not linked to a specific medical specialty.[1] This may partly explain why the scientific study of muscle-specific ailments in the sense of epidemiology, pathophysiology, and diagnostic and treatment options has not evolved until fairly recently. Articles and information on myofascial pain and trigger points are scattered over many disciplines and journals, with many of these journals not included in the more easily accessible literature databases that have become a cornerstone to current evidence-informed clinical practice. Despite these obstacles to professional discourse and scientific study, the last decade has seen a near-explosive increase in the literature discussing the nature, characteristics, and relevance of muscle pain.[2] We should note that the literature is far from uniform in the relevance it attaches to myofascial pain states. Some authors consider muscle pain as merely an epiphenomenon to tendonitis, joint degeneration, muscle strain, inflammation, or injuries to peripheral nerves or joints. Exercise-related muscle pain or delayed-onset muscle soreness is often summarily dismissed as temporary discomfort in the context of eccentric loading. Patients complaining about widespread muscle pain often noted in myofascial pain conditions are frequently regarded as most likely suffering from somatoform disorders.

Another likely reason knowledge with regard to myofascial trigger points has not permeated mainstream medicine and physical therapy to a greater degree is that historically manual physical therapists and physicians have directed their attention mostly to articular dysfunction. This occurred even though manual medicine pioneers, such as medical physicians James Cyriax and John Mennell, did include muscle dysfunction and myofascial trigger points in their thinking. Cyriax was strongly influenced by publications by Kellgren on pain referred from muscles[3,4] and advocated treating nodules and taut bands of abnormal muscle tissue with deep friction massage.[5] Cyriax is generally acknowledged as the founding father of modern manual medicine and orthopaedic manual physical therapy (OMPT) practice.[6] Mennell has been honored for his contributions to OMPT with an award named after him by the American Academy of Orthopaedic Manual Physical Therapy. Medical physician Janet Travell, who is generally credited with the introduction of the myofascial pain concepts and who documented common referred pain patterns from trigger points,[7] worked closely with Mennell. However, in contrast to Mennell, she is rarely mentioned in the manual medicine literature. In fact, in the history of OMPT, and perhaps contributing to the lack of emphasis within OMPT on the concepts she developed, Travell is mostly remembered for blocking physical therapists from membership in the North American Academy of Manipulative Medicine, an organization she founded in 1966 with Mennell.[6]

In the past decade, there has been an increased research emphasis on the neurobiology of pain and, with that, on the mechanisms of muscle-related pain. Muscle pain, and more specifically, trigger point pain have been shown to activate cortical structures, including the anterior cingulate gyrus.[8-10] Under normal circumstances, pain initiated from muscles is inhibited strongly by the descending pain-modulating pathways, with a dynamic balance between the degree of activation of dorsal horn neurons and the descending inhibitory systems. Prolonged nociceptive input from myofascial trigger points can be misinterpreted in the central nervous system and eventually can lead to allodynia and hyperalgesia and an expansion of receptive fields.[11,12] The scientific basis of trigger point therapies has evolved much beyond the empiric observations of many astute clinicians over the past five decades. The integrated trigger point hypothesis, introduced in 1999, is the best available model to explain the trigger point phenomena.[13] Several publications have since expanded upon this hypothesis based on more recent electrodiagnostic and histopathological studies and other related fields.[14-17]

We can all agree that the management of patients with musculoskeletal and myofascial trigger point–related pain should be based on a thorough understanding of the underlying mechanisms of motor, sensory, and autonomic dysfunction. Understanding the motor aspects of trigger points requires detailed knowledge of the motor endplate, the sarcomere assembly, the nature of the taut band, and the impact of trigger points on movement patterns. Recent studies have been able to visualize and explore characteristics of the taut bands, considered one diagnostic feature of myofascial trigger points, by way of magnetic resonance elastography.[18,19] Another study has demonstrated an objective topographical system that can be used to identify trigger points.[20] To better understand the sensory aspects of myofascial trigger points, including local and referred tenderness, pain, and paresthesiae, the mechanisms and function of muscle nociceptors, spinal cord mechanisms, and peripheral and central sensitization need to be explored. Recent studies at the National Institutes of Health in the United States have considerably advanced the basic science knowledge base with regard to the chemical milieu of trigger points.[21,22] We need to acknowledge here that the understanding of the autonomic components of trigger points is still rather unexplored.[23]

In consideration of the still limited incorporation of and at times outright resistance to myofascial pain concepts within the various health professions involved, we aim for this book to offer a current best-evidence review of the etiology, underlying mechanisms, pathophysiology, and clinical implications of myofascial trigger points. We have brought together a collection of both original work and chapters previously published or adapted from published papers with the intent of providing as comprehensive an overview as possible. Contributing authors from seven different countries and three different professional backgrounds (physical therapy, medicine, and osteopathy) highlight important scientific aspects of trigger points. Throughout the book, an emphasis is placed on the scientific merits of the literature. Rather than being a book that without critical evaluation introduces and discusses the trigger point concept, the contributing authors point out where scientific evidence is lacking. Hypothetical considerations are clearly identified as such, giving the reader a realistic perspective of our current understanding with regard to trigger points.

The book is divided into four main sections. The initial pathophysiology section includes three chapters. In Chapter 1, McPartland and Simons take the reader through a fascinating review of the integrated trigger point hypothesis. The main motor, sensory, and autonomic features of trigger points are highlighted within the context of clinical manual medicine and manual therapy. Chapter 2, prepared by Dommerholt, Bron, and Franssen, provides a brief historical review of early publications about trigger points and discusses in detail their clinical relevancy for current clinical practice. Emphasis is on the etiology of trigger points with a critical overview of current concepts. This chapter ends with a section of medical and metabolic perpetuating factors, upon which Dommerholt and Gerwin elaborate in great detail in Chapter 3. Physicians, physical therapists, and other clinicians seem not to consider metabolic perpetuating factors in their clinical practices despite a growing body of evidence supporting their importance.

The second section of the book deals primarily with the diagnosis of trigger points. The lack of accepted criteria for the identification of trigger points is reviewed in Chapter 4, where McEvoy and Huijbregts provide an in-depth overview of all published reliability studies with regard to the identification of myofascial trigger points. Bron, Franssen, Wensing, and Oostendorp discuss the interrater reliability of trigger point palpation in shoulder muscles in Chapter 5. Fernández-de-las-Peñas, Arendt-Nielsen, and Simons explore the contribution of myofascial trigger points in the etiology of chronic tension-type headaches in Chapter 6. This chapter also includes a detailed review of the proposed role of myofascial trigger points in peripheral and central sensitization.

The third section of the book discusses clinical management of patients with painful myofascial trigger points. In Chapter 7, Rickards provides a systematic analysis of the evidence with regard to effectiveness of noninvasive treatments. Dommerholt, Mayoral del Moral, and Gröbli review invasive therapies with specific attention to trigger point dry needling in Chapter 8. Issa and Huijbregts conclude this section with a detailed case history of a patient with chronic daily headache, emphasizing the integration of trigger point therapy into a broader therapeutic management approach.

The final section of the book contains only one chapter, but it is perhaps the most important and thought provoking. In this final chapter, Gerwin identifies many areas of interest where the scientific basis is lacking. This chapter will be of great benefit to any basic or clinical researcher looking for pertinent research projects addressing the etiology of trigger points, the epidemiology of myofascial pain, specific treatment issues, and the role of trigger points in various pain syndromes.

We hope that this book will bring the subject of myofascial trigger points closer for both clinicians and researchers. We have compiled objective reviews, studies, case studies, and critical commentaries, and we anticipate that an increasing number of clinicians will consider getting trained in the identification and management of myofascial trigger points. Only through a thorough understanding of the scientific literature will clinicians be able to develop evidence-informed management strategies. Eventually, our patients will benefit from we clinicians incorporating this exciting body of knowledge into our clinical practices.

# References

1. Simons DG. Orphan organ. *J Musculoskel Pain* 2007;15(2):7–9.
2. Graven-Nielsen T, Arendt-Nielsen L. Induction and assessment of muscle pain, referred pain, and muscular hyperalgesia. *Curr Pain Headache Rep* 2003;7(6):443–451.
3. Kellgren JH. Observations on referred pain arising from muscle. *Clin Sci* 1938;3:175–190.
4. Kellgren JH. A preliminary account of referred pains arising from muscle. *British Med J* 1938;1:325–327.
5. Cyriax J. *Massage, Manipulation and Local Anaesthesia*. London, UK: Hamish Hamilton; 1942.
6. Paris SV. A history of manipulative therapy through the ages and up to the current controversy in the United States. *J Manual Manipulative Ther* 2000;8:66–77.
7. Travell JG, Rinzler SH. The myofascial genesis of pain. *Postgrad Med* 1952;11:452–434.
8. Niddam DM, et al. Central modulation of pain evoked from myofascial trigger point. *Clin J Pain* 2007;23:440–448.
9. Niddam DM, et al. Central representation of hyperalgesia from myofascial trigger point. *Neuroimaging* 2008;39:1299–1306.
10. Svensson P, et al. Cerebral processing of acute skin and muscle pain in humans. *J Neurophysiol* 1997;78:450–460.
11. Arendt-Nielsen L, Graven-Nielsen T. Deep tissue hyperalgesia. *J Musculoskel Pain* 2002;10(1–2):97–119.
12. Mense S. The pathogenesis of muscle pain. *Curr Pain Headache Rep* 2003;7:419–425.
13. Simons DG, Travell JG, Simons LS. *Travell & Simons' Myofascial Pain and Dysfunction: The Trigger Point Manual*. 2nd ed. Vol. 1. Baltimore, MD: Lippincott Williams & Wilkins; 1999.
14. Gerwin RD, Dommerholt J, Shah JP. An expansion of Simons' integrated hypothesis of trigger point formation. *Curr Pain Headache Rep* 2004;8:468–475.
15. McPartland JM. Travell trigger points: Molecular and osteopathic perspectives. *J Am Osteopath Assoc* 2004;104:244–249.
16. McPartland JM, Simons DG. Myofascial trigger points: Translating molecular theory into manual therapy. *J Manual Manipulative Ther* 2006;14:232–239.
17. Simons DG. Review of enigmatic MTrPs as a common cause of enigmatic musculoskeletal pain and dysfunction. *J Electromyogr Kinesiol* 2004;14:95–107.
18. Chen Q, Basford J, An KN. Ability of magnetic resonance elastography to assess taut bands. *Clin Biomech* 2008;23:623–629.
19. Chen Q, et al. Identification and quantification of myofascial taut bands with magnetic resonance elastography. *Arch Phys Med Rehabil* 2007;88:1658–1661.
20. Ge HY, et al. Topographical mapping and mechanical pain sensitivity of myofascial trigger points in the infraspinatus muscle. *Eur J Pain* 2008;12:859–865.
21. Shah JP, et al. Biochemicals associated with pain and inflammation are elevated in sites near to and remote from active myofascial trigger points. *Arch Phys Med Rehabil* 2008;89:16–23.
22. Shah JP, et al. An in-vivo microanalytical technique for measuring the local biochemical milieu of human skeletal muscle. *J Appl Physiol* 2005;99:1977–1984.
23. Ge HY, Fernández-de-las-Peñas C, Arendt-Nielsen L. Sympathetic facilitation of hyperalgesia evoked from myofascial tender and trigger points in patients with unilateral shoulder pain. *Clin Neurophysiol* 2006;117:1545–1550.

# CONTRIBUTORS

**Lars Arendt-Nielsen, DMSci, PhD**
Laboratory for Experimental Pain Research
Center for Sensory-Motor Interaction
Department of Health Science and Technology
Aalborg University
Aalborg, Denmark

**Carel Bron, PT, MT**
Practice for Physical Therapy for Disorders of
    the Neck, Shoulder, and Upper Extremity
Groningen, The Netherlands
University Medical Center St. Radboud
Nijmegen, The Netherlands

**Jan Dommerholt, PT, DPT, MPS, DAAPM**
Bethesda Physiocare, Inc.
Bethesda, MD, USA
Myopain Seminars, LLC
Bethesda, MD, USA

**César Fernández-de-las-Peñas, PT, DO, PhD**
Department of Physical Therapy, Occupational
    Therapy, Physical Medicine, and Rehabilitation
Universidad Rey Juan Carlos
Alcorcón, Madrid, Spain
Esthesiology Laboratory
Universidad Rey Juan Carlos
Alcorcón, Madrid, Spain

Center for Sensory-Motor Interaction (SMI)
Department of Health Science and Technology
Aalborg University
Aalborg, Denmark

**Jo Franssen, PT**
Practice for Physical Therapy for Disorders of
    the Neck, Shoulder, and Upper Extremity
Groningen, The Netherlands

**Robert D. Gerwin, MD, FAAN**
Department of Neurology
Johns Hopkins University School of Medicine
Baltimore, MD, USA
Pain and Rehabilitation Medicine
Bethesda, MD, USA

**Christian Gröbli, PT**
David G. Simons Academy
Winterthur, Switzerland
Swiss PhysioCare
Winterthur, Switzerland

**Peter Huijbregts, PT, MSc, MHSc, DPT,
    OCS, FAAOMPT, FCAMT**
University of St. Augustine for Health Sciences
St. Augustine, FL, USA
Shelbourne Physiotherapy and Massage Clinic

Victoria, BC, Canada
North American Institute of Orthopaedic
    Manual Therapy
Eugene, OR, USA

**Tamer Issa, PT, BSc, DPT, OCS**
Issa Physical Therapy
Rockville, MD, USA
Myopain Seminars
Bethesda, MD, USA

**Orlando Mayoral del Moral, PT**
Hospital Provincial de Toledo
Toledo, Spain

**Johnson McEvoy, PT, BSc, MSc, DPT,
    MISCP, MCSP**
Private Practice Physiotherapy
Limerick, Ireland

**John M. McPartland, DO, MS**
Department of Family Practice
College of Medicine
University of Vermont
Middlebury, VT, USA

**Rob A. B. Oostendorp, PT, MT, PhD**
Radboud University Nijmegen Medical Centre
Centre for Quality of Care Research
Department of Allied Health Sciences
Nijmegen, The Netherlands

**Luke D. Rickards, BAppSc, MOsteo**
Kensington Osteopathy
Adelaide, SA, Australia

**David G. Simons, BSc, MD, DSc (Hon), DSc
    (Hon)**
Department of Physical Medicine and
    Rehabilitation
Emory University School of Medicine
Atlanta, GA, USA
School of Health Professions
Division of Physical Therapy
College of Health and Human Sciences
Georgia State University
Atlanta, GA, USA

**Michel J. P. Wensing, PhD**
Scientific Institute for Quality of Healthcare
Radboud University Nijmegen Medical Centre
The Netherlands

# Part 1

# Pathophysiology

# Chapter 1

# Myofascial Trigger Points: Translating Molecular Theory into Manual Therapy

*John M. McPartland, DO, MS*

*David G. Simons, BSc, MD, DSc (Hon), DSc (Hon)*

## Introduction

Simons, Travell, and Simons[1] defined the myofascial trigger point (MTrP) as ". . . a hyper-irritable spot in skeletal muscle that is associated with a hypersensitive palpable nodule in a taut band. The spot is tender when pressed, and can give rise to characteristic referred pain, motor dysfunction, and autonomic phenomena. . . ." Thus, each MTrP contains a sensory component, a motor component, and an autonomic component. These components comprise a new "integrated hypothesis" regarding the etiology of MTrPs.[1] This hypothesis involves local myofascial tissues, the central nervous system (CNS), and systemic biomechanical factors. The "integrated hypothesis" has changed our approach to treating MTrPs. The purpose of this chapter is to review new concepts concerning MTrPs and to describe our evolving approach to their treatment.

## The Motor Endplate: Epicenter of the Myofascial Trigger Point

Simons[2] implicated the motor endplate as the central etiology of MTrPs. The motor endplate is synonymous with the neuromuscular junction (the first term describes structure, the latter term describes function); it is the site where an $\alpha$-motor neuron synapses with its target muscle fibers. The $\alpha$-motor neuron terminates in multiple swellings termed presynaptic boutons. Each bouton contains many acetylcholine (ACh) vesicles, clustered around structures called dense bars (see **Figure 1-1**). Voltage-sensitive calcium channels (VsCCs, specifically P/Q-type VsCCs) also cluster near dense bars. When voltage running down an

Courtesy of John M. Medeiros, PT, PhD, Managing Editor of the *Journal of Manual and Manipulative Therapy*.

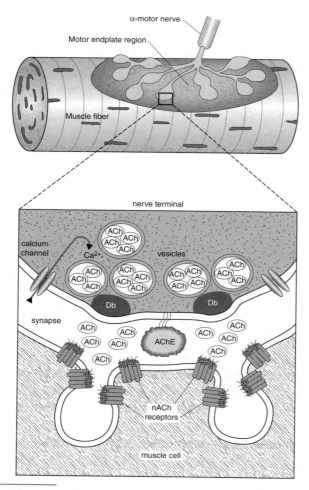

**Figure 1-1** The motor endplate—proposed site of trigger point dysfunction. Top illustration: The junction between the α-motor neuron and the muscle fiber. Bottom illustration: Presynaptic boutons are separated from the postsynaptic muscle cell by the synaptic cleft. Within each bouton are many vesicles containing ACh, clustered around dense bars (Db). Also clustered around the Db are calcium channels. The Db is the site of ACh release into the synaptic cleft. Across the synaptic cleft from the Db, the postsynaptic muscle cell membrane forms junctional folds that are lined with nicotinic ACh receptors (nACh). ACh released into the synaptic cleft activates nACh receptors, then is inactivated by the acetylcholinesterase enzyme (AChE).

*Source:* Redrawn with permission from: McPartland JM, Simons DG. Myofascial trigger points: Translating molecular theory into manual therapy. *J Manual Manipulative Ther* 2006;14:232–239.

α-motor neuron reaches VsCCs in the bouton, the VsCC channels open, leading to an influx of calcium ions ($Ca^{2+}$) into the bouton from the extracellular space. The influx of $Ca^{2+}$ causes the ACh vesicles to release their transmitter into the synaptic cleft (Figure 1-1).

Across the synaptic cleft, the postsynaptic muscle cell membrane forms junctional folds that are lined with nicotinic ACh receptors (nAChs). The nACh is a ligand-gated cation channel, and ACh is its ligand. Binding of ACh to nACh opens its channel, allowing sodium ions ($Na^+$) and potassium ions ($K^+$) to move in and out of the muscle cell membrane. Movement of $Na^+$ and $K^+$ depolarizes the postsynaptic cell, forming a miniature endplate potential (MEPP). A sufficient number of MEPPs activate VsCCs (specifically L-type VsCCs), which subsequently trigger another $Ca^{2+}$ channel, the ryanodine receptor. The ryanodine receptor is imbedded in the membrane of an intracellular structure called the sarcoplasmic reticulum, which houses intracellular stores of $Ca^{2+}$. Activation of the ryanodine receptor releases $Ca^{2+}$ from the sarcoplasmic reticulum into the cytoplasm of the muscle cell. This triggers the interaction between actin and myosin, and the sarcomere contracts.

Electromyography (EMG) studies of MTrPs have reported spontaneous electrical activity (SEA) in MTrPs, while adjacent muscle tissues are electrically silent.[3] Hubbard and Berkoff[3] originally attributed the source of SEA action potentials to sympathetically activated intrafusal muscle spindles. These researchers were unaware of previous work by Liley of New Zealand, who had demonstrated that SEA was a consequence of ACh release at motor endplates.[4] Simons[5] "connected the dots" by correlating SEA with "endplate noise" that had been described by electromyographers, and he linked SEA to excessive ACh release, which he proposed as the primary cause of MTrP development. This "motor endplate" hypothesis was tested in Hong's laboratory,[6] where MTrPs were injected with botulinum toxin type A, which blocks ACh release at the motor endplate. This treatment significantly decreased SEA activity. Mense et al[7] confirmed the hypothesis using a rat MTrP model. They injected diisopropylfluorophosphate (DFP), a drug that increases synaptic ACh, into the proximal half of the gastrocnemius muscle, and the motor nerve was electrically stimulated for 30–60 minutes to induce muscle contractions. The distal half of the muscle, which performed the same contractions, served as a control. Proximal and distal sections of the muscle were then examined for morphological changes. The DFP-injected proximal half exhibited significantly more contracted and torn muscle fibers compared to the distal half of the muscle.

Myofascial tension may play a role in excess ACh release. Chen and Grinnell[8] showed that a 1% increase in muscle stretch at the motor endplate evoked a 10% increase in ACh release. These researchers postulated that tension upon integrins (cell-surface proteins that bind connective tissues) in the presynaptic membrane was transduced mechanically into ACh vesicle release.

## Expanding the Endplate Hypothesis

Simons' description of a presynaptic dysfunction (excessive ACh release), however, is only one way to interpret the endplate hypothesis. We can expand the hypothesis to include presynaptic, intrasynaptic, and postsynaptic dysfunctions.[9] Intrasynaptic ACh must be deactivated; otherwise, it will continue to activate nAChRs in the muscle cell membrane. ACh is normally deactivated by the enzyme acetylcholinesterase (AChE), which is held in the synaptic cleft by a structural protein (collagen Q, ColQ) that anchors it to the plasma membrane (Figure 1-1). AChE deficiency permits excess ACh to accumulate in the synaptic cleft, tonically activating nAChRs. Several genetic mutations cause AChE deficiency, including mutations in ColQ. The gene for AChE expresses several splice variants,[10] which are alternative ways in which a gene's protein-coding sections (exons) are joined together to create a messenger RNA molecule and its translated protein. AChE splice variants are less effective at deactivating ACh, and the expression of these splice variants can be induced by psychological and physical stress.[10] Drugs and other chemicals may cause AChE deficiency. DFP, the drug used in the aforementioned experiment by Mense et al,[7] is an AChE antagonist. Organophosphate pesticides are AChE antagonists, and poisoning by these pesticides causes changes in motor endplates and MTrP-like pathology.[11-13] Muscle damage caused by AChE antagonists has been reduced by pretreatment with postsynaptic L-type VsCC blockers such as quinidine[12] and diltiazem.[13]

Postsynaptically, a "gain-of-function" defect of the nAChR may confer muscle hyperexcitability, a hallmark of MTrPs. Gain of function refers to an increased response by the nAChR, via several possible mechanisms: nAChR overexpression, constitutively active nAChRs,[14] nAChRs that gain responsiveness to choline (an ordinary serum metabolite),[14] or nACHRs whose channels remain open longer than normal.[15] The nAChR is an assembly of 5 subunits; at least 16 genes encode these subunits, so that the nAChR is particularly susceptible to mutational defects. Motor endplate nAChRs express a unique subunit assembly, whereas nAChRs in the central nervous system and in autonomic nerves express a different subunit configuration.[16]

The relative consequences of presynaptic, synaptic, and postsynaptic dysfunctions are under debate. Wang et al[17] used a variety of pharmacological tools to conclude that presynaptic mechanisms modulate the motor endplate rather than synaptic (AChE) or postsynaptic (nAChR density) mechanisms. Conversely, Nakanishi et al[18] determined that postsynaptic manipulation (using α-bungarotoxin, an nAChR antagonist) modulated motor endplates to a greater degree than presynaptic manipulation (using botulinum toxin, an inhibitor of ACh release).

## Motor Component

MTrPs have a motor component, whereas tender points found in patients with fibromyalgia do not. MTrPs have been biopsied and found to contain "contraction knots" described as "large, rounded, darkly staining muscle fibers and a statistically significant increase in the average diameter of muscle fibers...."[19] Thus, the structure of contraction knots differed from that of normal muscle fibers. Functionally, excessive motor activity initiates several perverse mechanisms that cause MTrPs to persist. Muscle contraction compresses local sensory nerves, which reduces the axoplasmic transport of molecules that normally inhibit ACh release.[20,21] Muscle contraction also compresses local blood vessels, reducing the local supply of oxygen. Reduced oxygen, combined with the metabolic demands generated by contracted muscles, results in a rapid depletion of local adenosine triphosphate (ATP).

The resultant "ATP energy crisis"[1] triggers a cascade of pre- and postsynaptic decompensations. Presynaptic ATP directly inhibits ACh release,[22] so depletion of ATP increases ACh release. Postsynaptic ATP powers the $Ca^{2+}$ pump that returns $Ca^{2+}$ to the sarcoplasmic reticulum. Hence, loss of ATP impairs the reuptake of $Ca^{2+}$, which increases contractile activity, creating a vicious cycle.[19] Excess $Ca^{2+}$ may snowball into "$Ca^{2+}$-induced $Ca^{2+}$ release," where $Ca^{2+}$ induces further $Ca^{2+}$ release from intracellular stores via ryanodine receptors, triggering actin and myosin, leading to muscle spasm.

Some controversy surrounds adenosine, a breakdown product of ATP. Adenosine normally decreases motor endplate activity by activating presynaptic adenosine A1 receptors, which reduce P/Q VsCC currents, thus reducing ACh release.[23] However, high levels of synaptic adenosine, from excess ATP breakdown (as is hypothesized to occur in the ATP energy crisis model), may activate postsynaptic adenosine A2 receptors, which recruit L-type VsCCs currents, thus triggering muscle contraction.[24]

MTrPs exert profound, yet unpredictable, influences upon motor function. MTrPs may excite or inhibit normal motor activity in their muscle of origin or in functionally related muscles. Latent MTrPs can be equally influential upon motor function. Motor inhibition is often identified clinically as muscle weakness, but treatment often focuses on strengthening exercises that only augment abnormal muscle substitution until the inhibiting MTrPs are inactivated. This inhibition can also cause poor coordination and muscle imbalances. These MTrP effects have gone largely unrecognized because of a lack of published research studies. Headley has explored these effects using surface electromyography, describing inhibition of the trapezius by MTrPs in the same muscle,[25] inhibition of anterior deltoid by MTrPs in the infraspinatus,[25] inhibition of gluteal muscles by MTrPs in the quadratus lumborum,[25] and excitation (referred spasm) of the paraspinals by MTrPs in the tensor fascia lata.[26,27]

## Sensory Component

MTrPs are painful. Pain begins in peripheral tissues as nociception, transmitted by Aδ- and C-fiber afferent sensory neurons (nociceptors). Mechanical pressure, thermal stimuli, and many chemicals activate nociceptors; potassium ions, protons, and free $O_2$ radicals are by-products of muscle metabolism and the hypothesized ATP energy crisis. Histamine is released from mast cells that migrate into injured tissues. Serotonin is released from platelets after they are exposed to platelet-activating factor (released from the mast cells). Bradykinin is cleaved from serum proteins. All of these chemical "activators" bind to receptors in the nociceptor and initiate an action potential. "Sensitizers" are also released from damaged tissue; examples include prostaglandins, leukotrienes, and substance P. Sensitizers decrease the activation threshold of a neuron, so that the nociceptor fires with less activation. This leads to peripheral sensitization and hyperalgesia.

Sensitizing substances may also generate a focal demyelination of sensory nerves. Demyelination creates abnormal impulse-generating sites (AIGS) capable of generating ectopic nociceptive impulses.[28] Shah et al[29] used a microdialysis needle to sample tissue fluids from the upper trapezius muscle in nine subjects; elevated concentrations of protons, bradykinin, serotonin, substance P, norepinephrine, calcitonin gene-related peptide, tumor necrosis factor-α, and interleukin-1b were detected in active MTrPs, compared to latent MTrPs and control subjects without MTrPs. The difference was statistically significant ($P < 0.01$) despite the small sample size.

A persistent barrage of nociceptive signals from MTrPs may eventually cause "central sensitization," a form of neural plasticity involving functional and/or structural change within the dorsal horn of the spinal cord. The sensitized dorsal horn becomes a "neurologic lens," consolidating other nociceptive signals that converge upon the same segment of the spinal cord, including other somatic dysfunctions and visceral dysfunctions.[1] As a result, postsynaptic spinal neurons exhibit decreased activation thresholds, increased response magnitudes, and increased recruitment of receptive field areas. They fire with increased frequency or fire spontaneously, transmitting nociceptive signals to supraspinal sites, such as the thalamus and cerebral cortex. Central sensitization may also modulate spinal interneurons and descending inhibitory pathways. Central sensitization is symptomatically expressed as allodynia (pain to normally nonpainful stimuli) and hyperalgesia (abnormally increased sensation of pain). Simons, Travell, and Simons[1] described the CNS as an "integrator" of MTrPs, akin to Korr's description[30] of the CNS as an "organizer" of somatic dysfunction.

## Autonomic Component

Autonomic phenomena associated with MTrPs include localized sweating, vasoconstriction or vasodilation, and pilomotor activity ("goose bumps").[1] MTrPs located in the head and neck may cause lacrimation, coryza (nasal discharge), and salivation.[1] The autonomic nervous system (ANS) is primarily involved in reflex arcs, exerting control of cardiac muscle and smooth muscle in blood vessels, glands, and visceral organs. Hubbard and Berkoff[3] reviewed the literature that demonstrated ANS involvement in skeletal muscles and MTrP formation. Sympathetic neurons innervating vessels in skeletal muscles may exit the perivascular space and terminate among intrafusal fibers within muscle spindles. Sympathetic neurons release norepinephrine, a neurotransmitter involved in the "fight-or-flight" response. Norepinephrine activates $\alpha_1$-adrenergic receptors in the intrafusal muscle cell membrane. Activation of $\alpha_1$-adrenergic receptors depresses the feedback control of muscle length, detrimentally affecting motor performance and possibly contributing to the ATP energy crisis.[31] Norepinephrine has been shown to augment the amplitude and duration of MEPPs in frog leg motor endplates.[32] Phentolamine, an antagonist of $\alpha_1$-adrenergic receptors, decreases SEA in MTrPs.[33] Similar effects have been seen with local intramuscular injections of phenoxybenzamine, another $\alpha_1$-adrenergic antagonist.[34]

The ANS may indirectly exacerbate MTrP formation via viscerosomatic reflexes. Visceral autonomic afferents from disturbed viscera carry signals to the dorsal horn.

Chronic input eventually facilitates neurotransmission at that spinal level.[35] This form of central sensitization accelerates in the presence of nociceptor AIGS and ephaptic crosstalk with neighboring autonomic nerves.[9] Ephaptic crosstalk (cross-excitation) is the nonsynaptic interaction between two nerves that are parallel and relatively close together so that their action potentials influence each other.

## Translating Theory to Therapy

The motor endplate and ATP energy crisis hypotheses have changed our approach to treating MTrPs. For example, the 1999 edition of *Travell and Simons' Myofascial Pain and Dysfunction: The Trigger Point Manual*,[1] abandoned the application of heavy ischemic compression upon MTrPs. Deep digital pressure that produces additional ischemia is not beneficial. Instead, Simons, Travell, and Simons[1] recommended applying *gentle* digital pressure to MTrPs to avoid exacerbating tissue hypoxia. They named their technique "'trigger point pressure release." A single finger pad palpates the MTrP while the affected muscle is passively lengthened to a point of tissue resistance. Next, the MTrP is pressed with slowly increasing pressure until the palpating finger encounters a barrier (local tissue resistance). The engaged barrier is held until a release of tension is palpated. The finger "follows" the released tissue by taking up tissue slack, engaging a new barrier, and repeating the sequence. This press and stretch is believed to restore abnormally contracted sarcomeres to their normal resting length. We hypothesize that press and stretch mechanically uncouples myosin from actin, a process that normally requires ATP, so that the technique reduces ATP demand and breaks the energy crisis cycle. Press and stretch may also help release the "stuck" spring function of the titin connection to the Z bands within sarcomeres.

Simons, Travell, and Simons' new manual[1] also emphasized the relationship between MTrPs and nearby articular dysfunctions. They correlated suboccipital MTrPs with occipito-atlantal dysfunction, semispinalis capitis MTrPs with occipito-atlantal and atlanto-axial dysfunctions, and splenius MTrPs with upper thoracic articular dysfunctions.[1] This close association between MTrPs and articular dysfunctions is the result of a positive feedback loop. Lewit has emphasized this close association in several publications.[36,37] An MTrP in a muscle that crosses an articulation reduces this articulation's full range of motion, and the MTrP taut band exerts continuous compression upon the articulation. Soft tissues surrounding the articulation cannot withstand chronic compression or tension, and they respond with increased sensitivity. When sufficiently sensitized, these structures send continuous nociceptive messages to the CNS, which responds by further activation of MTrPs, which in turn increases the muscle tension. This positive feedback loop aggravates the articular distress. Articular dysfunctions can be treated directly by muscle energy technique (similar to contract-relax or postisometric relaxation techniques), joint mobilization, and high-velocity, low-amplitude thrust techniques. Articular dysfunctions can be treated indirectly with techniques that address dysfunctional muscles or fascia that cross the articulations, such as strain-counterstrain and myofascial release. Indications and precautions for these techniques are the same as with any articular dysfunctions.

Methods for treating MTrPs and articular dysfunctions work best when combined with patient education.

## Patient Education

Postural training is paramount. Postural disorders often contribute to the perpetuation of MTrPs. For example, postural strain of the suboccipital muscles may cause MTrPs in these muscles,[1] thus leading to further deterioration in muscle structure and function, including radiating somatic pain and atrophic changes, such as muscle atrophy, fibrosis, and decreased tensile strength.[38] Suboccipital muscles contain a high density of proprioceptors,[39] so muscle atrophy leads to a loss in proprioceptive balance and a loss of proprioceptive "gate control" at the dorsal horn. This gives rise to chronic pain syndromes, including neck pain and headache.[38] In these patients, proprioceptive exercises can be very helpful, such as close-eyed balance training. Biomechanical factors that stress muscles, such as repetitive activities, must be avoided. Biomechanical stress of a *cold* muscle is a key factor in the formation of MTrPs.[1] Cooling the muscle apparently up-regulates nAChR activity at the motor endplate.[40]

Patients with MTrPs should avoid excess coffee[41]; caffeine up-regulates the motor endplate by acting as a ryanodine receptor agonist.[42] Tobacco should also be avoided, because nicotine up-regulates L-type VsCCs and nAChR expression, which may lead to muscle hyperexcitability.[43] Nicotine activates nAChRs in the CNS and autonomic nerves. Although nAChRs in motor endplates are not normally activated by nicotine, mutational defects may sensitize motor endplate nAChRs. One study indicated that ethanol also facilitates motor endplate activity, via a presynaptic mechanism.[44]

Simons, Travell, and Simons[1] recommended a diet adequate in vitamins and minerals for the prevention of MTrPs. Amazingly, in the more than 20 years since that recommendation, no well-designed study has been published concerning the effects of vitamin supplementation upon MTrPs. However, a wealth of clinical experience suggests that low-normal and subnormal levels of vitamins and minerals act as strong perpetuating factors of MTrPs. Many case histories attest to patients who responded weakly to manual and/or injection treatment, but adequate supplementation (the return of blood vitamin levels to within mid-normal range) brought about an effective response to the same treatment, and with continued supplementation the patients had no relapse. Interestingly, in two cases a VA hospital physician advised discontinuation of "unnecessary" vitamin supplements, and within a few months the patients returned to the myofascial pain clinic with active MTrPs as before. Reinstatement of their supplement regimen and a replication of previous treatment restored their health (Simons, unpublished data). Similarly, anemia is a perpetuating factor of MTrPs that must be corrected to achieve lasting results from treatment.[45] Inadequate hemoglobin perpetuates the hypoxia present in MTrPs.[46] The importance of calcium and magnesium for normal muscle function is well documented, and trace elements are well known to be essential for many body functions, including muscle function. Supplementing the diet with phosphatidyl choline has been recommended for the treatment of fibromyalgia,[47] but this may actually provoke MTrPs in some patients. Choline is a precursor to ACh, and an nAChR gain-of-function mutation may enable choline to directly activate the mutated receptors.[14] High doses of phosphatidyl choline are found in supplements containing lecithin, with lower amounts in raw egg yoke, organ meats, soybeans, peanuts, wheat germ, and brewer's yeast.

An estimated 50% of patients with chronic musculoskeletal pain take herbal remedies, so it behooves all health practitioners to understand the mechanisms of herbal medicines.[48] Clinical experience has shown that myofascial pain can be improved with many herbal remedies and essential oils,[47] including lavender (*Lavandula angustifolia*), lemon balm (*Melissa officinalis*), rosemary (*Rosmarinus officinalis*), kava kava (*Piper methysticum*), skullcap (*Scutellaria lateriflora*), passionflower (*Passiflora incarnata*), rose (*Rosa* species), and valerian (*Valeriana officinalis*). Nearly all these herbs contain linalool, a monoterpene that inhibits ACh release (a presynaptic mechanism) and nAChRs (a postsynaptic mechanism).[49] Marijuana (*Cannabis* species) also produces linalool, although the herb's efficacy may be due to tetrahydrocannabinol (THC), which inhibits P/Q-, N-, and L-type VsCCs via cannabinoid receptors found in the motor endplate.[50] Sativex, a standardized extract dispensed as an oromucosal spray, has been approved for the treatment of muscle spasticity and pain in Canada.[51] THC works by mimicking an endogenous neurotransmitter named anandamide.[50] Anandamide and THC bind to the same neuroreceptor, known as the cannabinoid receptor. Enhanced release of "endocannabinoids" may be one of the mechanisms of osteopathic manipulative treatment,[52] parallel to the effects of manipulative treatment upon serum endorphin levels.[53]

## Getting to the Point

Needling may be necessary to inactivate MTrPs. The motor endplate hypothesis led to the injection of MTrPs with botulinum toxin type A , which blocks ACh release.[54] A variety of VsCC blockers have also been injected. Recall that P/Q-type and L-type VsCCs are the primary pre- and postsynaptic $Ca^{2+}$ channels (respectively) in normal adult motor endplates. The P/Q-specific antagonist omega-agatoxin IVA (also known as omega-conotoxin GVIIC) has shown promise in rat studies,[55] while verapamil, a L-type VsCC blocker, reduced MTrP excitability in rabbits.[56] The drug had no effect on MEPP (a presynaptic measure), but it decreased postsynaptic currents.[57] Thus, verapamil may function as an nAChR antagonist, rather than by way of its known VsCC antagonism. Similarly, quinidine, another L-type antagonist, also downregulates nAChRs and may restore AChE activity.[12] Diltiazem also merits investigation. This L-type $Ca^{2+}$ channel blocker corrects myopathies caused by defects in AChE activity.[13] However, nifedipine, yet another L-type antagonist, unexpectedly increased ACh activity at motor endplates due to a unique effect upon ryanodine-sensitive intracellular $Ca^{2+}$ stores.[58] Hence, research with VsCC blockers has generated conflicting results, and recent clinical trials with botulinum toxin type A have produced mixed results.[59] Dry needling is usually as effective as injecting anything; if the procedure elicits a local twitch response, dry needling should be as effective as botulinum toxin type A and much less expensive.

Some nAChR antagonists and channel blockers can directly penetrate skin, so they need not be injected. Lidocaine patches have recently been suggested.[60] In 1983, Simons, Travell, and Simons[1] recommended dimethisoquin ointment for massaging MTrPs in superficial muscles such as the orbicularis oculi, frontalis, and occipitalis. Dimethisoquin, a local anesthetic, inhibits voltage-gated $Na^+$ channels (conferring its anesthetic effect), but it also acts as an nAChR antagonist.[61] Its potency is much greater than lidocaine and procaine, and dimethisoquin is uniquely selective for the motor endplate nAChR subtype. Massage with capsaicin cream (available over the counter as a 0.075% cream) is useful for treating MTrPs located in surgical scars,[62] which are particularly refractory to treatment.[1] This seems counterintuitive: Capsaicin is the primary active ingredient in hot peppers, and it activates the vanilloid receptor (TRPV1) in nociceptors. However, with repeated exposure to capsaicin, TRPV1 receptors become desensitized, which explains the seemingly paradoxical use of capsaicin as an analgesic.[63] Another massage treatment of MTrPs uses frequency-specific microcurrent (FSM), which delivers electromagnetic currents through graphite-conducting gloves. In relation to the MTrP ATP energy crisis model, studies have shown that FSM increases ATP production in muscle tissues as well as reducing cytokine levels.[64] To successfully treat MTrPs with FSM, a clinician must be skillful at finding MTrPs.

## Conclusion

The MTrP, according to our working hypothesis, centers upon dysregulated motor end-plates, sustained by a neural loop of sensory afferents and autonomic efferents. The resulting ATP energy crisis links with a spinal reflex disorder known as central sensitization. Treatment must simultaneously address the symptomatic trigger points and their underlying causes. Appropriate treatment includes dry needling (also know as acupuncture), vapocoolant spray-and-stretch, and thermal treatment (including ultrasound and infrared laser), some of which are discussed in other chapters of this book. New approaches described in this chapter, including manual techniques ("press-and-stretch" and articular methods), patient education, and ACh- or VsCC-attenuation techniques (e.g., medications, herbs, and nutrition), have evolved from our new etiological concepts.

## References

1. Simons DG, Travell JG, Simons LS. *Travell and Simons' Myofascial Pain and Dysfunction: The Trigger Point Manual. Volume 1: Upper Half of Body.* 2nd ed. Baltimore, MD: Williams & Wilkins; 1999.
2. Simons, DG. Clinical and etiological update of myofascial pain from trigger points. *J Musculoskel Pain* 1996;4:97–125.
3. Hubbard DR, Berkoff GM. Myofascial trigger points show spontaneous needle EMG activity. *Spine* 1993;18:1803–1807.
4. Liley AW. An investigation of spontaneous activity at the neuromuscular junction of the rat. *J Physiol (Lond)* 1956;132:650–666.
5. Simons DG. Review of enigmatic MTrPs as a common cause of enigmatic musculoskeletal pain and dysfunction. *J Electromyogr Kinesiol* 2004;14:95–107.

6. Kuan TS, Chen JT, Chen SM, Chien CH, Hong CZ. Effect of botulinum toxin on endplate noise in myofascial trigger spots of rabbit skeletal muscle. *Am J Phys Med Rehabil* 2002;81:512–520.

7. Mense S, Simons DG, Hoheisel U, Quenzer B. Lesions of rat skeletal muscle after local block of acetylcholinesterase and neuromuscular stimulation. *J Appl Physiol* 2003;94:2494–2501.

8. Chen BM, Grinnell AD. Kinetics, $Ca^{2+}$ dependence, and biophysical properties of integrin-mediated mechanical modulation of transmitter release from frog motor nerve terminals. *J Neurosci* 1997;17:904–916.

9. McPartland, JM. Travell trigger points: Molecular and osteopathic perspectives. *J Am Osteopath Assoc* 2002;104:244–249.

10. Grisaru D, Sternfeld M, Eldor A, Glick D, Soreq H. Structural roles of acetylcholinesterase variants in biology and pathology. *Eur J Biochem* 1999;264:672–686.

11. Wecker L, Mrak RE, Dettbarn WD. Evidence of necrosis in human intercostal muscle following inhalation of an organophosphate insecticide. *Fundam Appl Toxicol* 1986;6:172–174.

12. De Bleecker JL, Meire VI, Pappens S, Quinidine prevents paraoxon-induced necrotizing myopathy in rats. *Neurotoxicology* 1998;19:833–838.

13. Meshul CK. Calcium channel blocker reverses anticholinesterase-induced myopathy. *Brain Res* 1989;497:142–148.

14. Zhou M, Engel AG, Auerbach A. Serum choline activates mutant acetylcholine receptors that cause slow channel congenital myasthenic syndromes. *Proc Natl Acad Sci USA* 1999;96:10466–10471.

15. Shen XM, Ohno K, Sine SM, Engel AG. Subunit-specific contribution to agonist binding and channel gating revealed by inherited mutation in muscle acetylcholine receptor M3–M4 linker. *Brain* 2005;128:345–355.

16. Gentry CL, Lukas RJ. Local anesthetics noncompetitively inhibit function of four distinct nicotinic acetylcholine receptor subtypes. *J Pharmacol Exp Ther* 2001;299:1038–1048.

17. Wang X, Li Y, Engisch KL, Nakanishi ST, Dodson SE, Miller GW, Cope TC, Pinter MJ, Rich MM. Activity-dependent presynaptic regulation of quantal size at the mammalian neuromuscular junction in vivo. *J Neurosci* 2005;25:343–351.

18. Nakanishi ST, Cope TC, Rich MM, Carrasco DI, Pinter MJ. Regulation of motor neuron excitability via motor endplate acetylcholine receptor activation. *J Neurosci* 2005;25:2226–2232.

19. Mense S, Simons DG. *Muscle Pain: Understanding its Nature, Diagnosis, and Treatment*. Philadelphia, PA: Lippincott Williams & Wilkins; 2001.

20. Hohmann AG, Herkenham M. Cannabinoid receptors undergo axonal flow in sensory nerves. *Neuroscience* 1999;92:1171–1175.

21. Gessa GL, Casu MA, Carta G, Mascia MS. Cannabinoids decrease acetylcholine release in the medial-prefrontal cortex and hippocampus. *Eur J Pharmacol* 1998;355:119–124.

22. Giniatullin RA, Sokolova EM. ATP and adenosine inhibit transmitter release at the frog neuromuscular junction through distinct presynaptic receptors. *Br J Pharmacol* 1998;124:839–844.

23. Silinsky EM. Adenosine decreases both presynaptic calcium currents and neurotransmitter release at the mouse neuromuscular junction. *J Physiol* 2004;558:389–401.

24. Oliveira L, Timoteo MA, Correia-de-Sa P. Tetanic depression is overcome by tonic adenosine A(2A) receptor facilitation of L-type Ca(2+) influx into rat motor nerve terminals. *J Physiol* 2004;560:157–168.

25. Headley BJ. The use of biofeedback in pain management. *Orthop Phys Ther Pract* 1993;2(2):29–40.

26. Headley BJ. Evaluation and treatment of myofascial pain syndrome utilizing biofeedback. In: Cram JR, ed. *Clinical Electromyography for Surface Recordings*. Vol. 2. Nevada City, NV: Clinical Resources; 1990:235–254.

27. Headley BJ. Chronic pain management. In: O'Sullivan SB, Schmitz TS, eds. *Physical Rehabilitation: Assessment and Treatment.* Philadelphia, PA: F.A. Davis; 1994:577–600.

28. Butler DS. *The Sensitive Nervous System.* Adelaide, Australia: Noigroup Publications; 2000.

29. Shah JP, Phillips TM, Danoff JV, Gerber LH. An *in vivo* microanalytical technique for measuring the local biochemical milieu of human skeletal muscle. *J Appl Physiol* 2005;99:1977–1984.

30. Korr IM. The spinal cord as organizer of disease processes. In: Peterson B, ed. *The Collected Papers of Irvin M. Korr.* Newark, OH: American Academy of Osteopathy; 1979:207–221.

31. Roatta S, Windhorst U, Ljubisavljevic M, Johansson H, Passatore M. Sympathetic modulation of muscle spindle afferent sensitivity to stretch in rabbit jaw closing muscles. *J Physiol* 2002;540: 237–248.

32. Bukharaeva EA, Gainulov RKh, Nikol'skii EE. The effects of noradrenaline on the amplitude-time characteristics of multiquantum endplate currents and the kinetics of induced secretion of transmitter quanta. *Neurosci Behav Physiol* 2002;32:549–554.

33. Chen JT, Chen SM, Kuan TS, Chung KC, Hong CZ. Phentolamine effect on the spontaneous electrical activity of active loci in a myofascial trigger spot of rabbit skeletal muscle. *Arch Phys Med Rehabil* 1998;79:790–794.

34. Rivner MH. The neurophysiology of myofascial pain syndrome. *Curr Pain Headache Rep* 2001;5:432–440.

35. Kuchera ML, McPartland JM, Myofascial trigger points as somatic dysfunction. In *Foundations for Osteopathic Medicine.* 2nd ed. Baltimore, MD: Williams & Wilkins; 2002:1034–1050.

36. Lewit K. Chain reactions in disturbed function of the motor system. *Manual Medicine* 1987;3:27–29.

37. Lewit K. *Manipulative Therapy in Rehabilitation of the Locomotor System.* 2nd ed. Oxford, UK: Butterworth Heinemann; 1991.

38. McPartland JM, Brodeur R, Hallgren RC. Chronic neck pain, standing balance, and suboccipital muscle atrophy. *J Manipulative Physiol Ther* 1997;21:24–29.

39. Peck D, Buxton DF, Nitz A. A comparison of spindle concentrations in large and small muscles acting in parallel combinations. *J Morphology* 1984;180:243–252.

40. Foldes FF, Kuze S, Vizi ES, Deery A. The influence of temperature on neuromuscular performance. *J Neural Transm* 1978;43:27–45.

41. McPartland JM, Mitchell J. Caffeine and chronic back pain. *Arch Phys Med Rehab* 1997;78:61–63.

42. Hsu KS, Kang JJ, Lin-Shiau SY. Muscle contracture and twitch depression induced by arsenite in the mouse phrenic nerve-diaphragm. *Jpn J Pharmacol* 1993;62:161–168.

43. Katsura M, Mohri Y, Shuto K, Hai-Du Y, Amano T, Tsujimura A, Sasa M, Ohkuma S. Up-regulation of L-type voltage-dependent calcium channels after long-term exposure to nicotine in cerebral cortical neurons. *J Biol Chem* 2002;277:7979–7988.

44. Yu J, Lu G, Xu J. [The effects of ethanol on neuromuscular junctions of adult toad.] *Hua Xi Yi Ke Da Xue Xue Bao* 2001;32:274–276.

45. Gerwin R, Gevirtz R. Chronic myofascial pain: Iron insufficiency and coldness as risk factors. *J Musculoskel Pain* 1995;3(suppl 1):120 [abstract].

46. Brückle W, Suckfüll M, Fleckenstein W, Weiss C, Müller W. Gewebe-$pO_2$-Messung in der verspannten Rückenmuskulatur (m. erector spinae) [Tissue $pO_2$ measurement in hypertonic back muscles]. *Z Rheumatol* 1990;49:208–216.

47. Starlanyl D, Copeland M. *Fibromyalgia and Chronic Myofascial Pain Syndrome: A Survival Manual.* Oakland, CA: New Harbinger Publications; 1996.

48. Berger J. Vermont DO urges peers to learn about herbal medicine. *The DO* 1999;40(3):58–60.

49. Re L, Barocci S, Sonnino S, Mencarelli A, Vivani C, Paolucci G, Scarpantonio A, Rinaldi L, Mosca E. Linalool modifies the nicotinic receptor-ion channel kinetics at the mouse neuromuscular junction. *Pharmacol Res* 2000;42:177–182.

50. McPartland JM, Pruitt PP. Side effects of pharmaceuticals not elicited by comparable herbal medicines: The case of tetrahydrocannabinol and marijuana. *Alternative Therapies Health Medicine* 1999;5(4):57–62.

51. Barnes MP. Sativex: Clinical efficacy and tolerability in the treatment of symptoms of multiple sclerosis and neuropathic pain. *Expert Opin Pharmacother* 2006;7(5):607–615.

52. McPartland JM, Giuffrida A, King J, Skinner E, Scotter J, Musty RE. Cannabimimetic effects of osteopathic manipulative treatment. *J Am Osteopath Assoc* 2005;105:283–291.

53. Vernon HT, Dhami MS, Howley TP, Annett R. Spinal manipulation and beta-endorphin: A controlled study of the effect of a spinal manipulation on plasma beta-endorphin levels in normal males. *J Manipulative Physiol Ther* 1986;9:115–123.

54. Cheshire WP, Abashian SW, Mann JD. Botulinum toxin in the treatment of myofascial pain syndrome. *Pain* 1994;59:65–69.

55. Taguchi K, Shiina M, Shibata K, Utsunomiya I, Miyatake T. Spontaneous muscle action potentials are blocked by N-type and P/Q-calcium channel blockers in the rat spinal cord-muscle co-culture system. *Brain Res* 2005;1034:62–70.

56. Hou CR, Chung KC, Chen JT, Hong CZ. Effects of a calcium channel blocker on electrical activity in myofascial trigger spots of rabbits. *Am J Phys Med Rehabil* 2002;81:342–349.

57. Sharifullina ER, Afzalov RA, Talantova MV, Vyskochil F, Giniatullin RA. Pre- and postsynaptic effects of the calcium channel blocker verapamil at neuromuscular junctions. *Neurosci Behav Physiol* 2002;32:309–315.

58. Piriz J, Rosato Siri MD, Pagani R, Uchitel OD. Nifedipine-mediated mobilization of intracellular calcium stores increases spontaneous neurotransmitter release at neonatal rat motor nerve terminals. *J Pharmacol Exp Ther* 2003;306:658–663.

59. Ferrante FM, Bearn L, Rothrock R, King L. Evidence against trigger point injection technique for the treatment of cervicothoracic myofascial pain with botulinum toxin type A. *Anesthesiology* 2005;103:377–383.

60. Dalpiaz AS, Dodds TA. Myofascial pain response to topical lidocaine patch therapy: A case report. *J Pain Palliat Care Pharmacoth* 2002;16:99–104.

61. Gentry CL, Lukas RJ. Local anesthetics noncompetitively inhibit function of four distinct nicotinic acetylcholine receptor subtypes. *J Pharmacol Exp Ther* 2001;299:1038–1048.

62. McPartland JM. Use of capsaicin cream for abdominal wall scar pain. *Am Fam Phys* 2002;65:2211–2212.

63. McPartland JM, Pruitt PL. Sourcing the code: Searching for the evolutionary origins of cannabinoid receptors, vanilloid receptors, and anandamide. *J Canna Therapeut* 2002;2:73–103.

64. McMakin CR, Gregory WM, Phillips TM. Cytokine changes with microcurrent treatment of fibromyalgia associated with cervical spine trauma. *J Bodywork Movement Ther* 2005;9:169–176.

Chapter 2

# Myofascial Trigger Points: An Evidence-Informed Review

*Jan Dommerholt, PT, MPS, DPT, DAAPM*

*Carel Bron, PT*

*Jo Franssen, PT*

## Introduction

During the past few decades, myofascial trigger points (MTrPs) and myofascial pain syndrome (MPS) have received much attention in the scientific and clinical literature. Researchers worldwide are investigating various aspects of MTrPs, including their specific etiology, pathophysiology, histology, referred pain patterns, and clinical applications. Guidelines developed by the International Federation of Orthopaedic Manipulative Therapists (IFOMT) confirm the importance of muscle dysfunction for orthopedic manual therapy clinical practice. The IFOMT has defined *orthopedic manual therapy* as "a specialized area of physiotherapy/physical therapy for the management of neuromusculoskeletal conditions, based on clinical reasoning, using highly specific treatment approaches including manual techniques and therapeutic exercises." The IFOMT's educational standards require that skills be demonstrated in—among other areas—"analysis and specific tests for functional status of the muscular system," "a high level of skill in other manual and physical therapy techniques required to mobilize the articular, muscular or neural systems," and "knowledge of various manipulative therapy approaches as practiced within physical therapy, medicine, osteopathy and chiropractic."[1]

However, articles about muscle dysfunction in the manual therapy literature are sparse, and they generally focus on muscle injury and muscle repair mechanisms[2] or on muscle recruitment.[3] Until very recently, the current scientific knowledge and clinical implications of MTrPs were rarely included.[4-7] It appears that orthopedic manual therapists have not paid much attention to the pathophysiology and clinical manifestations of MTrPs.

Courtesy of John M. Medeiros, PT, PhD, Managing Editor of the *Journal of Manual and Manipulative Therapy*.

Manual therapy education programs in the United States seem to reflect this orientation and tend to place a strong emphasis on joint dysfunction, mobilizations, and manipulations, with only about 10–15% of classroom education devoted to muscle pain and muscle dysfunction.

This review of the MTrP literature is based on current best scientific evidence. The field of manual therapy has joined other medical disciplines by embracing evidence-based medicine, which proposes that the results of scientific research need to be integrated into clinical practice.[8] Evidence-based medicine has been defined as "the conscientious, explicit, and judicious use of current best evidence in making decisions about the care of individual patients."[9,10] Within the evidence-based medicine paradigm, evidence is not restricted to randomized controlled trials, systematic reviews, and meta-analyses, although this restricted view seems to be prevalent in the medical and physical therapy literature. Sackett et al[9,10] emphasized that external clinical evidence can inform but not replace individual clinical expertise. Clinical expertise determines whether external clinical evidence applies to an individual patient, and, if so, how it should be integrated into clinical decision making. Pencheon[11] shared this perspective and suggested that high-quality health care is about combining "wisdom produced by years of experience" with "evidence produced by generalizable research" in "ways with which patients are happy." He suggested shifting from evidence-based to evidence-informed medicine, where clinical decision making is informed by research evidence, but not driven by it, and always includes knowledge from experience. Evidence-informed manual therapy involves integrating the best available external scientific evidence with individual clinicians' judgments, expertise, and clinical decision making.[12] The purpose of this chapter is to provide a best–evidence-informed review of the current scientific understanding of MTrPs, including the etiology, pathophysiology, and clinical implications, against the background of extensive clinical experience.

## Brief Historical Review

While Dr. Janet Travell (1901–1997) is generally credited for bringing MTrPs to the attention of health-care providers, MTrPs have been described and rediscovered for several centuries by various clinicians and researchers.[13,14] As far back as the 16th century, de Baillou (1538–1616) described what is now known as myofascial pain syndrome (MPS).[15] MPS is defined as the "sensory, motor, and autonomic symptoms caused by MTrPs" and has become a recognized medical diagnosis among pain specialists.[16,17] In 1816, British physician Balfour described "nodular tumors and thickenings which were painful to the touch, and from which pains shot to neighboring parts."[18] In 1898, the German physician Strauss discussed "small, tender and apple-sized nodules and painful, pencil-sized to little-finger-sized palpable bands."[19] The first trigger-point manual was published in 1931 in Germany, nearly a decade before Travell became interested in MTrPs.[20] Although these early descriptions may appear a bit archaic and unusual—for example, in clinical practice one does not encounter "apple-sized nodules"—these and other historic papers did illustrate the basic features of MTrPs quite accurately.[14]

In the late 1930s, Travell, who at that time was a cardiologist and medical researcher, became particularly interested in muscle pain following the publication of several articles on referred pain.[21] Kellgren's descriptions of referred pain patterns of many muscles and spinal ligaments after injecting these tissues with hypertonic saline[22-25] eventually moved Travell to shift her medical career from cardiology to musculoskeletal pain. During the 1940s, she published several articles on injection techniques of MTrPs.[26-28] In 1952, she described the myofascial genesis of pain, with detailed referred pain patterns for 32 muscles.[29] Other clinicians also became interested in MTrPs. European physicians Lief and Chaitow developed a treatment method, which they referred to as "neuromuscular technique."[30] German physician Gutstein described the characteristics of MTrPs and effective manual therapy treatments in several papers under the names of Gutstein, Gutstein-Good, and Good.[31-34] In Australia, Kelly produced a series of articles about fibrositis, which paralleled Travel's writings.[35-38]

In the United States, chiropractors Nimmo and Vannerson[39] described muscular "noxious generative points," which were thought to produce nerve impulses and eventually result in "vasoconstriction, ischemia, hypoxia, pain, and cellular degeneration." Later in his career, Nimmo adopted the term "trigger point" after having been introduced to Travell's writings. Nimmo maintained that hypertonic muscles are always painful to pressure, a statement that later became known as "Nimmo's law." Like Travell, Nimmo described distinctive referred pain patterns and recommended releasing these dysfunctional points by applying the proper degree of manual pressure. Nimmo's "receptor-tonus control method" continues to be popular among chiropractic physicians.[39,40] According to a 1993 report by the National Board of Chiropractic Economics, over 40% of chiropractors in the United States frequently apply Nimmo's techniques.[41] Two spinoffs of Nimmo's work are the St. John Neuromuscular Therapy (NMT) method and the NMT American version, which have become particularly popular among massage therapists.[30]

In 1966, Travell founded the North American Academy of Manipulative Medicine together with Dr. John Mennell, who also published several articles about MTrPs.[42,43] Throughout her career, Travell promoted integrating myofascial treatments with articular treatments.[16] One of her earlier papers described a technique for reducing sacroiliac displacement.[44] However, Paris reported that Travell[45] maintained the opinion that manipulations were the exclusive domain of physicians, and she rejected membership in the North American Academy of Manipulative Medicine by physical therapists.

In the early 1960s, Dr. David Simons was introduced to Travell and her work, which became the start of a fruitful collaboration eventually resulting in several publications, including the *Trigger Point Manuals*, consisting of a 1983 first volume (upper half of the body) and a 1992 second volume (lower half of the body).[46,47] The first volume has since been revised and updated, and a second edition was released in 1999.[16] The *Trigger Point Manuals* are the most comprehensive review of nearly 150 muscle referred pain patterns based on Travell's clinical observations, and they include an extensive review of the scientific basis of MTrPs. Both volumes have been translated into several foreign languages, including Russian, German, French, Italian, Japanese, and Spanish. Several other clinicians worldwide have also published their own trigger point manuals.[48-54]

## Clinical Aspects of Myofascial Trigger Points

An MTrP is described as "a hyperirritable spot in skeletal muscle that is associated with a hypersensitive palpable nodule in a taut band."[16] Myofascial trigger points are classified into active and latent trigger points.[16] An active MTrP is a symptom-producing MTrP and can trigger local or referred pain or other paresthesiae. A latent MTrP does not trigger pain without being stimulated. Myofascial trigger points are the hallmark characteristics of MPS and feature motor, sensory, and autonomic components. Motor aspects of active and latent MTrPs may include disturbed motor function, muscle weakness as a result of motor inhibition, muscle stiffness, and restricted range of motion.[55,56] Sensory aspects may include local tenderness, referral of pain to a distant site, and peripheral and central sensitization. Peripheral sensitization can be described as a reduction in threshold and an increase in responsiveness of the peripheral ends of nociceptors, whereas central sensitization is an increase in the excitability of neurons within the central nervous system. Signs of peripheral and central sensitization are allodynia (pain due to a stimulus that does not normally provoke pain) and hyperalgesia (an increased response to a stimulus that is normally painful). Both active and latent MTrPs are painful on compression. Vecchiet et al[57-59] described specific sensory changes over MTrPs. They observed significant lowering of the pain threshold over active MTrPs when measured by electrical stimulation, not only in the muscular tissue, but also in the overlying cutaneous and subcutaneous tissues. In contrast, with latent MTrPs the sensory changes did not involve the cutaneous and subcutaneous tissues.[57-59] Autonomic aspects of MTrPs may include, among others, vasoconstriction, vasodilatation, lacrimation, and piloerection.[16,60-63]

A detailed clinical history, examination of movement patterns, and consideration of muscle referred pain patterns assist clinicians in determining which muscles may harbor clinically relevant MTrPs.[64] Muscle pain is perceived as aching and poorly localized. At present, no laboratory or imaging tests are available for use in the clinic that can confirm the presence of MTrPs. Myofascial trigger points are identified through either a flat palpation technique (**Figure 2-1**) in which a clinician applies finger or thumb pressure to muscle against underlying bone tissue, or a pincer palpation technique (**Figure 2-2**) in which a particular muscle is palpated between the clinician's fingers.

By definition, MTrPs are located within a taut band of contractured muscle fibers (**Figure 2-3**), and palpating for MTrPs starts with identifying this taut band by palpating perpendicular to the fiber direction. Once the taut band is located, the clinician moves along the taut band to find a discrete area of intense pain and hardness.

Two studies have reported good overall interrater reliability for identifying taut bands, MTrPs, referred pain, and local twitch responses.[65,66] The minimum criteria that must be satisfied in order to distinguish an MTrP from any other tender area in muscle are a taut band and a tender point in that taut band.[65] Although Janda maintained that systematic palpation can differentiate between myofascial taut bands and general muscle spasms, electromyography is the gold standard to differentiate taut bands from contracted muscle fibers associated with general muscle spasms.[67,68] Spasms can be defined as electromyographic

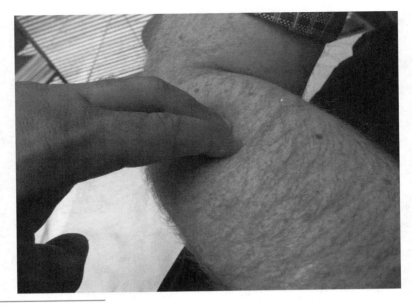

**Figure 2-1**   Flat palpation.

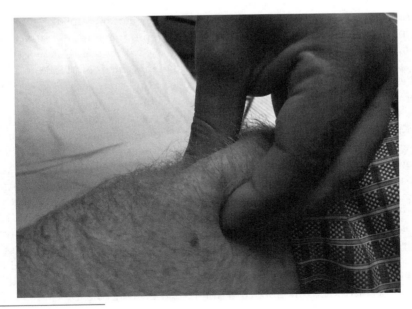

**Figure 2-2**   Pincer palpation.

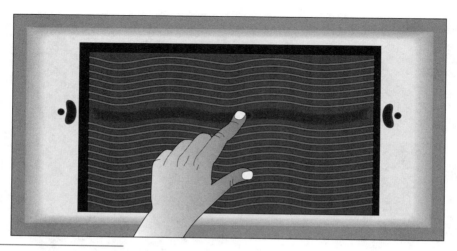

**Figure 2-3** Palpation of a trigger point within a taut band.

*Source:* Adapted from: H-W Weisskircher: "Head Pains Due to Myofascial Trigger Points," CD-ROM, www.trigger-point.com, 1997.

(EMG) activity as the result of increased neuromuscular tone of the entire muscle, and they are the result of nerve-initiated contractions. A taut band is an endogenous localized contracture within the muscle without activation of the motor endplate.[69] From a physiological perspective, the term "contracture" is more appropriate than "contraction" when describing chronic involuntary shortening of a muscle without EMG activity. In clinical practice, surface EMG is used in the diagnosis and management of MTrPs, in addition to manual examinations.[67,70,71] Diagnostically, surface EMG can assist in assessing muscle behavior during rest and during functional tasks. Clinicians use the MTrP referred pain patterns in determining which muscles to examine with surface EMG. Muscles that harbor MTrPs responsible for the patient's pain complaint are examined first. EMG assessments guide the clinician with postural training, ergonomic interventions, and muscle awareness training.[67]

The patient's recognition of the elicited pain further guides the clinician. The presence of a so-called local twitch response (LTR), referred pain, or reproduction of the person's symptomatic pain increases the certainty and specificity of the diagnosis of MPS. Local twitch responses are spinal reflexes that appear to be unique to MTrPs. They are characterized by a sudden contraction of muscle fibers within a taut band when the taut band is strummed manually or needled. The sudden contractions can be observed visually, can be recorded electromyographically, or can be visualized with diagnostic ultrasound.[72] When an MTrP is needled with a monopolar teflon-coated EMG needle, LTRs appear as high-amplitude polyphasic EMG discharges.[73-78]

In clinical practice, there is no benefit in using needle EMG or sonography, and its utility is limited to research studies. For example, Audette et al[79] established that in 61.5% of active MTrPs in the trapezius and levator scapulae muscles, dry needling an active MTrP elicited an LTR in the same muscle on the opposite side of the body. Needling of latent MTrPs resulted in unilateral LTRs only. In this study, LTRs were used to research the nature of active versus latent MTrPs. Studies have shown that clinical outcomes are significantly improved when LTRs are elicited in the treatment of patients with dry needling or injection therapy.[74,80,81] The taut band, MTrP, and LTR (**Figure 2-4**) are objective criteria, identified solely by palpation, that do not require a verbal response from the patient.[82]

Active MTrPs usually refer pain to a distant site. The referred pain patterns (**Figure 2-5**) are not necessarily restricted to single segmental pathways or to peripheral nerve distributions. Although typical referred pain patterns have been established, there is considerable variation between patients.[16,48]

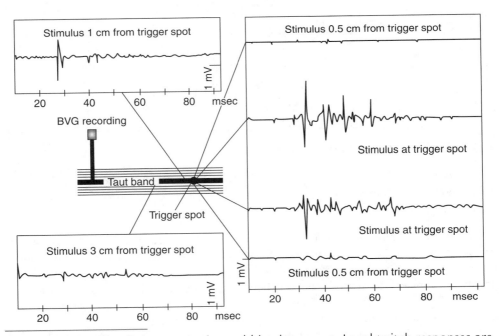

**Figure 2-4**  Local twitch response in a rabbit trigger spot. Local twitch responses are elicited only when the needle is placed accurately within the trigger spot. Moving as little as 0.5 cm away from the trigger spot virtually eliminates the local twitch response.

*Source:* Adapted from: Hong C-Z, Torigoe Y. Electrophysiological characteristics of localized twitch responses in responsive taut bands of rabbit skeletal muscle. *J Musculoskeletal Pain* 1994;2:17–43.

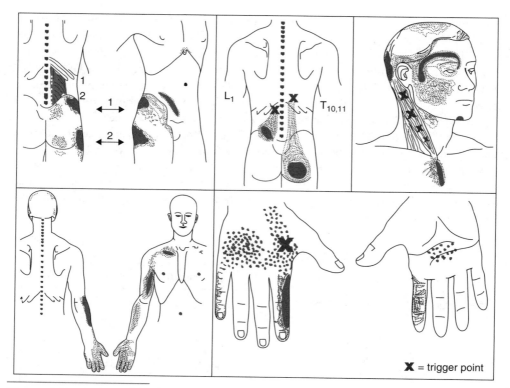

**Figure 2-5** MTrP referred pain patterns.

*Source:* Reproduced with permission from MEDICLIP, Manual Medicine 1 & 2, Version 1.0a, 1997, Williams & Wilkins.

The pain in reference zones usually is described as "deep tissue pain" of a dull and aching nature. Occasionally, patients may report burning or tingling sensations, especially in superficial muscles such as the platysma muscle.[83,84] By mechanically stimulating active MTrPs, patients may report the reproduction of their pain, either immediately or after a 10- to 15-second delay. Skeletal muscle nociceptors normally require high intensities of stimulation, and they do not respond to moderate local pressure, contractions, or muscle stretches.[85]

However, MTrPs cause persistent noxious stimulation, which results in increasing the number and size of the receptive fields to which a single dorsal horn nociceptive neuron responds, and the experience of spontaneous and referred pain.[86] Several recent studies have determined previously unrecorded referred pain patterns of different muscles and MTrPs.[87-90] Referred pain is not specific to MPS, but it is relatively easy to elicit over MTrPs.[91] Normal muscle tissue and other body tissues, including the skin, zygapophyseal joints, or internal organs, may also refer pain to distant regions with mechanical pressure, making referred pain elicited by stimulation of a tender location a nonspecific finding.[84,92-95] Gibson et al[96] found that referred pain is actually easier to elicit in tendon–bone junctions and tendon than in the muscle belly. However, after exposing the muscle to eccentric exercise, significantly higher referred pain frequency and enlarged pain areas were found at the muscle belly and the tendon–bone junction sites following injection with hypotonic saline. The authors suggested that central sensitization may explain the referred pain frequency and enlarged pain areas.[97]

Although a survey of members of the American Pain Society showed general agreement that MTrPs and MPS exist as distinct clinical entities, MPS continues to be one of the most commonly missed diagnoses.[17,98] In a recent study of 110 adults with low back pain, myofascial pain was the most common finding, affecting 95.5% of patients, even though myofascial pain was poorly defined as muscle pain in the paraspinal muscles, piriformis, or tensor fasciae latae.[99] A study of adults with frequent migraine headaches diagnosed according to the International Headache Society criteria showed that 94% of the patients reported migrainous pain with manual stimulation of cervical and temporal MTrPs, compared with only 29% of controls.[100,101] In 30% of the migraine group, palpation of MTrPs elicited a "full-blown migraine attack that required abortive treatment." The researchers found a positive relationship between the number of MTrPs and the frequency of migraine attacks and duration of the illness.[100] Several studies have confirmed that MTrPs are common not only in persons attending pain management clinics, but also in those seeking help through internal medicine and dentistry.[102-107] In fact, MTrPs have been identified with nearly every musculoskeletal pain problem, including radiculopathies,[104] joint dysfunction,[108] disk pathology,[109] tendonitis,[110] craniomandibular dysfunction,[111-113] migraines,[100,114] tension-type headaches,[7,87] carpal tunnel syndrome,[115] computer-related disorders,[116] whiplash-associated disorders,[60,117] spinal dysfunction,[118] and pelvic pain and other urologic syndromes.[119-122] Myofascial trigger points are associated with many other pain syndromes[123] including, for example, postherpetic neuralgia,[124,125] complex regional pain syndrome,[126,127] nocturnal cramps,[128] phantom pain,[129,130] and other relatively uncommon diagnoses, such as Barré-Liéou syndrome[131] and neurogenic pruritus.[132] A recent study suggested that there might be a relationship between MTrPs in the upper trapezius muscle and cervical spine dysfunction at the C3 and C4 vertebrae, although a cause-and-effect relationship was not established in this correlational study.[133] Another study described that persons with mechanical neck pain had significantly more clinically relevant MTrPs in the upper trapezius, sternocleidomastoid, levator scapulae, and suboccipital muscles as compared to healthy controls.[5]

## Etiology of Myofascial Trigger Points

Several possible mechanisms can lead to the development of MTrPs, including low-level muscle contractions, uneven intramuscular pressure distribution, direct trauma, unaccustomed eccentric contractions, eccentric contractions in unconditioned muscle, and maximal or submaximal concentric contractions.

## Low-Level Muscle Contractions

Of particular interest in the etiology of MTrPs are low-level muscle exertions and the so-called Cinderella hypothesis developed by Hägg in 1988.[134] The Cinderella hypothesis postulates that occupational myalgia is caused by selective overloading of the earliest recruited and last de-recruited motor units according to the ordered recruitment principle or Henneman's "size principle."[134,135] Smaller motor units are recruited before and de-recruited after larger ones; as a result, the smaller type 1 fibers are continuously activated during prolonged motor tasks.[135] According to the Cinderella hypothesis, muscular force generated at submaximal levels during sustained muscle contractions engages only a fraction of the motor units available without the normally occurring substitution of motor units during higher force contractions, which in turn can result in metabolically overloaded motor units, prone to loss of cellular $Ca^{2+}$ homeostasis, subsequent activation of autogenic destructive processes, and muscle pain.[136,137] The other pillar of the Cinderella hypothesis is the finding of an excess of ragged red fibers in myalgic patients.[136] Indeed, several researchers have demonstrated the presence of ragged red fibers and moth-eaten fibers in subjects with myalgia, which are indications of structural damage to the cell membrane and mitochondria and a change in the distribution of mitochondria or the sarcotubular system, respectively.[138-142]

There is growing evidence that low-level static muscle contractions or exertions can result in degeneration of muscle fibers.[143] Gissell[144,145] has shown that low-level exertions can result in an increase of $Ca^{2+}$ release in skeletal muscle cells, muscle membrane damage due to leakage of the intracellular enzyme lactate dehydrogenase, structural damage, energy depletion, and myalgia. Low-level muscle stimulation can also lead to the release of interleukin-6 (IL-6) and other cytokines.[146,147]

Several studies have confirmed the Cinderella hypothesis and support the idea that in low-level static exertions, muscle fiber recruitment patterns tend to be stereotypical with continuous activation of smaller type 1 fibers during prolonged motor tasks.[148-152] As Hägg indicated, the continuous activity and metabolic overload of certain motor units does not occur in all subjects.[136] The Cinderella hypothesis was recently applied to the development of MTrPs.[116] In a well-designed study, Treaster et al[116] established that sustained low-level muscle contractions during continuous typing for as little as 30 minutes commonly resulted in the formation of MTrPs. They suggested that MTrPs might provide a useful explanation for muscle pain and injury that can occur from low-level static exertions.[116] Myofascial trigger points are common in office workers, musicians, dentists, and other occupational groups exposed to low-level muscle exertions.[153] Chen et al[154] also suggested that low-level muscle exertions can lead to sensitization and development of MTrPs. Forty piano students showed significantly reduced pressure thresholds over latent MTrPs after only 20 minutes of continuous piano playing.[154]

## Intramuscular Pressure Distribution

Otten[155] has suggested that circulatory disturbances secondary to increased intramuscular pressure may also lead to the development of myalgia. Based on mathematical modeling applied to a frog gastrocnemius muscle, Otten confirmed that during static low-level muscle contractions, capillary pressures increase dramatically, especially near the muscle insertions (**Figure 2-6**). In other words, during low-level exertions the intramuscular pressure near the muscle insertions might increase rapidly, leading to excessive capillary pressure, decreased circulation, and localized hypoxia and ischemia.[155] With higher-level contractions between 10–20% of maximum voluntary effort, the intramuscular pressure also increases in the muscle belly.[156,157] According to Otten, the increased pressure gradients during low-level exertions may contribute to the development of pain at the musculotendinous junctions, and eventually to the formation of MTrPs (personal communication, 2005).

In 1999, Simons introduced the concept of "attachment trigger points" to explain pain at the musculotendinous junctions in persons with MTrPs, based on the assumption that taut bands would generate sufficient sustained force to induce localized enthesopathies.[16,158] More recently, Simons concluded that there is no convincing evidence that the tension generated in shortened sarcomeres in a muscle belly would indeed be able to generate passive or resting force throughout an entire taut band resulting in enthesopathies, even though there

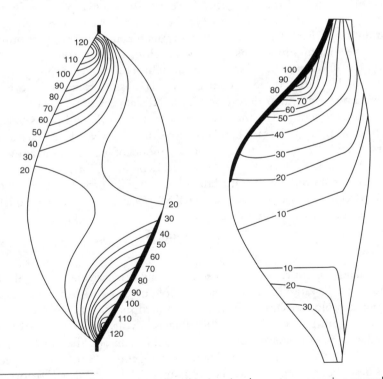

**Figure 2-6**    Intramuscular pressure distribution in the gastrocnemius muscle of the toad.

*Source:* Reproduced with permission from E. Otten, 2006.

may be certain muscles or conditions where this could occur (personal communication, 2005). To the contrary, force generated by individual motor units is always transmitted laterally to the muscle's connective tissue matrix, involving at least two protein complexes containing vinculin and dystrophin, respectively.[159] There is also considerable evidence that the assumption that muscle fibers pass from tendon to tendon is without basis.[160] Trotter[160] has demonstrated that skeletal muscle is composed of in-series fibers. In other words, evidence suggests that a single muscle fiber does not run from tendon to tendon. The majority of fibers are in series with inactive fibers, which makes it even more unlikely that the whole muscle length–tension properties would be dictated by the shortest contractured fibers in the muscle.[161]

In addition, it is important to consider the mechanical and functional differences between fast and slow motor units.[162,163] Slow motor units are always stiffer than fast units, although fast units can produce more force. If there were any transmission of force along the muscle fiber, as Simons initially suggested, fast fibers would be better suited to accomplish this. Yet fast motor units have larger series of elastic elements, which would absorb most of the force displacement.[164,165] Fast fibers show a progressive decrease in cross-sectional area and end in a point within the muscle fascicle, making force transmission even more unlikely.[163] Fast fibers rely on transmitting a substantial proportion of their force to the endomysium, transverse cytoskeleton, and adjacent muscle fibers.[162,163] In summary, the development of so-called "attachment trigger points" as a result of increased tension by contractured sarcomeres in MTrPs is not clear, and more research is needed to explain the clinical observation that MTrPs appear to be linked to pain at the musculotendinous junction. The increased tension in the muscle belly is likely to dissipate across brief sections of the taut band on both sides of the MTrP and laterally through the transverse cytoskeleton.[166-168] Instead, Otten's model of increased intramuscular pressure, decreased circulation, localized hypoxia, and ischemia at the muscle insertions provides an alternative model for the clinically observed pain near the musculotendinous junction and osseous insertions in persons with MTrPs, even though the model does not explain why taut bands are commonly present.[155]

## Direct Trauma

There is general agreement that acute muscle overload can activate MTrPs, although systematic studies are lacking.[169] For example, people involved in whiplash injuries commonly experience prolonged muscle pain and dysfunction.[170-173] In a retrospective review, Schuller et al[174] found that 80% of 1,096 subjects involved in low-velocity collisions demonstrated evidence of muscle pain, with myogeloses among the most common findings. Although Schuller et al did not define these myogeloses, Simons has suggested that a myogelosis describes the same clinical entity as an MTrP.[174,175] Baker[117] reported that the splenius capitis, semispinalis capitis, and sternocleidomastoid muscles developed symptomatic MTrPs in 77%, 62%, and 52% of 52 whiplash patients, respectively. In a retrospective review of 54 consecutive chronic whiplash patients, Gerwin and Dommerholt[176] reported that clinically relevant MTrPs were found in every patient, with the trapezius muscle involved most often. Following treatment emphasizing the inactivation of MTrPs and restoration of normal muscle length, approximately 80% of patients experienced little or no pain, even though the average time following the initiating injury was 2.5 years at the beginning of the treatment regimen. All patients had been seen previously by other physicians and physical therapists who apparently had not considered MTrPs in their thought process and clinical management.[176] Fernández-de-las-Peñas et al[177,178] confirmed that inactivation of MTrPs should be included in the management of persons suffering from whiplash-associated disorders. In their research-based treatment protocol, the combination of cervical and thoracic spine manipulations with MTrP treatments proved superior to more "conventional" physical therapy consisting of massage, ultrasound, home exercises, and low-energy high-frequency pulsed electromagnetic therapy.[177]

Direct trauma may create a vicious cycle of events wherein damage to the sarcoplasmic reticulum or the muscle cell membrane may lead to an increase of the calcium concentration, a subsequent activation of actin and myosin, a relative shortage of adenosine triphosphate (ATP), and an impaired calcium pump, which in turn will increase the intracellular calcium concentration even more, completing the cycle. The calcium pump is responsible for returning intracellular $Ca^{2+}$ to the sarcoplasmic reticulum against a concentration gradient, which requires a functional energy supply. Simons and Travell[179] considered this sequence in the development of the so-called "energy crisis hypothesis" introduced in 1981. Sensory and motor system dysfunction have been shown to develop rapidly after injury and actually may persist in those who develop chronic muscle pain and in individuals who have recovered or continue to have persistent mild symptoms.[172,180] Scott et al[181] determined that individuals with chronic whiplash pain develop more widespread hypersensitivity to mechanical pressure and thermal stimuli than those with chronic idiopathic neck pain. Myofascial trigger points are a likely source of ongoing peripheral nociceptive input, and they contribute to both peripheral and central sensitization, which may explain the observation of widespread allodynia and hypersensitivity.[60,62,63] In addition to being caused by whiplash injury, acute muscle overload can occur with direct impact, lifting injuries, sports performance, and so on.[182]

## Eccentric and (Sub)Maximal Concentric Contractions

Many patients report the onset of pain and activation of MTrPs following either acute, repetitive, or chronic muscle overload.[183] Gerwin et al[184] suggested that likely mechanisms relevant for the development of MTrPs included either unaccustomed eccentric exercise, eccentric exercise in unconditioned muscle, or maximal or submaximal concentric exercise. A brief review of pertinent aspects of exercise follows, preceding linking this body of research to current MTrP research.

Eccentric exercise is associated with myalgia, muscle weakness, and destruction of muscle fibers, partially because eccentric contractions cause an irregular and uneven lengthening of muscle fibers.[185-187] Muscle soreness and pain occur because of local ultrastructural damage, the release of sensitizing algogenic substances, and the subsequent onset of peripheral and central sensitization.[85,188-190] Muscle damage occurs at the cytoskeletal level and frequently involves disorganization of the A-band, streaming of the Z-band, and disruption of cytoskeletal proteins, such as titin, nebulin, and desmin, even after very short bouts of eccentric exercise.[186,189-194] Loss of desmin can occur within 5 minutes of eccentric loading, even in muscles that routinely contract eccentrically during functional activities, but does not occur after isometric or concentric contractions.[193,195] Lieber and Fridén[193] suggested that the rapid loss of desmin might indicate a type of enzymatic hydrolysis or protein phosphorylation as a likely mechanism.

One of the consequences of muscle damage is muscle weakness.[196-198] Furthermore, concentric and eccentric contractions are linked to contraction-induced capillary constrictions, impaired blood flow, hypoperfusion, ischemia, and hypoxia, which in turn contribute to the development of more muscle damage, a local acidic milieu, and an excessive release of protons ($H^+$), potassium ($K^+$), calcitonin-gene-related-peptide (CGRP), bradykinin (BK), and substance P (SP) and sensitization of muscle nociceptors.[184,188] There are striking similarities with the chemical environment of active MTrPs established with microdialysis, suggesting an overlap between the research on eccentric exercise and MTrP research.[184,199] However, at this time it is premature to conclude that there is solid evidence that eccentric and submaximal concentric exercise are absolute precursors to the development of MTrPs. In support of this hypothesized causal relation, Itoh et al[200] demonstrated in a recent study that eccentric exercise can lead to the formation of taut and tender ropy bands in exercised muscle, and they hypothesized that eccentric exercise may indeed be a useful model for the development of MTrPs.

Eccentric and concentric exercise and MTrPs have been associated with localized hypoxia, which appears to be one of the most important precursors for the development of MTrPs.[201] As mentioned, hypoxia leads to the release of multiple algogenic substances. In this context, recent research by Shah et al[199] at the U.S. National Institutes of Health is particularly relevant. Shah et al analyzed the chemical milieu of latent and active MTrPs and normal muscles. They found significantly increased concentrations of BK, CGRP, SP, tumor necrosis factor-$\alpha$ (TNF-$\alpha$), interleukin-1$\beta$ (IL-1$\beta$), serotonin, and norepinephrine in the immediate milieu of active MTrPs only.[199] These substances are well-known stimulants for various muscle nociceptors and bind to specific receptor molecules of the nerve endings, including the so-called purinergic and vanilloid receptors.[85,202]

Muscle nociceptors are dynamic structures whose receptors can change depending on the local tissue environment. When a muscle is damaged it releases ATP, which stimulates purinergic receptors, which are sensitive to ATP, adenosine diphosphate, and adenosine. They bind ATP, stimulate muscle nociceptors, and cause pain. Vanilloid receptors are sensitive to heat and respond to an increase in $H^+$ concentration, which is especially relevant under conditions with a lowered pH, such as ischemia, inflammation, or prolonged and exhaustive muscle contractions.[85] Shah et al[199] determined that the pH at active MTrP sites is significantly lower than at latent MTrP sites. A lowered pH can initiate and maintain muscle pain and mechanical hyperalgesia through activation of acid-sensing ion channels.[203,204]

Neuroplastic changes in the central nervous system facilitate mechanical hyperalgesia even after the nociceptive input has been terminated (central sensitization).[203,204] Any noxious stimulus sufficient to cause nociceptor activation causes bursts of SP and CGRP to be released into the muscle, which have a significant effect on the local biochemical milieu and microcirculation by stimulating "feed-forward" neurogenic inflammation. Neurogenic inflammation can be described as a continuous cycle of increasing production of inflammatory mediators and neuropeptides and an increasing barrage of nociceptive input into wide dynamic-range neurons in the spinal cord dorsal horn.[184]

## The Integrated Trigger Point Hypothesis

The integrated trigger point hypothesis (**Figure 2-7**) has evolved since its first introduction as the "energy crisis hypothesis" in 1981. It is based on a combination of electrodiagnostic and histopathological evidence.[179,183]

Already in 1957, Weeks and Travell[205] had published a report that outlined a characteristic electrical activity of an MTrP. It was not until 1993 that Hubbard and Berkoff[206] confirmed that this EMG discharge consists of low-amplitude discharges in the order of 10–50 μV and intermittent high-amplitude discharges (up to 500 μV) in painful MTrPs. Initially, the electrical activity was termed "spontaneous electrical activity" (SEA) and was thought to be related to dysfunctional muscle spindles.[206] Best available evidence now suggests that the SEA is in fact endplate noise (EPN), which is found much more commonly in the endplate zone near

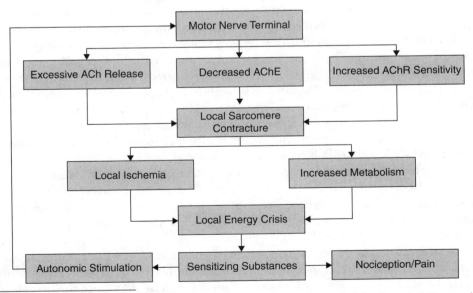

**Figure 2-7**  The integrated trigger point hypothesis. Ach–acetylcholine; AchE–acetylcholinesterase; AchR–acetylcholine receptor.

MTrPs than in an endplate zone outside MTrPs.[207-209] The electrical discharges occur with frequencies that are 10 to 1,000 times that of normal endplate potentials, and they have been found in humans, rabbits, and recently even in horses.[209,210] The discharges are most likely the result of an abnormally excessive release of acetylcholine (ACh) and indicative of dysfunctional motor endplates, contrary to the commonly accepted notion among electromyographers that endplate noise arises from normal motor endplates.[183] The effectiveness of botulinum toxin in the treatment of MTrPs provides indirect evidence of the presence of excessive ACh.[211] Botulinum toxin is a neurotoxin that blocks the release of ACh from presynaptic cholinergic nerve endings. A recent study in mice demonstrated that the administration of botulinum toxin resulted in a complete functional repair of dysfunctional endplates.[212] There is some early evidence that muscle stretching and hypertonicity may also enhance the excessive release of ACh.[213,214] Tension on the integrins in the presynaptic membrane at the motor nerve terminal is hypothesized to mechanically trigger an ACh release that does not require $Ca^{2+}$.[213-215] Integrins are receptor proteins in the cell membrane involved in attaching individual cells to the extracellular matrix.

Excessive ACh affects voltage-gated sodium channels of the sarcoplasmic reticulum and increases the intracellular calcium levels, which triggers sustained muscle contractures. It is conceivable that in MTrPs myosin filaments literally get stuck in the Z-band of the sarcomere. During sarcomere contractions, titin filaments are folded into a gel-like structure at the Z-band. In MTrPs, the gel-like titin may prevent the myosin filaments from detaching. The myosin filaments may actually damage the regular motor assembly and prevent the sarcomere from restoring its resting length.[216] Muscle contractures are also maintained because of the relative shortage of ATP in an MTrP, because ATP is required to break the cross-bridges between actin and myosin filaments. The question remains whether sustained contractures require an increase of oxygen availability.

At the same time, the shortened sarcomeres compromise the local circulation, causing ischemia. Studies of oxygen saturation levels have demonstrated severe hypoxia in MTrPs.[201] Hypoxia leads to the release of sensitizing substances and activates muscle nociceptors as reviewed earlier. The combined decreased energy supply and possible increased metabolic demand would also explain the common finding of abnormal mitochondria in the nerve terminal and the previously mentioned ragged red fibers. In mice, the onset of hypoxia led to an immediate increased ACh release at the motor endplate.[217]

The combined high-intensity mechanical and chemical stimuli may cause activation and sensitization of the peripheral nerve endings and autonomic nerves; activate second-order neurons, including so-called "sleeping" receptors; cause central sensitization; and lead to the formation of new receptive fields, referred pain, a long-lasting increase in the excitability of nociceptors, and a more generalized hyperalgesia beyond the initial nociceptive area. An expansion of a receptive field means that a dorsal horn neuron receives information from areas it has not received information from previously.[218] Sensitization of peripheral nerve endings can also cause pain through SP activating the neurokin-1 receptors and glutamate activating N-methyl-D-aspartate receptors, which opens postsynaptic channels through which $Ca^{2+}$ can enter the dorsal horn and activate many enzymes involved in the sensitization.[85]

Several histological studies offer further support for the integrated trigger point hypothesis. In 1976, Simons and Stolov published the first biopsy study of MTrPs in a canine muscle and reported multiple contraction knots in various individual muscle fibers (**Figure 2-8**).[219] The knots featured a combination of severely shortened sarcomeres in the center and lengthened sarcomeres outside the immediate MTrP region.[219]

Reitinger et al[220] reported pathologic alterations of the mitochondria as well as increased width of A-bands and decreased width of I-bands in muscle sarcomeres of MTrPs in the gluteus medius muscle. Windisch et al[221] determined similar alterations in a postmortem histological study of MTrPs completed within 24 hours of time of death. Mense et al[222] studied the effects of electrically induced muscle contractions and a cholinesterase blocker on muscles with experimentally induced contraction knots and found evidence of localized contractions, torn fibers, and longitudinal stripes. Pongratz and Späth[223,224] demonstrated evidence of a contraction disk in a region of an MTrP using light microscopy. New MTrP histopathological studies are currently being conducted at the Friedrich Baur Institute in Munich, Germany. Gariphianova[225] described pathological changes with biopsy studies of MTrPs, including a decrease in quantity of mitochondria, possibly indicating metabolic distress. Several older histological studies are often quoted, but it is not clear to what extent those findings are specific for MTrPs. In 1951, Glogowsky and Wallraff[226] reported damaged fibril structures. Fassbender[227] observed degenerative

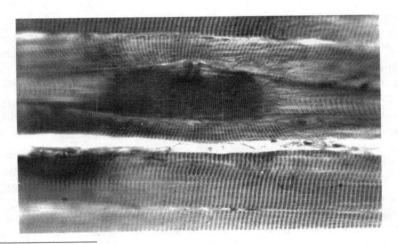

**Figure 2-8** Longitudinal section of a contraction knot in a canine gracilis muscle.

*Source:* Adapted from: Simons DG and Stolov WC, Microscopic features and transient contraction of palpable bands in canine muscle. *Am J Phys Med* 1976;55(2):65–88.

changes of the I-bands in addition to capillary damage, a focal accumulation of glycogen, and a disintegration of the myofibrillar network.

There is growing evidence for the integrated trigger point hypothesis with regard to the motor and sensory aspects of MTrPs, but many questions remain about the autonomic aspects. Several studies have shown that MTrPs are influenced by the autonomic nervous system. Exposing subjects with active MTrPs in the upper trapezius muscles to stressful tasks consistently increased the electrical activity in MTrPs in the upper trapezius muscle but not in control points in the same muscle, while autogenic relaxation was able to reverse the effects.[228-231] The administration of the sympathetic blocking agent phentolamine significantly reduced the electrical activity of an MTrP.[228,232,233] The interactions between the autonomic nervous system and MTrPs need further investigation. Hubbard[228] maintained that the autonomic features of MTrPs are evidence that MTrPs may be dysfunctional muscle spindles. Gerwin et al[184] have suggested that the presence of α- and β-adrenergic receptors at the endplate provide a possible mechanism for autonomic interaction. In a rodent, stimulation of the α- and β-adrenergic receptors stimulated the release of ACh in the phrenic nerve.[234] In a recent study, Ge et al[61] provided, for the first time, experimental evidence of sympathetic facilitation of mechanical sensitization of MTrPs, which they attributed to a change in the local chemical milieu at the MTrPs due to increased vasoconstriction, an increased sympathetic release of norepinephrine, or an increased sensitivity to norepinephrine. Another intriguing possibility is that the cytokine interleukin-8 (IL-8) found in the immediate milieu of active MTrPs may contribute to the autonomic features of MTrP. IL-8 can induce mechanical hypernociception, which is inhibited by β-adrenergic receptor antagonists.[235] Shah et al found significantly increased levels of IL-8 in the immediate milieu of active MTrPs (Shah, 2006, personal communication).

The findings of Shah et al[199] mark a major milestone in the understanding and acceptance of MTrPs and support parts of the integrated trigger point hypothesis.[183] The possible consequences of several of the chemicals present in the immediate milieu of active MTrPs have been explored by Gerwin et al.[184] As stated, Shah et al found significantly increased concentrations of H+, BK, CGRP, SP, TNF-α, IL-1β, serotonin, and norepinephrine in active MTrPs only. There are many interactions between these chemicals that all can contribute to the persistent nature of MTrPs through various vicious feedback cycles.[236] For example, BK is known to activate and sensitize muscle nociceptors, which leads to inflammatory hyperalgesia, an activation of high-threshold nociceptors associated with C-fibers, and even an increased production of BK itself. Furthermore, BK stimulates the release of TNF-α, which activates the production of the interleukins IL-1β, IL-6, and IL-8. Especially IL-8 can cause hyperalgesia that is independent from prostaglandin mechanisms. Via a positive feedback loop, IL-1β can also induce the release of BK.[237] Release of BK, K+, H+, and cytokines from injured muscle activates the muscle nociceptors, thereby causing tenderness and pain.[184]

Calcitonin gene-related peptide can enhance the release of ACh from the motor endplate and simultaneously decrease the effectiveness of acetylcholinesterase (AChE) in the synaptic cleft, which decreases the removal of ACh.[238,239] Calcitonin gene-related peptide also up-regulates the

ACh-receptors (AChR) at the muscle and thereby creates more docking stations for ACh. Miniature endplate activity depends on the state of the AChR and on the local concentration of ACh, which is the result of ACh release, reuptake, and breakdown by AChE. In summary, increased concentrations of CGRP lead to a release of more ACh and increase the impact of ACh by reducing AChE effectiveness and increasing AChR efficiency. Miniature endplate potential frequency is increased as a result of greater ACh effect. The observed lowered pH has several implications as well. Not only does a lower pH enhance the release of CGRP, it also contributes to a further down-regulation of AChE. The multiple chemicals and lowered pH found in active MTrPs can contribute to the chronic nature of MTrPs, enhance the segmental spread of nociceptive input into the dorsal horn of the spinal cord, activate multiple receptive fields, and trigger referred pain, allodynia, hypersensitivity, and peripheral and central sensitization that are characteristic of active myofascial MTrPs.[184] There is no other evidence-based hypothesis that explains the phenomena of MTrPs in as much detail and clarity as the expanded integrated trigger point hypothesis (**Figure 2-9**).

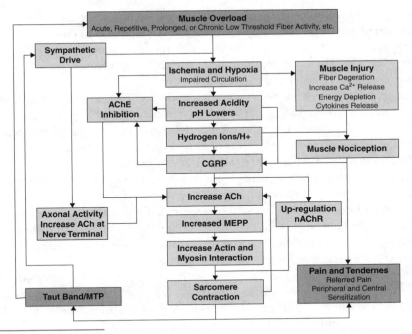

**Figure 2-9**   The expanded MTrP hypothesis.

*Source:* Adapted from: Gerwin RD, Dommerholt J, Shah J. An expansion of Simons' integrated hypothesis of trigger point formation. *Curr Pain Headache Rep* 2004;8:468–475.

## Perpetuating Factors

Several precipitating or perpetuating factors need to be identified and, if present, adequately managed to successfully treat persons with chronic myalgia. Even though several common perpetuating factors are more or less outside the direct scope of manual physical therapy, familiarity with these factors is critical, especially considering the development of increasingly autonomous physical therapy practice. Simons, Travell, and Simons[16] identified mechanical, nutritional, metabolic, and psychological categories of perpetuating factors. Mechanical factors are familiar to manual therapists and include the commonly observed forward head posture, structural leg length inequalities, scoliosis, pelvic torsion, joint hypermobility, ergonomic stressors, poor body mechanics, and so on.[16,102,116,240]

In recent review articles, Gerwin[241,242] provided a comprehensive update with an emphasis on nonstructural perpetuating factors, which has been updated in Chapter 3. Management of these factors usually requires an interdisciplinary approach, including medical and psychological intervention.[64,82] Common nutritional deficiencies or insufficiencies involve vitamin $B_1$, $B_6$, $B_{12}$, folic acid, vitamin C, vitamin D, iron, magnesium, and zinc, among others. The term "insufficiency" is used to indicate levels in the lower range of normal, such as those associated with biochemical or metabolic abnormalities or with subtle clinical signs and symptoms. Nutritional or metabolic insufficiencies are frequently overlooked and not necessarily considered clinically relevant by physicians unfamiliar with MTrPs and chronic pain conditions. Yet any inadequacy that interferes with the energy supply of muscle is likely to aggravate MTrPs.[242] The most common deficiencies and insufficiencies will be reviewed briefly here and in more detail in the next chapter.

Vitamin $B_{12}$ deficiencies are rather common and may affect as many as 15–20% of the elderly and approximately 16% of persons with chronic MTrPs.[103,243] $B_{12}$ deficiencies can result in cognitive dysfunction, degeneration of the spinal cord, and peripheral neuropathy, which is most likely linked to complaints of diffuse myalgia seen in some patients. Serum levels of vitamin $B_{12}$ as high as 350 pg/ml may be associated with a metabolic deficiency, manifested by elevated serum or urine methylmalonic acid or homocysteine and may be clinically symptomatic.[244] However, there are patients with normal levels of methylmalonic acid and homocysteine who do present with abnormal metabolic abnormalities of $B_{12}$ function.[242] Folic acid is closely linked to vitamin $B_{12}$ and should be measured as well. Although folic acid is able to correct the pernicious anemia associated with vitamin $B_{12}$ deficiency, it does not influence the neuromuscular aspects.

Iron deficiency in muscle occurs when ferritin is depleted. Ferritin represents the tissue-bound nonessential iron stores in muscle, liver, and bone marrow that supply the essential iron for oxygen transport and iron-dependent enzymes. Iron is critical for the generation of energy through the cytochrome oxidase enzyme system, and a lack of iron may be a factor in the development and maintenance of MTrPs.[242] Interestingly, lowered levels of cytochrome oxidase are common in patients with myalgia.[140] Serum levels of 15–20 ng/ml indicate a depletion of ferritin. Common symptoms are chronic tiredness, coldness, extreme fatigue with exercise, and muscle pain. Anemia is common at levels of

10 ng/ml or less. Although optimal levels of ferritin are unknown, Gerwin[242] suggested that levels below 50 ng/ml may be clinically significant.

Close to 90% of patients with chronic musculoskeletal pain may have vitamin D deficiency.[245] Vitamin D deficiencies are identified by measuring 25-OH vitamin D levels. Levels above 20 ng/ml are considered normal, but Gerwin[242] suggested that levels below 34 ng/ml may represent insufficiencies. Correction of insufficient levels of vitamin $B_{12}$, vitamin D, and iron levels may take many months, during which patients may not see much improvement.

Even when active MTrPs have been identified in a particular patient, clinicians must always consider that MTrPs may be secondary to metabolic insufficiencies or other medical diagnoses. It is questionable whether physical therapy and—as an integral part of physical therapy management—manual therapy intervention can be successful when patients have nutritional or metabolic insufficiencies or deficiencies. A close working relationship with physicians familiar with this body of literature is essential. Therapists should consider the possible interactions between arthrogenic or neurogenic dysfunction and MTrPs.[4,5,118,133,246,247]

Clinically, physical therapists should address all aspects of the dysfunction. Many other conditions feature muscle pain and MTrPs, including hypothyroidism, systemic lupus erythematosis, Lyme disease, babesiosis, ehrlichiosis, *Candida albicans* infections, myoadenylate deaminase deficiency, hypoglycemia, and parasitic diseases such as fascioliasis, amoebiasis, and giardia.[64,242] Therapists should be familiar with the symptoms associated with these medical diagnoses.[64]

Psychological stress may activate MTrPs. Electromyographic activity in MTrPs has been shown to increase dramatically in response to mental and emotional stress, whereas adjacent non-trigger-point muscle EMG activity remained normal.[229,230] Relaxation techniques, such as autogenic relaxation, can diminish the electrical activity.[231] In addition, many patients with persistent MTrPs are dealing with depression, anxiety, anger, and feelings of hopelessness.[248] Pain-related fear and avoidance can lead to the development and maintenance of chronic pain.[249] Sleep disturbance can also be a major factor in the perpetuation of musculoskeletal pain and must be addressed. Sleep problems may be related to pain, apnea, or to mood disorders such as depression or anxiety. Management can be both pharmacologic and nonpharmacologic. Pharmacologic treatment utilizes drugs that promote normal sleep patterns and induce and maintain sleep through the night without causing daytime sedation. Nonpharmacologic treatment emphasizes sleep hygiene, such as using the bed only for sleep and sex, and not for reading, television viewing, and eating.[250] Therapists must be sensitive to the impact of psychological and emotional distress and refer patients to clinical social workers or psychologists when appropriate.

## The Role of Manual Therapy

Although the various management approaches are beyond the scope of this chapter, manual therapy is one of the basic treatment options, and the role of orthopedic manual physical therapists cannot be overemphasized.[82,158] Myofascial trigger points are treated with manual techniques, spray and stretch, dry needling, or injection therapy. Dry needling is within the scope of physical therapy practice in many countries, including Canada, Spain, Ireland, South Africa, Australia, the Netherlands, and Switzerland. In the United States, the physical therapy boards of 12 states have ruled that physical therapists can engage in the practice of dry needling: New Hampshire, Maryland, Virginia, South Carolina, Georgia, Kentucky, New Mexico, Colorado, Alabama, Oregon, Texas, and Ohio.[80] A promising new development used in the diagnosis and treatment of MTrPs involves shockwave therapy, but as of yet there are no controlled studies substantiating its use.[251,252]

## Conclusion

Although MTrPs are a common cause of pain and dysfunction in persons with musculoskeletal injuries and diagnoses, the importance of MTrPs is not obvious from reviewing the orthopedic manual therapy literature. Current scientific evidence strongly supports that awareness and a working knowledge of muscle dysfunction—in particular, MTrPs—should be incorporated into manual physical therapy practice, consistent with the IFOMT guidelines for clinical practice. Although there are still many unanswered questions with regard to explaining the etiology of MTrPs, this chapter provides manual therapists with an up-to-date evidence-informed review of the current scientific knowledge.

## References

1. IFOMT. Available at: http://www.ifomt.org/ifomt/about/standards. Accessed November 15, 2006.
2. Huijbregts PA. Muscle injury, regeneration, and repair. *J Manual Manipulative Ther* 2001;9:9–16.
3. Urquhart DM, Hodges PW, Allen TJ, Story IH. Abdominal muscle recruitment during a range of voluntary exercises. *Man Ther* 2005;10:144–153.
4. Fernández-de-las-Peñas C, Alonso-Blanco C, Alguacil-Diego IM, Miangolarra-Page JC. Myofascial trigger points and postero-anterior joint hypomobility in the mid-cervical spine in subjects presenting with mechanical neck pain: A pilot study. *J Manual Manipulative Ther* 2006;14:88–94.
5. Fernández-de-las-Peñas C, Alonso-Blanco C, Miangolarra JC. Myofascial trigger points in subjects presenting with mechanical neck pain: A blinded, controlled study. *Man Ther* 2007;13:29–33.
6. Lew PC, Lewis J, Story I. Inter-therapist reliability in locating latent myofascial trigger points using palpation. *Man Ther* 1997;2:87–90.
7. Fernández-de-las-Peñas C, Alonso-Blanco C, Cuadrado ML, Pareja JA. Myofascial trigger points in the suboccipital muscles in episodic tension-type headache. *Man Ther* 2006;11:225–230.
8. Moore A, Petty N. Evidence-based practice: Getting a grip and finding a balance. *Man Ther* 2001;6:195–196.
9. Sackett DL, Rosenberg WM. The need for evidence-based medicine. *J R Soc Med* 1995;88:620–624.
10. Sackett DL, Rosenberg WM, Gray JA, Haynes RB, Richardson WS. Evidence-based medicine: What it is and what it isn't. *BMJ* 1996;312:71–72.
11. Pencheon D. What's next for evidence-based medicine? *Evidenced-Based Healthcare Public Health* 2005;9:319–321.

12. Cicerone KD. Evidence-based practice and the limits of rational rehabilitation. *Arch Phys Med Rehabil* 2005;86:1073–1074.
13. Baldry PE. *Acupuncture, Trigger Points and Musculoskeletal Pain*. Edinburgh, UK: Churchill Livingstone; 2005.
14. Simons DG. Muscle pain syndromes. Part 1. *Am J Phys Med* 1975;54:289–311.
15. Ruhmann W. The earliest book on rheumatism. *Br J Rheumatism* 1940;11:140–162.
16. Simons DG, Travell JG, Simons LS. *Travell and Simons' Myofascial Pain and Dysfunction: The Trigger Point Manual*. Vol. 1. 2nd ed. Baltimore, MD: Williams & Wilkins; 1999.
17. Harden RN, Bruehl SP, Gass S, Niemiec C, Barbick B. Signs and symptoms of the myofascial pain syndrome: A national survey of pain management providers. *Clin J Pain* 2000;16:64–72.
18. Stockman R. The causes, pathology, and treatment of chronic rheumatism. *Edinburgh Med J* 1904;15:107–116.
19. Strauss H. Über die sogenannten 'rheumatische Muskelschwiele' [German; With regard to the so-called myogelosis]. *Klin Wochenschr* 1898;35:89–91,121–123.
20. Lange M. *Die Muskelhärten (Myogelosen)* [German; The Muscle Hardenings (Myogeloses)]. Munich, Germany: J.F. Lehmann's Verlag; 1931.
21. Travell J. *Office Hours: Day and Night. The Autobiography of Janet Travell, MD*. New York, NY: World Publishing; 1968.
22. Kellgren JH. Deep pain sensibility. *Lancet* 1949;1:943–949.
23. Kellgren JH. Observations on referred pain arising from muscle. *Clin Sci* 1938;3:175–190.
24. Kellgren JH. A preliminary account of referred pains arising from muscle. *British Med J* 1938;1:325–327.
25. Simons DG. Cardiology and myofascial trigger points: Janet G. Travell's contribution. *Tex Heart Inst J* 2003;30(1):3–7.
26. Travell J. Basis for the multiple uses of local block of somatic trigger areas (procaine infiltration and ethyl chloride spray). *Miss Valley Med* 1949;71:13–22.
27. Travell J, Bobb AL. Mechanism of relief of pain in sprains by local injection techniques. *Fed Proc* 1947;6:378.
28. Travell JG, Rinzler S, Herman M. Pain and disability of the shoulder and arm: Treatment by intramuscular infiltration with procaine hydrochloride. *JAMA* 1942;120:417–422.
29. Travell JG, Rinzler SH. The myofascial genesis of pain. *Postgrad Med* 1952;11:452–434.
30. Chaitow L, DeLany J. Neuromuscular techniques in orthopedics. *Techniques in Orthopedics* 2003;18(1):74–86.
31. Good MG. Five hundred cases of myalgia in the British army. *Ann Rheum Dis* 1942;3:118–138.
32. Good MG. The role of skeletal muscle in the pathogenesis of diseases. *Acta Medica Scand* 1950;138:285–292.
33. Gutstein M. Common rheumatism and physiotherapy. *Br J Phys Med* 1940;3:46–50.
34. Gutstein M. Diagnosis and treatment of muscular rheumatism. *Br J Phys Med* 1938;1:302–321.
35. Kelly M. The nature of fibrositis. I. The myalgic lesion and its secondary effects: A reflex theory. *Ann Rheum Dis* 1945;5:1–7.
36. Kelly M. The nature of fibrositis. II. A study of the causation of the myalgic lesion (rheumatic, traumatic, infective). *Ann Rheum Dis* 1946;5:69–77.
37. Kelly M. The relief of facial pain by procaine (Novocaine) injections. *J Am Geriatr Soc* 1963;11:586–596.
38. Kelly M. The treatment of fibrositis and allied disorders by local anesthesia. *Med J Aust* 1941;1:294–298.

39. Schneider M, Cohen J, Laws S. *The Collected Writings of Nimmo & Vannerson: Pioneers of Chiropractic Trigger Point Therapy*. Pittsburgh, PA: Schneider; 2001.
40. Cohen JH, Gibbons RW. Raymond L. Nimmo and the evolution of trigger point therapy, 1929–1986. *J Manipulative Physiol Ther* 1998;21:167–172.
41. National Board of Chiropractic Economics. *Chiropractic Treatment Procedures*. Greely, CO, 1993.
42. Mennell J. Spray-stretch for the relief of pain from muscle spasm and myofascial trigger points. *J Am Podiatry Assoc* 1976;66:873–876.
43. Mennell J. Myofascial trigger points as a cause of headaches. *J Manipulative Physiol Ther*, 1989;12:308–313.
44. Travell W, Travell JG. Technic for reduction and ambulatory treatment of sacroiliac displacement. *Arch Phys Ther* 1942;23:222–232.
45. Paris, SV. A history of manipulative therapy through the ages and up to the current controversy in the United States. *J Manual Manipulative Ther* 2000;8(2):66–77.
46. Travell JG, Simons DG. *Myofascial Pain and Dysfunction: The Trigger Point Manual*. Vol. 2. Baltimore, MD: Williams & Wilkins; 1992.
47. Travell JG, Simons DG. *Myofascial Pain and Dysfunction: The Trigger Point Manual*. Vol. 1. Baltimore, MD: Williams & Wilkins; 1983.
48. Dejung B, Gröbli C, Colla F, Weissmann R. *Triggerpunkttherapie* [German; Trigger Point Therapy]. Bern, Switzerland: Hans Huber; 2003.
49. Ferguson LW, Gerwin R. *Clinical Mastery in the Treatment of Myofascial Pain*. Philadelphia, PA: Lippincott Williams & Wilkins; 2005.
50. Kostopoulos D, Rizopoulos K. *The Manual of Trigger Point and Myofascial Therapy*. Thorofare, NJ: Slack; 2001.
51. Prateepavanich P. *Myofascial Pain Syndrome: A Common Problem in Clinical Practice*. Bangkok, Thailand: Ammarind; 1999.
52. Rachlin ES, Rachlin IS. *Myofascial Pain and Fibromyalgia: Trigger Point Management*. St. Louis, MO: Mosby; 2002.
53. Cardinal S. *Points Détente et Acupuncture: Approche Neurophysiologique* [French; Trigger Points and Acupuncture: Neurophysiological Approach]. Montreal, Canada: Centre Collégial de Dévelopement de Matériel Didactique; 2004.
54. Jonckheere PDM. *Spieren en Dysfuncties, Trigger punten, Basisprincipes van de Myofasciale Therapie* [Dutch; Muscles and Dysfunctions, Basic Principles of Myofascial Therapy]. Brussels, Belgium: Satas; 1993.
55. Lucas KR, Polus BI, Rich PS. Latent myofascial trigger points: Their effect on muscle activation and movement efficiency. *J Bodywork Movement Ther* 2004;8:160–166.
56. Weissmann RD. Überlegungen zur Biomechanik in der Myofaszialen Triggerpunkttherapie [German; Considerations with regard to the biomechanics related to myofascial triggerpoint therapy]. *Physiotherapie* 2000;35(10):13–21.
57. Vecchiet L, Giamberardino MA, De Bigontina P. Comparative sensory evaluation of parietal tissues in painful and nonpainful areas in fibromyalgia and myofascial pain syndrome. In: Gebhart GF, Hammond DL, Jensen TS, eds. *Proceedings of the 7th World Congress on Pain (Progress in Pain Research and Management)*. Seattle, WA: IASP Press; 1994:177–185.
58. Vecchiet L, Giamberardino MA, Dragani L. Latent myofascial trigger points: Changes in muscular and subcutaneous pain thresholds at trigger point and target level. *J Manual Medicine* 1990;5:151–154.
59. Vecchiet L, Pizzigallo E, Iezzi S, Affaitati G, Vecchiet J, Giamberardino MA. Differentiation of sensitivity in different tissues and its clinical significance. *J Musculoskel Pain* 1998;6:33–45.
60. Dommerholt J. Persistent myalgia following whiplash. *Curr Pain Headache Rep* 2005;9:326–330.

61. Ge HY, Fernández-de-las-Peñas C, Arendt-Nielsen L. Sympathetic facilitation of hyperalgesia evoked from myofascial tender and trigger points in patients with unilateral shoulder pain. *Clin Neurophysiol* 2006;117:1545–1550.

62. Lidbeck J. Central hyperexcitability in chronic musculoskeletal pain: A conceptual break-through with multiple clinical implications. *Pain Res Manag* 2002;7(2):81–92.

63. Munglani R. Neurobiological mechanisms underlying chronic whiplash associated pain: The peripheral maintenance of central sensitization. *J Musculoskel Pain* 2000;8:169–178.

64. Dommerholt J, Issa TS. Differential diagnosis: Myofascial pain. In Chaitow L, ed. *Fibromyalgia Syndrome; A Practitioner's Guide to Treatment.* Edinburgh, UK: Churchill Livingstone. 2010: 179–213.

65. Gerwin RD, Shannon S, Hong CZ, Hubbard D, Gevirtz R. Interrater reliability in myofascial trigger point examination. *Pain* 1997;69(1–2):65–73.

66. Sciotti VM, Mittak VL, DiMarco L, Ford LM, Plezbert J, Santipadri E, Wigglesworth J, Ball K. Clinical precision of myofascial trigger point location in the trapezius muscle. *Pain* 2001;93(3):259–266.

67. Franssen JLM. *Handboek Oppervlakte Elektromyografie* [Dutch; Manual Surface Electromyography]. Utrecht, The Netherlands: De Tijdstroom; 1995.

68. Janda V. Muscle spasm: A proposed procedure for differential diagnosis. *J Manual Med* 1991;6:136–139.

69. Mense S. Pathophysiologic basis of muscle pain syndromes. In: Fischer AA, ed. *Myofascial Pain: Update in Diagnosis and Treatment.* Philadelphia, PA: W.B. Saunders Company; 1997:23–53.

70. Headly BJ. Evaluation and treatment of myofascial pain syndrome utilizing biofeedback. In: Cram JR, ed. *Clinical Electromyography for Surface Recordings.* Nevada City, NV: Clinical Resources; 1990:235–254.

71. Headley BJ. Chronic pain management. In: O'Sullivan SB, Schmitz TS, eds. *Physical Rehabilitation: Assessment and Treatment.* Philadelphia, PA: F.A. Davis Company; 1994:577–600.

72. Gerwin RD, Duranleau D. Ultrasound identification of the myofascial trigger point. *Muscle Nerve* 1997;20:767–768.

73. Hong CZ. Persistence of local twitch response with loss of conduction to and from the spinal cord. *Arch Phys Med Rehabil* 1994;75:12–16.

74. Hong C-Z, Torigoe Y. Electrophysiological characteristics of localized twitch responses in responsive taut bands of rabbit skeletal muscle. *J Musculoskel Pain* 1994;2:17–43.

75. Hong C-Z, Yu J. Spontaneous electrical activity of rabbit trigger spot after transection of spinal cord and peripheral nerve. *J Musculoskele Pain* 1998;6(4):45–58.

76. Fricton JR, Auvinen MD, Dykstra D, Schiffman E. Myofascial pain syndrome: Electromyographic changes associated with local twitch response. *Arch Phys Med Rehabil* 1985;66:314–317.

77. Simons DG, Dexter JR. Comparison of local twitch responses elicited by palpation and needling of myofascial trigger points. *J Musculoskel Pain* 1995;3:49–61.

78. Wang F, Audette J. Electrophysiological characteristics of the local twitch response with active myofascial pain of neck compared with a control group with latent trigger points. *Am J Phys Med Rehabil* 2000;79:203.

79. Audette JF, Wang F, Smith H. Bilateral activation of motor unit potentials with unilateral needle stimulation of active myofascial trigger points. *Am J Phys Med Rehabil* 2004;83:368–374.

80. Dommerholt J. Dry needling in orthopedic physical therapy practice. *Orthop Phys Ther Pract* 2004;16(3):15–20.

81. Hong C-Z. Lidocaine injection versus dry needling to myofascial trigger point: The importance of the local twitch response. *Am J Phys Med Rehabil* 1994;73:256–263.

82. Gerwin RD, Dommerholt J. Treatment of myofascial pain syndromes. In: Boswell MV, Cole BE, eds. *Weiner's Pain Management: A Practical Guide for Clinicians.* Boca Raton, FL: CRC Press; 2006:477–492.

83. Vecchiet L, Dragani L, De Bigontina P, Obletter G, Giamberardino MA. Experimental referred pain and hyperalgesia from muscles in humans. In: Vecchiet L, et al, eds. *New Trends in Referred Pain and Hyperalgesia*. Amsterdam, The Netherlands: Elsevier Science; 1993:239–249.

84. Vecchiet L, Giamberardino MA. Referred pain: Clinical significance, pathophysiology and treatment. In: Fischer AA, ed. *Myofascial Pain: Update in Diagnosis and Treatment*. Philadelphia, PA: W.B. Saunders Company; 1997:119–136.

85. Mense S. The pathogenesis of muscle pain. *Curr Pain Headache Rep* 2003;7:419–425.

86. Mense S. Referral of muscle pain: New aspects. *Amer Pain Soc J* 1994;3:1–9.

87. Fernández-de-las-Peñas CF, Cuadrado ML, Gerwin RD, Pareja JA. Referred pain from the trochlear region in tension-type headache: A myofascial trigger point from the superior oblique muscle. *Headache* 2005;45:731–737.

88. Fernández-de-las-Peñas C, Cuadrado ML, Gerwin RD, Pareja JA. Myofascial disorders in the trochlear region in unilateral migraine: A possible initiating or perpetuating factor. *Clin J Pain* 2006;22:548–553.

89. Hwang M, Kang YK, Kim DH. Referred pain pattern of the pronator quadratus muscle. *Pain* 2005;116:238–242.

90. Hwang M, Kang YK, Shin JY, Kim DH. Referred pain pattern of the abductor pollicis longus muscle. *Am J Phys Med Rehabil* 2005;84:593–597.

91. Hong CZ, Kuan TS, Chen JT, Chen SM. Referred pain elicited by palpation and by needling of myofascial trigger points: A comparison. *Arch Phys Med Rehabil* 1997;78:957–960.

92. Dwyer A, Aprill C, Bogduk N. Cervical zygapophyseal joint pain patterns. I: A study in normal volunteers. *Spine* 1990;15:453–457.

93. Giamberardino MA, Vecchiet L. Visceral pain, referred hyperalgesia and outcome: New concepts. *Eur J Anaesthesiol* 1995;10(suppl):61–66.

94. Scudds RA, Landry M, Birmingham T, Buchan J, Griffin K. The frequency of referred signs from muscle pressure in normal healthy subjects (abstract). *J Musculoskel Pain* 1995;3(suppl 1):99.

95. Torebjörk HE, Ochoa JL, Schady W. Referred pain from intraneural stimulation of muscle fascicles in the median nerve. *Pain* 1984;18:145–156.

96. Gibson W, Arendt-Nielsen L, Graven-Nielsen T. Referred pain and hyperalgesia in human tendon and muscle belly tissue. *Pain* 2006;120(1–2):113–123.

97. Gibson W, Arendt-Nielsen L, Graven-Nielsen T. Delayed onset muscle soreness at tendon-bone junction and muscle tissue is associated with facilitated referred pain. *Exp Brain Res* 2006;174(2):351–60.

98. Hendler NH, Kozikowski JG. Overlooked physical diagnoses in chronic pain patients involved in litigation. *Psychosomatics* 1993;34:494–501.

99. Weiner DK, Sakamoto S, Perera S, Breuer P. Chronic low back pain in older adults: Prevalence, reliability, and validity of physical examination findings. *J Am Geriatr Soc* 2006;54:11–20.

100. Calandre EP, Hidalgo J, Garcia-Leiva JM, Rico-Villademoros F. Trigger point evaluation in migraine patients: An indication of peripheral sensitization linked to migraine predisposition? *Eur J Neurol* 2006;13:244–249.

101. Headache Classification Subcommittee of the International Headache Society: The international classification of headache disorders. *Cephalalgia* 2004;24(suppl 1):9–160.

102. Fricton JR, Kroening R, Haley D, Siegert R. Myofascial pain syndrome of the head and neck: A review of clinical characteristics of 164 patients. *Oral Surg Oral Med Oral Pathol* 1985;60:615–623.

103. Gerwin R. A study of 96 subjects examined both for fibromyalgia and myofascial pain (abstract). *J Musculoskel Pain* 1995;3(suppl 1):121.

104. Rosomoff HL, Fishbain DA, Goldberg N, Rosomoff RS. Myofascial findings with patients with chronic intractable benign pain of the back and neck. *Pain Management* 1989;3:114–118.

105. Skootsky SA, Jaeger B, Oye RK. Prevalence of myofascial pain in general internal medicine practice. *West J Med* 1989;151:157–160.

106. Chaiamnuay P, Darmawan J, Muirden KD, Assawatanabodee P. Epidemiology of rheumatic disease in rural Thailand: A WHO-ILAR COPCORD study. Community Oriented Programme for the Control of Rheumatic Disease. *J Rheumatol* 1998;25:1382–1387.

107. Graff-Radford B. Myofascial trigger points: Their importance and diagnosis in the dental office. *J Dent Assoc S Afr* 1984;39:249–253.

108. Bajaj P, Bajaj P, Graven-Nielsen T, Arendt-Nielsen L. Trigger points in patients with lower limb osteoarthritis. *J Musculoskel Pain* 2001;9(3):17–33.

109. Hsueh TC, Yu S, Kuan TS, Hong C-Z. Association of active myofascial trigger points and cervical disc lesions. *J Formosa Med Assoc* 1998;97(3):174–180.

110. Wang C-F, Chen M, Lin M-T, Kuan T-S, Hong C-Z. Teres minor tendinitis manifested with chronic myofascial pain syndrome in the scapular muscles: A case report. *J Musculoskel Pain* 2006;14(1):39–43.

111. Fricton JR. Etiology and management of masticatory myofascial pain. *J Musculoskel Pain* 1999;7(1–2):143–160.

112. Teachey WS. Otolaryngic myofascial pain syndromes. *Curr Pain Headache Rep* 2004;8:457–462.

113. Dommerholt J. El sindrome de dolor miofascial en la region craneomandibular. [Spanish; Myofascial pain syndrome in the craniomandibular region]. In: Padrós Serrat E, ed. *Bases diagnosticas, terapeuticas y posturales del functionalismo craniofacial.* Madrid, Spain: Ripano; 2006:564–581.

114. Hesse J, Mogelvang B, Simonsen H. Acupuncture versus metoprolol in migraine prophylaxis: A randomized trial of trigger point inactivation. *J Intern Med* 1994;235:451–456.

115. Skubick DL, Clasby R, Donaldson CC, Marshall WM. Carpal tunnel syndrome as an expression of muscular dysfunction in the neck. *J Occupational Rehab* 1993;3:31–43.

116. Treaster D, Marras WS, Burr D, Sheedy JE, Hart D. Myofascial trigger point development from visual and postural stressors during computer work. *J Electromyogr Kinesiol* 2006;16:115–124.

117. Baker BA. The muscle trigger: Evidence of overload injury. *J Neurol Orthop Med Surg* 1986;7:35–44.

118. Fruth SJ. Differential diagnosis and treatment in a patient with posterior upper thoracic pain. *Phys Ther* 2006;86:254–268.

119. Doggweiler-Wiygul R. Urologic myofascial pain syndromes. *Curr Pain Headache Rep* 2004;8:445–451.

120. Jarrell J. Myofascial dysfunction in the pelvis. *Curr Pain Headache Rep* 2004;8:452–456.

121. Jarrell JF, Vilos GA, Allaire C, Burgess S, Fortin C, Gerwin R, Lapensee L, Lea RH, Leyland NA, Martyn P, Shenassa H, Taenzer P, Abu-Rafea B. Consensus guidelines for the management of chronic pelvic pain. *J Obstet Gynaecol Can* 2005;27:869–887

122. Weiss JM. Pelvic floor myofascial trigger points: Manual therapy for interstitial cystitis and the urgency-frequency syndrome. *J Urol* 2001;166:2226–2231.

123. Dommerholt J. Muscle pain syndromes. In: Cantu RI, Grodin AJ, eds. *Myofascial Manipulation.* Gaithersburg, MD: Aspen; 2001:93–140.

124. Weiner DK, Schmader KE. Postherpetic pain: More than sensory neuralgia? *Pain Med* 2006;7:243–249.

125. Chen SM, Chen JT, Kuan TS, Hong C-Z. Myofascial trigger points in intercostal muscles secondary to herpes zoster infection of the intercostal nerve. *Arch Phys Med Rehabil* 1998;79:336–338.

126. Dommerholt J. Complex regional pain syndrome. Part 1: History, diagnostic criteria and etiology. *J Bodywork Movement Ther* 2004;8:167–177.

127. Rashiq S, Galer BS. Proximal myofascial dysfunction in complex regional pain syndrome: A retrospective prevalence study. *Clin J Pain*,1999;15:151–153.

128. Prateepavanich P, Kupniratsaikul VC. The relationship between myofascial trigger points of gastrocnemius muscle and nocturnal calf cramps. *J Med Assoc Thailand* 1999;82:451–459.

129. Kern KU, Martin C, Scheicher S, Muller H. Auslosung von Phantomschmerzen und-sensationen durch Muskuläre Stumpftriggerpunkte nach Beinamputationen [German; Referred pain from amputation stump trigger points into the phantom limb]. *Schmerz* 2006;20:300–306.

130. Kern U, Martin C, Scheicher S, Müller H. Does botulinum toxin A make prosthesis use easier for amputees? *J Rehabil Med* 2004;36:238–239.

131. Longbottom J. A case report of postulated "Barré Liéou syndrome." *Acupunct Med* 2005;23:34–38.

132. Stellon A. Neurogenic pruritus: An unrecognized problem? A retrospective case series of treatment by acupuncture. *Acupunct Med* 2002;20:186–190.

133. Fernández-de-las-Peñas C, Fernández-Carnero J, Miangolarra-Page JC. Musculoskeletal disorders in mechanical neck pain: Myofascial trigger points versus cervical joint dysfunction. *J Musculoskel Pain* 2005;13(1):27–35.

134. Hägg GM. Ny förklaringsmodell för muskelskador vid statisk belastning i skuldra och nacke [Swedish; New explanation for muscle damage as a result of static loads in the neck and shoulder]. *Arbete Människa Miljö* 1988;4:260–262.

135. Henneman E, Somjen G, Carpenter DO. Excitability and inhibitability of motoneurons of different sizes. *J Neurophysiol* 1965;28:599–620.

136. Hägg GM. The Cinderella Hypothesis. In: Johansson H, et al, eds. *Chronic Work-Related Myalgia*. Gävle, Sweden: Gävle University Press; 2003:127–132.

137. Armstrong RB. Initial events in exercise-induced muscular injury. *Med Sci Sports Exerc* 1990;22:429–435.

138. Hägg GM. Human muscle fibre abnormalities related to occupational load. *Eur J Appl Physiol* 2000;83(2–3):159–165.

139. Kadi F, Hagg G, Hakansson R, Holmner S, Butler-Browne GS, Thornell LE. Structural changes in male trapezius muscle with work-related myalgia. *Acta Neuropathol (Berl)* 1998;95:352–360.

140. Kadi F, Waling K, Ahlgren C, Sundelin G, Holmner S, Butler-Browne GS, Thornell LE. Pathological mechanisms implicated in localized female trapezius myalgia. *Pain*,1998;78:191–196.

141. Larsson B, Bjork J, Kadi F, Lindman R, Gerdle B. Blood supply and oxidative metabolism in muscle biopsies of female cleaners with and without myalgia. *Clin J Pain* 2004;20:440–446.

142. Henriksson KG, Bengtsson A, Lindman R, Thornell LE. Morphological changes in muscle in fibromyalgia and chronic shoulder myalgia. In: Værøy H, Merskey H, eds. *Progress in Fibromyalgia and Myofascial Pain*. Amsterdam, The Netherlands: Elsevier; 1993:61–73.

143. Lexell J, Jarvis J, Downham D, Salmons S. Stimulation-induced damage in rabbit fast-twitch skeletal muscles: A quantitative morphological study of the influence of pattern and frequency. *Cell Tissue Res* 1993;273:357–362.

144. Gissel H. $Ca^{2+}$ accumulation and cell damage in skeletal muscle during low frequency stimulation. *Eur J Appl Physiol* 2000;83(2–3):175–180.

145. Gissel H, Clausen T. Excitation-induced $Ca^{(2+)}$ influx in rat soleus and EDL muscle: Mechanisms and effects on cellular integrity. *Am J Physiol Regul Integr Comp Physiol* 2000;279:R917–R924.

146. Febbraio MA, Pedersen BK. Contraction-induced myokine production and release: Is skeletal muscle an endocrine organ? *Exerc Sport Sci Rev* 2005;33(3):114–119.

147. Pedersen BK, Febbraio M. Muscle-derived interleukin-6: A possible link between skeletal muscle, adipose tissue, liver, and brain. *Brain Behav Immun* 2005;19:371–376.

148. Forsman M, Birch L, Zhang Q, Kadefors R. Motor unit recruitment in the trapezius muscle with special reference to coarse arm movements. *J Electromyogr Kinesiol* 2001;11:207–216.

149. Forsman M, Kadefors R, Zhang Q, Birch L, Palmerud G. Motor-unit recruitment in the trapezius muscle during arm movements and in VDU precision work. *Int J Ind Ergon* 1999;24:619–630.

150. Forsman M, Taoda K, Thorn S, Zhang Q. Motor-unit recruitment during long-term isometric and wrist motion contractions: A study concerning muscular pain development in computer operators. *Int J Ind Ergon* 2002;30:237–250.

151. Zennaro D, Laubli T, Krebs D, Klipstein A, Krueger H. Continuous, intermittent and sporadic motor unit activity in the trapezius muscle during prolonged computer work. *J Electromyogr Kinesiol* 2003;13:113–124.

152. Zennaro D, Laubli T, Krebs D, Krueger H, Klipstein A. Trapezius muscle motor unint activity in symptomatic participants during finger tapping using properly and improperly adjusted desks. *Hum Factors* 2004;46:252–266.

153. Andersen JH, Kærgaard A, Rasmussen K. Myofascial pain in different occupational groups with monotonous repetitive work (abstract). *J Musculoskel Pain* 1995;3(suppl 1):57.

154. Chen S-M, Chen J-T, Kuan T-S, Hong J, Hong C-Z. Decrease in pressure pain thresholds of latent myofascial trigger points in the middle finger extensors immediately after continuous piano practice. *J Musculoskel Pain* 2000;8(3):83–92.

155. Otten E. Concepts and models of functional architecture in skeletal muscle. *Exerc Sport Sci Rev* 1988;16:89–137.

156. Sjogaard G, Lundberg U, Kadefors R. The role of muscle activity and mental load in the development of pain and degenerative processes at the muscle cell level during computer work. *Eur J Appl Physiol* 2000;83(2–3):99–105.

157. Sjogaard G, Sogaard K. Muscle injury in repetitive motion disorders. *Clin Orthop* 1998;351:21–31.

158. Simons DG. Understanding effective treatments of myofascial trigger points. *J Bodywork Movement Ther* 2002;6:81–88.

159. Proske U, Morgan DL. Stiffness of cat soleus muscle and tendon during activation of part of muscle. *J Neurophysiol* 1984;52:459–468.

160. Trotter JA. Functional morphology of force transmission in skeletal muscle: A brief review. *Acta Anat (Basel)* 1993;146(4):205–222.

161. Monti RJ, Roy RR, Hodgson JA, Edgerton VR. Transmission of forces within mammalian skeletal muscles. *J Biomech* 1999;32:371–380.

162. Bodine SC, Roy RR, Eldred E, Edgerton VR. Maximal force as a function of anatomical features of motor units in the cat tibialis anterior. *J Neurophysiol* 1987;57:1730–1745.

163. Ounjian M, Roy RR, Eldred E, Garfinkel A, Payne JR, Armstrong A, Toga AW, Edgerton VR. Physiological and developmental implications of motor unit anatomy. *J Neurobiol* 1991;22:547–559.

164. Petit J, Filippi GM, Emonet-Denand F, Hunt CC, Laporte Y. Changes in muscle stiffness produced by motor units of different types in peroneus longus muscle of cat. *J Neurophysiol* 1990;63:190–197.

165. Petit J, Filippi GM, Gioux M, Hunt CC, Laporte Y. Effects of tetanic contraction of motor units of similar type on the initial stiffness to ramp stretch of the cat peroneus longus muscle. *J Neurophysiol* 1990;64:1724–1732.

166. Altringham JD, Bottinelli R. The descending limb of the sarcomere length-force relation in single muscle fibres of the frog. *J Muscle Res Cell Motil* 1985;6:585–600.

167. Street SF. Lateral transmission of tension in frog myofibers: A myofibrillar network and transverse cytoskeletal connections are possible transmitters. *J Cell Physiol* 1983;114:346–364.

168. Denoth J, Stussi E, Csucs G, Danuser G. Single muscle fiber contraction is dictated by inter-sarcomere dynamics. *J Theor Biol* 2002;216(1):101–122.
169. Dommerholt J, Royson MW, Whyte-Ferguson L. Neck pain and dysfunction following whiplash. In: Whyte-Ferguson L, Gerwin RD, eds. *Clinical Mastery of Myofascial Pain Syndrome*. Baltimore, MD: Lippincott, Williams & Wilkins; 2005:57–89.
170. Jull GA. Deep cervical flexor muscle dysfunction in whiplash. *J Musculoskel Pain* 2000;8(1–2): 143–154.
171. Kumar S, Narayan Y, Amell T. Analysis of low velocity frontal impacts. *Clin Biomech* 2003;18:694–703.
172. Sterling M, Jull G, Vicenzino B, Kenardy J, Darnell R. Development of motor system dysfunction following whiplash injury. *Pain* 2003;103(1–2):65–73.
173. Sterling M, Jull G, Vicenzino B, Kenardy J, Darnell R. Physical and psychological factors predict outcome following whiplash injury. *Pain* 2005;114(1–2):141–148.
174. Schuller E, Eisenmenger W, Beier G. Whiplash injury in low speed car accidents. *J Musculoskel Pain* 2000;8(1–2):55–67.
175. Simons DG. Triggerpunkte und Myogelose [German; Trigger points and myogeloses]. *Manuelle Medizin* 1997;35:290–294.
176. Gerwin RD, Dommerholt J. Myofascial trigger points in chronic cervical whiplash syndrome. *J Musculoskel Pain* 1998;6(suppl. 2):28.
177. Fernández-de-las-Peñas C, Fernández-Carnero J, Palomeque-del-Cerro L, Miangolarra-Page JC. Manipulative treatment vs. conventional physiotherapy treatment in whiplash injury: A randomized controlled trial. *J Whiplash Rel Disord* 2004;3(2):73–90.
178. Fernández-de-las-Peñas C, Palomeque-del-Cerro L, Fernández-Carnero J. Manual treatment of post-whiplash injury. *J Bodywork Movement Ther* 2005;9:109–119.
179. Simons DG, Travell J. Myofascial trigger points: A possible explanation. *Pain* 1981;10:106–109.
180. Sterling M, Jull G, Vicenzino B, Kenardy J. Sensory hypersensitivity occurs soon after whiplash injury and is associated with poor recovery. *Pain* 2003;104:509–517.
181. Scott D, Jull G, Sterling M. Widespread sensory hypersensitivity is a feature of chronic whiplash-associated disorder but not chronic idiopathic neck pain. *Clin J Pain* 2005;21: 175–181.
182. Vecchiet L, Vecchiet J, Bellomo R, Giamberardino MA. Muscle pain from physical exercise. *J Musculoskel Pain* 1999;7(1–2):43–53.
183. Simons DG. Review of enigmatic MTrPs as a common cause of enigmatic musculoskeletal pain and dysfunction. *J Electromyogr Kinesiol* 2004;14:95–107.
184. Gerwin RD, Dommerholt J, Shah J. An expansion of Simons' integrated hypothesis of trigger point formation. *Curr Pain Headache Rep* 2004;8:468–475.
185. Newham DJ, Jones DA, Clarkson PM. Repeated high-force eccentric exercise: Effects on muscle pain and damage. *J Appl Physiol* 1987;63:1381–1386.
186. Fridén J, Lieber RL. Segmental muscle fiber lesions after repetitive eccentric contractions. *Cell Tissue Res* 1998;293:165–171.
187. Stauber WT, Clarkson PM, Fritz VK, Evans WJ. Extracellular matrix disruption and pain after eccentric muscle action. *J Appl Physiol* 1990;69:868–874.
188. Graven-Nielsen T, Arendt-Nielsen L. Induction and assessment of muscle pain, referred pain, and muscular hyperalgesia. *Curr Pain Headache Rep* 2003;7:443–451.
189. Lieber RL, Shah S, Fridén J. Cytoskeletal disruption after eccentric contraction-induced muscle injury. *Clin Orthop* 2002;403:S90–S99.
190. Lieber RL, Thornell LE, Fridén J. Muscle cytoskeletal disruption occurs within the first 15 min of cyclic eccentric contraction. *J Appl Physiol* 1996;80:278–284.

191. Barash IA, Peters D, Fridén J, Lutz GJ, Lieber RL. Desmin cytoskeletal modifications after a bout of eccentric exercise in the rat. *Am J Physiol Regul Integr Comp Physiol* 2002;283:R958–R963.

192. Thompson JL, Balog EM, Fitts RH, Riley DA. Five myofibrillar lesion types in eccentrically challenged, unloaded rat adductor longus muscle: A test model. *Anat Rec* 1999;254:39–52.

193. Lieber RL, Fridén J. Mechanisms of muscle injury gleaned from animal models. *Am J Phys Med Rehabil* 2002;81(11 suppl):S70–S79.

194. Peters D, Barash IA, Burdi M, Yuan PS, Mathew L, Fridén J, Lieber RL. Asynchronous functional, cellular and transcriptional changes after a bout of eccentric exercise in the rat. *J Physiol* 2003;553(Pt 3):947–957.

195. Bowers EJ, Morgan DL, Proske U. Damage to the human quadriceps muscle from eccentric exercise and the training effect. *J Sports Sci* 2004;22(11–12):1005–1014.

196. Byrne C, Twist C, Eston R. Neuromuscular function after exercise-induced muscle damage: Theoretical and applied implications. *Sports Med* 2004;34(1):49–69.

197. Hamlin MJ, Quigley BM. Quadriceps concentric and eccentric exercise. 2: Differences in muscle strength, fatigue and EMG activity in eccentrically-exercised sore and non-sore muscles. *J Sci Med Sport* 2001;4(1):104–115.

198. Pearce AJ, Sacco P, Byrnes ML, Thickbroom GW, Mastaglia FL. The effects of eccentric exercise on neuromuscular function of the biceps brachii. *J Sci Med Sport* 1998;1(4):236–244.

199. Shah JP, Phillips TM, Danoff JV, Gerber LH. An *in-vivo* microanalytical technique for measuring the local biochemical milieu of human skeletal muscle. *J Appl Physiol* 2005;99:1980–1987.

200. Itoh K, Okada K, Kawakita K. A proposed experimental model of myofascial trigger points in human muscle after slow eccentric exercise. *Acupunct Med* 2004;22(1):2–12.

201. Brückle W, Sückfull M, Fleckenstein W, Weiss C, Müller W. Gewebe-pO$_2$-Messung in der verspannten Rückenmuskulatur (m. erector spinae) [German; Tissue pO$_2$ in hypertonic back muscles]. *Z Rheumatol* 1990;49:208–216.

202. McCleskey EW, Gold MS. Ion channels of nociception. *Annu Rev Physiol* 1999;61:835–856.

203. Sluka KA, Kalra A, Moore SA. Unilateral intramuscular injections of acidic saline produce a bilateral, long-lasting hyperalgesia. *Muscle Nerve* 2001;24:37–46.

204. Sluka KA, Price MP, Breese NM, Stucky CL, Wemmie JA, Welsh MJ. Chronic hyperalgesia induced by repeated acid injections in muscle is abolished by the loss of ASIC3, but not ASIC1. *Pain* 2003;106:229–239.

205. Weeks VD. Travell J. How to give painless injections. In: *AMA Scientific Exhibits*. New York, NY: Grune & Stratton; 1957:318–322.

206. Hubbard DR, Berkoff GM. Myofascial trigger points show spontaneous needle EMG activity. *Spine* 1993;18:1803–1807.

207. Couppé C, Midttun A, Hilden J, Jørgensen U, Oxholm P, Fuglsang-Frederiksen A. Spontaneous needle electromyographic activity in myofascial trigger points in the infraspinatus muscle: A blinded assessment. *J Musculoskel Pain* 2001;9(3):7–17.

208. Simons DG. Do endplate noise and spikes arise from normal motor endplates? *Am J Phys Med Rehabil* 2001;80:134–140.

209. Simons DG, Hong C-Z, Simons LS. Endplate potentials are common to midfiber myofascial trigger points. *Am J Phys Med Rehabil* 2002;81:212–222.

210. Macgregor J, Graf von Schweinitz D. Needle electromyographic activity of myofascial trigger points and control sites in equine cleidobrachialis muscle: An observational study. *Acupunct Med* 2006;24(2):61–70.

211. Mense S. Neurobiological basis for the use of botulinum toxin in pain therapy. *J Neurol* 2004;251(suppl 1):I1–I7.

212. De Paiva A, Meunier FA, Molgo J, Aoki KR, Dolly JO. Functional repair of motor endplates after botulinum neurotoxin type A poisoning: Biphasic switch of synaptic activity between nerve sprouts and their parent terminals. *Proc Natl Acad Sci USA* 1999;96:3200–3205.

213. Chen BM, Grinnell AD. Kinetics, $Ca^{2+}$ dependence, and biophysical properties of integrin-mediated mechanical modulation of transmitter release from frog motor nerve terminals. *J Neurosci* 1997;17:904–916.

214. Grinnell AD, Chen BM, Kashani A, Lin J, Suzuki K, Kidokoro Y. The role of integrins in the modulation of neurotransmitter release from motor nerve terminals by stretch and hypertonicity. *J Neurocytol* 2003;32(5-8):489–503.

215. Kashani AH, Chen BM, Grinnell AD. Hypertonic enhancement of transmitter release from frog motor nerve terminals: $Ca^{2+}$ independence and role of integrins. *J Physiol* 2001;530(Pt 2):243–252.

216. Wang K, Yu L. Emerging concepts of muscle contraction and clinical implications for myofascial pain syndrome (abstract). In: *Focus on Pain*. Mesa, AZ: Janet G. Travell, MD Seminar Series; 2000.

217. Bukharaeva EA, Salakhutdinov RI, Vyskocil F, Nikolsky EE. Spontaneous quantal and non-quantal release of acetylcholine at mouse endplate during onset of hypoxia. *Physiol Res* 2005;54:251–255.

218. Hoheisel U, Mense S, Simons D, Yu X-M. Appearance of new receptive fields in rat dorsal horn neurons following noxious stimulation of skeletal muscle: A model for referral of muscle pain? *Neurosci Lett* 1993;153:9–12.

219. Simons DG, Stolov WC. Microscopic features and transient contraction of palpable bands in canine muscle. *Am J Phys Med* 1976;55:65–88.

220. Reitinger A, Radner H, Tilscher H, Hanna M, Windisch A, Feigl W. Morphologische Untersuchung an Triggerpunkten [German; Morphological investigation of trigger points]. *Manuelle Medizin* 1996;34:256–262.

221. Windisch A, Reitinger A, Traxler H, Radner H, Neumayer C, Feigl W, Firbas W. Morphology and histochemistry of myogelosis. *Clin Anat* 1999;12:266–271.

222. Mense S, Simons DG, Hoheisel U, Quenzer B. Lesions of rat skeletal muscle after local block of acetylcholinesterase and neuromuscular stimulation. *J Appl Physiol* 2003;94:2494–2501.

223. Pongratz D. Neuere Ergebnisse zur Pathogenese Myofaszialer Schmerzsyndrom [German; New findings with regard to the etiology of myofascial pain syndrome]. *Nervenheilkunde* 2002;21(1):35–37.

224. Pongratz DE, Späth M. Morphologic aspects of muscle pain syndromes. In: Fischer AA, ed. *Myofascial Pain: Update in Diagnosis and Treatment*. Philadelphia, PA: W.B. Saunders Company; 1997:55–68.

225. Gariphianova MB. The ultrastructure of myogenic trigger points in patients with contracture of mimetic muscles (abstract). *J Musculoskel Pain* 1995;3(suppl 1):23.

226. Glogowsky C, Wallraff J. Ein Beitrag zur Klinik und Histologie der Muskelhärten (Myogelosen) [German; A contribution on clinical aspects and histology of myogeloses]. *Z Orthop* 1951;80:237–268.

227. Fassbender HG. Morphologie und Pathogenese des Weichteilrheumatismus [German; Morphology and etiology of soft tissue rheumatism]. *Z Rheumaforsch* 1973;32:355–374.

228. Hubbard DR. Chronic and recurrent muscle pain: Pathophysiology and treatment, and review of pharmacologic studies. *J Musculoskel Pain* 1996;4:123–143.

229. Lewis C, Gevirtz R, Hubbard D, Berkoff G. Needle trigger point and surface frontal EMG measurements of psychophysiological responses in tension-type headache patients. *Biofeedback & Self-Regulation* 1994;3:274–275.

230. McNulty WH, Gevirtz RN, Hubbard DR, Berkoff GM. Needle electromyographic evaluation of trigger point response to a psychological stressor. *Psychophysiology* 1994;31:313–316.

231. Banks SL, Jacobs DW, Gevirtz R, Hubbard DR. Effects of autogenic relaxation training on electromyographic activity in active myofascial trigger points. *J Musculoskel Pain* 1998;6(4):23–32.

232. Chen JT, Chen SM, Kuan TS, Chung KC, Hong C-Z. Phentolamine effect on the spontaneous electrical activity of active loci in a myofascial trigger spot of rabbit skeletal muscle. *Arch Phys Med Rehabil* 1998;79:790–794.

233. Chen SM, Chen JT, Kuan TS, Hong C-Z. Effect of neuromuscular blocking agent on the spontaneous activity of active loci in a myofascial trigger spot of rabbit skeletal muscle. *J Musculoskel Pain* 1998;6(suppl. 2):25.

234. Bowman WC, Marshall IG, Gibb AJ, Harborne AJ. Feedback control of transmitter release at the neuromuscular junction. *Trends Pharmacol Sci* 1988;9(1):16–20.

235. Cunha FQ, Lorenzetti BB, Poole S, Ferreira SH. Interleukin-8 as a mediator of sympathetic pain. *Br J Pharmacol* 1991;104:765–767.

236. Verri WA, Jr., Cunha TM, Parada CA, Poole S, Cunha FQ, Ferreira SH. Hypernociceptive role of cytokines and chemokines: Targets for analgesic drug development? *Pharmacol Ther* 2006; 112(1):116–38.

237. Poole S, de Queiroz Cunha F, Ferreira SH. Hyperalgesia from subcutaneous cytokines. In: Watkins LR, Maier SF, eds. *Cytokines and Pain*. Basel, Switzerland: Birkhaueser; 1999:59–87.

238. Fernandez HL, Hodges-Savola CA. Physiological regulation of G4 AChE in fast-twitch muscle: Effects of exercise and CGRP. *J Appl Physiol* 1996;80:357–362.

239. Hodges-Savola CA, Fernandez HL. A role for calcitonin gene-related peptide in the regulation of rat skeletal muscle G4 acetylcholinesterase. *Neurosci Lett* 1995;190(2):117–120.

240. Fernandez-de-las-Penas C, Alonso-Blanco C, Cuadrado ML, Gerwin RD, Pareja JA. Trigger points in the suboccipital muscles and forward head posture in tension-type headache. *Headache* 2006;46:454–460.

241. Gerwin RD. Factores que promueven la persistencia de mialgia en el síndrome de dolor miofascial y en la fibromyalgia [Spanish; Factors that promote the continued existence of myalgia in myofascial pain syndrome and fibromyalgia]. *Fisioterapia* 2005;27(2):76–86.

242. Gerwin RD. A review of myofascial pain and fibromyalgia: Factors that promote their persistence. *Acupunct Med* 2005;23(3):121–134.

243. Andres E, Loukili NH, Noel E, Kaltenbach G, Abdelgheni MB, Perrin AE, Noblet-Dick M, Maloisel F, Schlienger JL, Blickle JF. Vitamin $B_{12}$ (cobalamin) deficiency in elderly patients. *CMAJ* 2004;171:251–259.

244. Pruthi RK, Tefferi A. Pernicious anemia revisited. *Mayo Clin Proc* 1994;69:144–150.

245. Plotnikoff GA, Quigley JM. Prevalence of severe hypovitaminosis D in patients with persistent, nonspecific musculoskeletal pain. *Mayo Clin Proc* 2003;78:1463–1470.

246. Bogduk N, Simons DG. Neck pain: Joint pain or trigger points. In: Værøy H, Merskey H, eds. *Progress in Fibromyalgia and Myofascial Pain*. Amsterdam, The Netherlands: Elsevier; 1993:267–273.

247. Padamsee M, Mehta N, White GE. Trigger point injection: A neglected modality in the treatment of TMJ dysfunction. *J Pedod* 1987;12(1):72–92.

248. Linton SJ. A review of psychological risk factors in back and neck pain. *Spine* 2000;25: 1148–1156.

249. Vlaeyen JW, Linton SJ. Fear-avoidance and its consequences in chronic musculoskeletal pain: A state of the art. *Pain* 2000;85:317–332.

250. Menefee LA, Cohen MJ, Anderson WR, Doghramji K, Frank ED, Lee H. Sleep disturbance and nonmalignant chronic pain: A comprehensive review of the literature. *Pain Med* 2000;1:156–172.

251. Bauermeister W. Diagnose und Therapie des Myofaszialen Triggerpunkt Syndroms durch Lokalisierung und Stimulation sensibilisierter Nozizeptoren mit fokussierten elektrohydraulische Stosswellen [German; Diagnosis and therapy of myofascial trigger point symptoms by localization and stimulation of sensitized nociceptors with focused ultrasound shockwaves]. *Medizinisch-Orthopädische Technik* 2005;5:65–74.

252. Müller-Ehrenberg H, Licht G. Diagnosis and therapy of myofascial pain syndrome with focused shock waves (ESWT). *Medizinisch-Orthopädische Technik* 2005;5:1–6.

# Chapter 3

# Nutritional and Metabolic Perpetuating Factors in Myofascial Pain

*Jan Dommerholt, PT, MPS, DPT, DAAPM*

*Robert D. Gerwin, MD, FAAN*

## Introduction

In the clinical management of patients with chronic myofascial pain, it is critical to consider any probable underlying cause or contributing factor. Chronic pain is very common and has a major impact on patients, clinicians, and society as a whole. Between 20–25% of the U.S. population has regional chronic muscle pain, and 10–15% has chronic widespread pain.[1] A recent survey in 15 European countries and Israel showed that 19% of adults suffered from significant long-lasting pain.[2] In a similar study, 56% of patients with cancer suffered moderate to severe pain at least monthly.[3] Considering all different types of chronic pain, including cancer pain, musculoskeletal pain is the most prevalent type of pain.[4]

Chronic muscle pain may not improve until underlying perpetuating or precipitating factors are managed.[5,6] In some cases, the pain problem can even be totally resolved when these perpetuating factors are corrected. In the context of myofascial pain, Travell and Simons[7] identified structural or mechanical perpetuating factors, such as scoliosis, leg length discrepancies, localized or widespread joint hypermobility, and nutritional, metabolic, or systemic perpetuating factors, including vitamin insufficiencies or hormonal imbalances, such as seen with hypothyroidism. A comprehensive medical evaluation is indicated to identify any conditions that may feature diffuse myalgia. In this era of direct access and often limited contact time between physicians and patients, nonmedical clinicians also need to be familiar with the most common perpetuating factors and communicate with patients' physicians when they suspect any underlying problems. There is a lack of randomized controlled double-blind studies or even epidemiological correlational studies verifying the clinical observations that certain metabolic and nutritional factors are relevant in the treatment of patients with myofascial pain. Yet considering the accepted hierarchy of evidence-based medicine, clinical evidence is a valid parameter and, especially in the absence of higher-level evidence, should be included as evidence.[8–10]

As mentioned in Chapter 2, an important distinction needs to be made between deficiencies and insufficiencies, although these terms are often used interchangeably. A deficiency is a value outside the normal range, which is easily recognized and usually associated with a clinical syndrome. For example, a vitamin C deficiency is associated with scurvy. An insufficiency is within the normal range, but may be suboptimal for a given individual. Insufficiencies are often associated with symptoms and can be rather challenging to recognize, but they may cause serious problems for individual patients. This chapter will review common nutritional and metabolic perpetuating factors of myofascial pain, including hypothyroidism, iron and vitamin insufficiencies, as well as the effects of statin drugs.

## Hypothyroidism

Although no epidemiological studies have shown a definitive relationship between hypothyroidism and myofascial pain, clinical observations of patients with chronic myalgia would seem to suggest that they are causally linked. A thyroid-stimulating hormone (TSH) level in the upper range of normal (3.5 ISU or higher) combined with complaints of muscle pain and additional complaints of coldness, dry skin or dry hair, constipation, and fatigue suggest that a patient may be hypothyroid and should be given a trial of thyroid hormone supplementation. The normal TSH range is 0.5–5.5 ISU; however, the individual optimal range is quite narrow. A person may have a TSH value within the normal laboratory range, but it can be outside of that individual's optimal range and, as such, can be abnormal for that individual, as shown by thyroid releasing hormone (TRH) stimulation tests.[6] In one study, 10% of patients with myofascial pain were diagnosed with hypothyroidism.[11] Thyroid supplementation that lowers the TSH to levels of 2.25 or less will often improve these symptoms, and patients will show marked improvement in endurance and also experience a drastic decrease in pain. Muscle pain and trigger points become more readily responsive to manual and needling methods of trigger point inactivation and restoration of function. Without thyroid therapy, it is our clinical observation that patients may not improve in spite of being treated with appropriate physical therapy interventions.

Thyroid hormone plays an essential role in the regulation of $Na^+/K^+$-ATPase pumping, ion cycling, and other functions, including thermogenesis.[12,13] Underactive thyroid function is a form of hypometabolism and can occur as a result of insufficient production of tetraiodothyronine (T4), which in turn may be due to a variety of reasons, including failure of the pituitary gland to produce TSH, insufficient synthesis and secretion of TRH, lack of hypothalamic responsiveness, or because of thyroid disease itself, such as Hashimoto thyroiditis. It can also occur because of impaired conversion of inactive T4 to active triiodothyronine (T3), which takes place by the iron-dependent 5'-deiodination of T4 in the liver.[14] Pro-inflammatory cytokines IL-6 and tumor necrosis factor-α can also reduce TSH production and impair thyroid function.[15,16]

The hypothalamic-pituitary-adrenal axis is sensitive to acute and chronic stress, which may result in suppression of TSH, decreased release of T4, or inhibition of T3 and T4 binding proteins and 5'-deiodinase-I, which may further decrease the peripheral conversion of inactive T4 to active T3.[17-19] Chronic stress can result in hypo-activation or suppression of the hypothalamic-pituitary-adrenal axis, causing a decrease in cortisol releasing hormone (CRH) and glucocorticoid. Reverse T3 (rT3) is increased in the acute stress response. Increased levels of T4 and rT3 and decreased levels of T3 are associated with hypothyroidism,[20] although the role of rT3 is not entirely clear. In one study, subjects with high rT3 concentrations had decreased physical performance scores and lower grip strength.[20]

TSH and T4 levels are poor measures of tissue thyroid levels, and clinicians should not rely solely on these measures to determine tissue thyroid levels. The best estimate of the tissue thyroid effect may be the rT3 level and the T3/rT3 ratio.[20] Controversy exists over whether rT3 is metabolically active and whether it is a functional inhibitor of T3, capable of producing a hypometabolic state. Changes in rT3 may be a marker of nonspecific response to stress without biological activity.[21] In nonmyalgic pathology, rT3 may be biologically active,[22,23] but it is still not entirely clear whether it can play a role in producing hypothyroidism and, if so, whether its effect can be overcome by administering large doses of T3. There is no conclusive evidence that so-called hormone-resistant hypothyroidism due to the peripheral blocking of T3 activity by rT3 plays a role in the development of myalgia. TSH may be normal in states where T3 activity is blocked by rT3, making the determination of hormone-resistant hypothyroidism problematic. There are conflicting data regarding the metabolic activity of rT3 and its actions as an inhibitor of T3, creating a peripheral hypothyroidism unrelated to hypothalamic, pituitary, or thyroid dysfunction. One view is that it is capable of functionally blocking T3, but a contrasting view is that it is metabolically inactive, acting only as a marker of down-regulation of the thyroid axis. In the latter view, elevation of rT3 indicates that there is an impairment of the feedback mechanism whereby TSH rises when T3 concentrations decrease.

The relationship of hypothyroidism to muscle pain is rather complicated. Several authors have suggested that fibromyalgia may be associated with hypothyroidism.[24,25] Thyroid autoimmunity has been described in fibromyalgia and in rheumatoid arthritis at higher rates than in controls.[26] Myalgia is also one of the soft-tissue manifestations of autoimmune thyroiditis.[27] Vitamin D deficiency impairs the immune system and can lead to thyroiditis, linking the two conditions. A person with myofascial pain associated with a vitamin D deficiency or hypothyroidism caused by thyroiditis should always be evaluated for both conditions. Clinical hypothyroidism with normal levels of T3, T4, and TSH, but characterized by a peripheral suppression of thyroid hormone activity, occurs in the "nonthyroidal illness syndrome," seen in chronic illness and in prolonged critical illness. Nonthyroidal illness syndrome was previously referred to as "sick euthyroid syndrome." Tissue thyroid levels are reduced in prolonged critical illness, which appears to be relevant to the presumed hypometabolic state postulated to be a factor in the development of myofascial pain and the generation of trigger points. Evidence suggests that there is a central neuroendocrine failure at the level of the hypothalamus.[28] Nonthyroidal illness with low levels of T3 and T4 can also be a response to stress.

Patients with hypothyroidism are commonly managed with medications such as levothyroxine.[29,30] However, not all tissues are equally able to convert thyroxine to T3, and the addition of T3 to thyroxine has been shown to result in an improved sense of well-being, an improvement in cognitive function and mood, and an increase in serum levels of sex-hormone-binding globulins, a sensitive marker of thyroid hormone function.[31,32]

## Iron Insufficiency

Similarly to hypothyroidism, the relationship between iron deficiency or insufficiency and myofascial trigger points has not been clearly established in clinical studies. Improvement in endurance, lessening of an abnormal sense of coldness, and a decrease in muscle pain is commonly seen when iron insufficiency is treated with iron supplementation in patients with myofascial pain, either orally or via intravenous infusion. Iron deficiency in muscle is a common condition and occurs when muscle ferritin is depleted. The prevalence of iron deficiency in females is 9–16%, but may be as high as 19–22% in African American and Hispanic women.[33] Low iron levels are associated with excessive menstrual iron loss, chronic intake of nonsteroidal anti-inflammatory drugs, and bowel cancer. It may also be seen in vegans or in people with iron-poor diets. Iron levels vary with age and gender and are low in adolescence, during periods of increased growth, and with the onset of menstrual blood loss in girls and young women. Iron levels rise again in adulthood and when women become postmenopausal. This variability is important when assessing iron stores in persons with muscle pain, particularly adolescent girls and premenopausal women. Although at this time unrelated to reported myofascial pain in this particular population, of note is that worldwide an estimated 25% of infants have iron-deficiency anemia and at least that many have iron deficiencies without anemia, which may have long-lasting effects on sleep patterns and motor activity planning.[34,35]

Ferritin represents the tissue-bound nonessential iron stores in the body that supply the essential iron for oxygen transport and iron-dependent enzymes. Serum ferritin levels of 15 ng/ml mark the first stage of iron deficiency, which means that storage sites for iron in muscle, liver, and bone marrow that are normally freely mobilized are depleted of ferritin. The second stage of iron deficiency is microcytosis. The third stage of iron deficiency is anemia, by which time iron bone marrow stores are undetectable. Anemia is associated with ferritin levels of less than 10 ng/ml. Early detection of ferritin depletion is important and should be suspected when patients present with complaints of muscle aching, chronic tiredness, unusual fatigue with exercise, and a sense of coldness. Measuring microcytic hypochromic anemia is an inadequate indicator of iron deficiency in persons with myalgia, because it does not identify the first stage of iron deficiency. Iron insufficiencies in chronic myofascial pain suggest that iron-requiring enzymatic reactions, such as the cytochrome oxidase and NAD(H) dehydrogenase reactions, may be limited, possibly resulting in a local energy crisis when muscles are exposed to excessive mechanical stress.[6]

Iron is essential for the generation of energy through the cytochrome oxidase system. According to Simons' integrated trigger point hypothesis, myofascial trigger points may develop as a result of an energy crisis within muscle.[36] A deficiency of freely accessible iron in muscle creates an energy crisis by limiting cytochrome oxidase energy-producing reactions. Cytochrome oxidase reactions can also be blocked when nitric oxide binds to ferrous heme iron.[37] Brigham and Beard found that norepinephrine and energy metabolism were altered in iron-deficient rats,[38] which was also noted in human subjects exposed to cold.[39] Iron-deficient rats were also found to have a low plasma levels of active thyroid hormone T3, an impaired ability to convert inactive T4 to active T3, low levels of T4-5′ deiodinase activity, low levels of TSH, and an attenuated TSH response to TRH.[13,40] The disposal rate of T4 and T3 is lower in iron-deficient rats. Interestingly, thyroid hormone kinetics are normalized with thyroxine replacement in the absence of changes in serum iron indices.[13] Brigham and Beard have postulated that the effect on thyroid hormone turnover might be caused by impaired thermoregulatory responses in iron-deficient states.[41]

Iron-deficient rats are hypothermic, which is related to the impaired conversion of T4 to T3.[42] Iron deficiency can adversely affect thyroid hormone metabolism,[43] but studies in humans give differing results, even though iron-deficient individuals often complain of feeling cold. Goiter can be associated with iron deficiency,[44] but thyroid hormone levels and TSH responses have not been shown to be significantly different in iron-deficient populations.[45,46] On the contrary, T3 augmentation can up-regulate ferritin levels and increase iron-dependent functions.[47]

Because iron is essential for the cytochrome oxidase system and iron insufficiency appears to be a significant factor in the development or maintenance of myofascial trigger points, iron supplementation is often indicated. Unfortunately, optimum ferritin levels for normal muscle function have not been established. Although restless leg syndrome (RLS) is a different condition, which can also be caused by iron deficiency, the serum ferritin levels associated with RLS may give some guidance in determining optimal ferritin levels. RLS is associated with serum ferritin levels below 50 ng/ml.[48] In adolescents and children with RLS, the serum ferritin level was below 20 ng/ml in 50% of cases and below 50 ng/ml in 83% of cases. Serum ferritin levels less than 45 ng/ml were correlated with an increased risk for sleep–wake transition disorders, including abnormal sleep movements, in children with attention-deficit/hyperactivity disorder.[49] This suggests that not only serum ferritin levels below 45–50 g/ml are clinically significant in RLS, but also that levels below 50 ng/ml are likely to be suboptimal from a general perspective. A significant association was found between blood donation and the occurrence of RLS in males, especially with five or more annual donations.[50]

RLS causes a sleep disturbance with sleep deprivation and reduced or absent levels of deep sleep. Sleep deprivation has been associated with muscle pain, including, in our experience, myofascial pain. Thus, iron insufficiency associated with RLS can indirectly contribute to muscle pain. Fortunately, iron supplementation can correct RLS[51] and is also important in correcting myofascial pain.[52] For further guidance, the upper limit of normal ferritin in premenopausal women is 150 ng/ml, and in men and postmenopausal women it is 300 ng/ml.

## Statin-Class Drugs

Statins, or 3-hydroxy-3-methylglutaryl-CoA (HMG-CoA) reductase inhibitors, are cholesterol-lowering drugs. They may cause myopathy, rhabdomyolysis, and myalgia associated with elevated creatine phosphokinase (CPK) in more severe cases. Fortunately, significant increases of CPK are infrequent, and rhabdomyolysis is very rare.[53] Myalgia can occur in the absence of elevated CPK levels. It is estimated that 1–7% of persons receiving statins develop muscle pain and weakness. In patients with initial complaints of widespread muscle pain shortly after an increased dose or after initiating any of the statin drugs, statins could be responsible for the pain complaint.[53,54] Although some have hypothesized that statin-induced coenzyme Q10 (CoQ10) deficiencies may be responsible for statin myopathy, recent studies have not confirmed the role of CoQ10 in causing myopathies.[55,56] Statin drugs block the production of farnesyl pyrophosphate, which is an intermediate in the synthesis of ubiquinone, or CoQ10, and important in mitochondrial energy production. Some evidence indicates that statins may impair the mitochondria, resulting in a mitochondrial calcium leak and an altered regulation of the sarcoplasmic reticulum.[54]

Hypothyroidism, diabetes mellitus, and the use of certain medications, such as gemfibrozil, which increase statin plasma concentrations, heighten the risk for the development of myalgia. Elevations of CPK are more common in patients with hypothyroidism receiving statins than in persons with euthyroid activity receiving statins.[57] No literature relates statin class drugs specifically to the development of myofascial pain syndromes, and even the role of statins in producing chronic myalgia, irrespective of trigger point formation, has been questioned, because chronic myalgias have not been confirmed by many blinded placebo-controlled trials.[58] Nevertheless, in a large meta-analysis involving 36,062 patients receiving a statin-class drug compared to 35,046 receiving a placebo, the most common adverse events were myalgia and liver function elevations; these adverse events were seen in two-thirds of the subjects receiving statins.[53] Irrespective of the underlying mechanism, these patients usually can be treated successfully by reducing the dosage of the medication or by switching to another cholesterol-lowering drug.[5]

## Vitamin D Insufficiency

Vitamin D deficiencies are endemic in northern Europe and America and are commonly associated with chronic nonspecific musculoskeletal pain.[59-62] Symptoms include muscle weakness, myofibrillar protein degradation, reduced muscle mass, osteoporosis, and decreased functional ability.[63-68] There are no high-quality correlational studies examining the association between vitamin D deficiencies or insufficiencies and myofascial pain. Vitamin D insufficiencies were, however, commonly observed in an observational study of patients with myofascial pain in a community pain management center, suggesting that such a deficiency might play a role in the etiology and maintenance of chronic myofascial pain.[6] Serum 25(OH)D levels above 30 ng/ml are considered optimal. Vitamin D deficiency in adults is defined as serum 25(OH)D levels below 20 ng/ml, while in vitamin D insufficiency serum 25(OH)D levels fall between 20 and 30 ng/ml.[69] In one study, almost 90% of 150 patients with musculoskeletal pain had vitamin D levels less than 20 ng/ml and 28% had less than 8 ng/ml.[62]

We should consider that vitamin D is not a true vitamin, because vitamin D metabolites play an active role in the gene transcription of hundreds, if not thousands, of genes.

Marshall[70] has challenged the notion that vitamin D deficiencies would cause or contribute to disease processes and proposes that low values of vitamin D may not be the cause, but the result, of the disease process. According to Marshall,[70] the idea that exogenous modulation of metabolism could provide a simple clinical solution is not only naïve, but could pose significant risks.

## Vitamin B$_{12}$ Insufficiency

Vitamin B$_{12}$ deficiencies were discussed in Chapter 2, but are included here as well for the sake of completeness. Vitamin B$_{12}$ deficiencies are very common and may affect as many as 15–20% of the elderly and persons with chronic myofascial pain.[11,71] Patients with serum levels of vitamin B$_{12}$ below 350 pg/ml may be clinically symptomatic, although clinical laboratory reports usually indicate that the normal range for vitamin B$_{12}$ levels falls between 200 and 1,200 pg/ml.[72] Low levels of vitamin B$_{12}$ are associated with a metabolic insufficiency manifested by elevated serum or urine methylmalonic acid or homocysteine, although some patients with normal levels of methylmalonic acid and homocysteine do present with metabolic abnormalities of B$_{12}$ function.[6,72] Vitamin B$_{12}$ insufficiencies can result in cognitive dysfunction, degeneration of the spinal cord, peripheral neuropathy, and widespread myalgia. Vitamin B$_{12}$ and folic acid are closely related and function not only in erythropoiesis, but also in nerve formation in both the central and peripheral nervous system. Gerwin[6,11] found that 16% of patients with chronic myofascial pain were either deficient in vitamin B$_{12}$ or had insufficient levels of vitamin B$_{12}$. Ten percent of those patients also had low serum folate levels. In a study of patients with low back pain, subjects who received intramuscular injections of B$_{12}$ demonstrated significant improvements in pain levels and function compared to a placebo group.[73] There is, however, no evidence of any advantage of administering trigger point injections with vitamin B$_{12}$.[74]

## Conclusion

The clinician should consider that there are several other possible perpetuating factors of myofascial pain and myalgia in general not discussed in this chapter.[5] Parasitic and infectious diseases, including fascioliasis, amoebiasis, and giardia, may all cause widespread myalgia, as can infectious diseases, such as Lyme disease and polymyalgia rheumatica.[75–80] Patients with these diagnoses are frequently erroneously diagnosed with fibromyalgia. Disturbed sleep, psychological issues, and mechanical problems can also contribute to the development of muscle pain and trigger points.

Although admittedly the correlations between the metabolic and nutritional insufficiencies described in this chapter and the development of myofascial trigger points have as of yet not been confirmed by double-blind controlled studies or even correlational studies, clinical experience with thousands of patients in our community-based pain management centers have, in our opinion, lent significant credence to Travell and Simons' initial notions expressed in their textbooks on myofascial pain.[36,81] It is clear that higher-quality scientific studies are needed to further expand the knowledge base and clinical management of persons suffering from myofascial pain beyond the anecdotal, experience-based evidence.

## References

1. Clauw DJ, Crofford LJ. Chronic widespread pain and fibromyalgia: What we know, and what we need to know. *Best Pract Res Clin Rheumatol* 2003;17:685–701.
2. Breivik H, et al. Survey of chronic pain in Europe: Prevalence, impact on daily life, and treatment. *Eur J Pain* 2006;10:287–333.
3. Breivik H, et al. Cancer-related pain: A pan-European survey of prevalence, treatment, and patient attitudes. *Ann Oncol* 2009;doi:10.1093/annonc/mdp001.
4. Gran JT. The epidemiology of chronic generalized musculoskeletal pain. *Best Pract Res Clin Rheumatol* 2003;17:547–561.
5. Dommerholt J, Issa T. Differential diagnosis: Myofascial pain. In Chaitow L, ed. *Fibromyalgia Syndrome: A Practitioner's Guide to Treatment.* Edinburgh, UK: Churchill Livingstone; 2009:179–213.
6. Gerwin RD. A review of myofascial pain and fibromyalgia: Factors that promote their persistence. *Acupunct Med* 2005;23:121–134.
7. Travell JG, Simons DG. *Myofascial Pain and Dysfunction: The Trigger Point Manual.* Vol. 1. Baltimore, MD: Williams & Wilkins; 1983.
8. Moore A, McQuay H, Gray JAM. Evidence-based everything. *Bandolier* 1995;1(12):1.
9. Pencheon D. What's next for evidence-based medicine? *Evidenced-Based Healthcare Public Health* 2005;9:319–321.
10. Sackett DL, et al. Evidence-based medicine: What it is and what it isn't. *BMJ* 1996;312:71–72.
11. Gerwin R. A study of 96 subjects examined both for fibromyalgia and myofascial pain (abstract). *J Musculoskel Pain* 1995;3(suppl 1):121.
12. Guernsey DL, Edelman IS. Loss of thyroidal inducibility of Na, K-ATPase with neoplastic transformation in tissue culture. *J Biol Chem* 1986;261:11956–11961.
13. Beard JL, et al. Plasma thyroid hormone kinetics are altered in iron-deficient rats. *J Nutr* 1998;128:1401–1408.
14. Sorvillo F, et al. Increased serum reverse triiodothyronine levels at diagnosis of hepatocellular carcinoma in patients with compensated HCV-related liver cirrhosis. *Clin Endocrinol* 2003;58: 207–212.
15. Witzke O, et al. Transient stimulatory effects on pituitary-thyroid axis in patients treated with interleukin-2. *Thyroid* 2001;11:665–670.
16. Jakobs TC, et al. Proinflammatory cytokines inhibit the expression and function of human type I 5'-deiodinase in HepG2 hepatocarcinoma cells. *Eur J Endocrinol* 2002;146:559–566.
17. Tsigos C, Chrousos GP. Hypothalamic-pituitary-adrenal axis, neuroendocrine factors and stress. *J Psychosom Res* 2002;53:865–871.
18. Feelders RA, et al. Characteristics of recovery from the euthyroid sick syndrome induced by tumor necrosis factor alpha in cancer patients. *Metabolism* 1999;48:324–329.
19. Michalaki M, et al. Dissociation of the early decline in serum T(3) concentration and serum IL-6 rise and TNF-alpha in nonthyroidal illness syndrome induced by abdominal surgery. *J Clin Endocrinol Metab* 2001;86:4198–4205.
20. Van den Beld AW, et al. Thyroid hormone concentrations, disease, physical function, and mortality in elderly men. *J Clin Endocrinol Metab* 2005;90:6403–6409.

21. Lange U, et al. Thyroid disorders in female patients with ankylosing spondylitis. *Eur J Med Res* 1999;4:468–474.
22. Friberg L, et al. Association between increased levels of reverse triiodothyronine and mortality after acute myocardial infarction. *Am J Med* 2001;111:699–703.
23. Martin JV, et al. Inhibition of the activity of the native gamma-aminobutyric acid A receptor by metabolites of thyroid hormones: Correlations with molecular modeling studies. *Brain Res* 2004;1004(1–2):98–107.
24. Garrison RL, Breeding PC. A metabolic basis for fibromyalgia and its related disorders: The possible role of resistance to thyroid hormone. *Med Hypotheses* 2003;61:182–189.
25. Lowe JC. Thyroid status of 38 fibromyalgia patients: Implications for the etiology of fibromyalgia. *Clin Bull Myofascial Therapy* 1996;2(1):36–40.
26. Pamuk ON, Cakir N. The frequency of thyroid antibodies in fibromyalgia patients and their relationship with symptoms. *Clin Rheumatol* 2007;26:55–59.
27. Punzi L, Betterle C. Chronic autoimmune thyroiditis and rheumatic manifestations. *Joint Bone Spine* 2004;71:275–283.
28. Van den Berghe G, et al. Neuroendocrinology of prolonged critical illness: Effects of exogenous thyrotropin-releasing hormone and its combination with growth hormone secretagogues. *J Clin Endocrinol Metab* 1998;83:309–319.
29. Singh N, Singh PN, Hershman JM. Effect of calcium carbonate on the absorption of levothyroxine. *JAMA* 2000;283:2822–2825.
30. Woeber KA. Update on the management of hyperthyroidism and hypothyroidism. *Arch Fam Med* 2000;9:743–747.
31. Bunevicius R, et al. Effects of thyroxine as compared with thyroxine plus triiodothyronine in patients with hypothyroidism. *N Engl J Med* 1999;340:424–429.
32. Bunevicius R, Prange AJ. Mental improvement after replacement therapy with thyroxine plus triiodothyronine: Relationship to cause of hypothyroidism. *Int J Neuropsychopharmacol* 2000;3:167–174.
33. Seaverson EL, et al. Poor iron status is more prevalent in Hispanic than in non-Hispanic white older adults in Massachusetts. *J Nutr* 2007;137:414–420.
34. Peirano, PD, et al. Sleep and neurofunctions throughout child development: Lasting effects of early iron deficiency. *J Pediatr Gastroenterol Nutr* 2009;48(suppl 1):S8–S15.
35. Peirano PD, et al. Iron deficiency anemia in infancy is associated with altered temporal organization of sleep states in childhood. *Pediatr Res* 2007;62:715–719.
36. Simons DG, Travell JG, Simons LS. *Travell and Simons' Myofascial Pain and Dysfunction: The Trigger Point Manual.* 2nd ed. Vol. 1. Baltimore, MD: Williams & Wilkins; 1999.
37. Cooper CE. Nitric oxide and iron proteins. *Biochem Biophys Acta* 1999;1411(2–3):290–309.
38. Brigham DE, Beard JL. Effect of thyroid hormone replacement in iron-deficient rats. *Am J Physiol* 1995;269 (5 Pt 2):R1140–R1147.
39. Martinez-Torres C, et al. Effect of exposure to low temperature on normal and iron-deficient subjects. *Am J Physiol* 1984;246(3 Pt 2):R380–R383.
40. Chiraseveenuprapund P, et al. Conversion of L-thyroxine to triiodothyronine in rat kidney homogenate. *Endocrinology* 1978;102:612–622.
41. Brigham D, Beard J. Iron and thermoregulation: A review. *Crit Rev Food Sci Nutr* 1996;36:747–763.
42. Dillman E, et al. Hypothermia in iron deficiency due to altered triiodothyronine metabolism. *Am J Physiol* 1980;239:R377–R381.
43. Arthur JR, Beckett GJ. Thyroid function. *Br Med Bull* 1999;55:658–668.

44. Azizi F, et al. The relation between serum ferritin and goiter, urinary iodine and thyroid hormone concentration. *Int J Vitam Nutr Res* 2002;72:296–299.
45. Yavuz O, et al. The relationship between iron status and thyroid hormones in adolescents living in an iodine deficient area. *J Pediatr Endocrinol Metab* 2004;17:1443–1449.
46. Tienboon P, Unachak K. Iron deficiency anaemia in childhood and thyroid function. *Asia Pac J Clin Nutr* 2003;12:198–202.
47. Leedman PJ, et al. Thyroid hormone modulates the interaction between iron regulatory proteins and the ferritin mRNA iron-responsive element. *J Biol Chem* 1996;271:12017–12023.
48. Wang J, et al. Efficacy of oral iron in patients with restless legs syndrome and a low-normal ferritin: A randomized, double-blind, placebo-controlled study. *Sleep Med* 2009 (in press).
49. Cortese S, et al. Sleep disturbances and serum ferritin levels in children with attention-deficit/hyperactivity disorder. *Eur Child Adolesc Psychiatry* 2009;18:393–399.
50. Gamaldo CE, et al. Childhood and adult factors associated with restless legs syndrome (RLS) diagnosis. *Sleep Med* 2007;8(7–8):716–722.
51. Gorder V, Kuntz S, Khosla S. Treatment of restless legs syndrome with iron infusion therapy. *JAAPA* 2009;22(3):29–32.
52. Gerwin RD, Gevirtz R. Chronic myofascial pain: Iron insufficieny and coldness as risk factors. *J Musculoskel Pain* 1995;3(suppl 1):120.
53. Silva MA, et al. Statin-related adverse events: A meta-analysis. *Clin Ther* 2006;28:26–35.
54. Sirvent P, Mercier J, Lacampagne A. New insights into mechanisms of statin-associated myotoxicity. *Curr Opin Pharmacol* 2008;8:333–338.
55. Marcoff L, Thompson PD. The role of coenzyme Q10 in statin-associated myopathy: A systematic review. *J Am Coll Cardiol* 2007;49:2231–2237.
56. Young JM, et al. Effect of coenzyme Q(10) supplementation on simvastatin-induced myalgia. *Am J Cardiol* 2007;100:1400–1403.
57. Tokinaga K, et al. HMG-CoA reductase inhibitors (statins) might cause high elevations of creatine phosphokinase (CK) in patients with unnoticed hypothyroidism. *Endocr J* 2006;53:401–405.
58. Brown WV. Safety of statins. *Curr Opin Lipidol* 2008;19:558–562.
59. Gordon CM, et al. Prevalence of vitamin D deficiency among healthy adolescents. *Arch Pediatr Adolesc Med* 2004;158:531–537.
60. Huh SY, Gordon CM. Vitamin D deficiency in children and adolescents: Epidemiology, impact and treatment. *Rev Endocr Metab Disord* 2008;9:161–170.
61. MacFarlane GD, et al. Hypovitaminosis D in a normal, apparently healthy urban European population. *J Steroid Biochem Mol Biol* 2004;89–90(1–5):621–622.
62. Plotnikoff GA, Quigley JM. Prevalence of severe hypovitaminosis D in patients with persistent, nonspecific musculoskeletal pain. *Mayo Clin Proc* 2003;78:1463–1470.
63. Bischoff HA, et al. In situ detection of 1,25-dihydroxyvitamin D3 receptor in human skeletal muscle tissue. *Histochem J* 2001;33:19–24.
64. Bischoff HA, et al. Relationship between muscle strength and vitamin D metabolites: Are there therapeutic possibilities in the elderly? *Z Rheumatol* 2000;59(suppl 1):39–41.
65. Bischoff HA, et al. Muscle strength in the elderly: Its relation to vitamin D metabolites. *Arch Phys Med Rehabil* 1999;80:54–58.
66. Dukas L, et al. Better functional mobility in community-dwelling elderly is related to D-hormone serum levels and to daily calcium intake. *J Nutr Health Aging* 2005;9:347–351.
67. Holick MF. High prevalence of vitamin D inadequacy and implications for health. *Mayo Clin Proc* 2006;81:353–373.

68. Wassner SJ, et al. Vitamin D Deficiency, hypocalcemia, and increased skeletal muscle degradation in rats. *J Clin Invest* 1983;72:102–112.
69. Vieth R, et al. The urgent need to recommend an intake of vitamin D that is effective. *Am J Clin Nutr* 2007;85:649–650.
70. Marshall TG. Vitamin D discovery outpaces FDA decision making. *Bioessays* 2008;30:173–182.
71. Andres E, et al. Vitamin B$_{12}$ (cobalamin) deficiency in elderly patients. *CMAJ* 2004;171:251–259.
72. Pruthi RK, Tefferi A. Pernicious anemia revisited. *Mayo Clin Proc* 1994;69:144–150.
73. Mauro GL, et al. Vitamin B$_{12}$ in low back pain: a randomised, double-blind, placebo-controlled study. *Eur Rev Med Pharmacol Sci* 2000;4(3):53–58.
74. Dommerholt J, Gerwin RD. *Neurophysiological effects of trigger point needling therapies.* In: Fernández-de-las-Peñas C, Arendt-Nielsen L, Gerwin RD, Eds. *Diagnosis and Management of Tension-Type and Cervicogenic Headache.* Sudbury, MA: Jones & Bartlett; 2010:247–259.
75. De Gorgolas M, et al. Infestacion por Fasciola hepatica: Biopatologia y nuevos aspectos diagnosticos y terapeuticos. *Enferm Infecc Microbiol Clin* 1992;10:514–519.
76. Lim JH, Kim SY, Park CM. Parasitic diseases of the biliary tract. *AJR Am J Roentgenol* 2007;188:1596–1603.
77. Jamaiah I, Shekhar KC. Amoebiasis: A 10-year retrospective study at the University Hospital, Kuala Lumpur. *Med J Malaysia* 1999;54:296–302.
78. Qureshi H, et al. Efficacy of a combined diloxanide furoate-metronidazole preparation in the treatment of amoebiasis and giardiasis. *J Int Med Res* 1997;25:167–170.
79. Ogrinc K, Ruzic-Sabljic E, Strle F. Clinical assessment of patients with suspected Lyme borreliosis. *Int J Med Microbiol* 2008;298(suppl1):356–260.
80. Reilly PA. The differential diagnosis of generalized pain. *Baillieres Best Pract Res Clin Rheumatol* 1999;13:391–401.
81. Travell JG, Simons DG. *Myofascial Pain and Dysfunction: The Trigger Point Manual.* Vol. 2. Baltimore, MD: Williams & Wilkins; 1992.

Part 2

# Diagnosis

# Chapter 4

# Reliability of Myofascial Trigger Point Palpation: A Systematic Review

*Johnson McEvoy, PT, BSc, MSc, DPT, MISCP, MCSP*

*Peter A. Huijbregts, PT, MSc, MHSc, DPT, OCS,*
*FAAOMPT, FCAMT*

## Introduction

Myofascial pain syndrome (MPS) refers to a clinical syndrome in which pain arises from myofascial trigger points (MTrPs). Prevalence of MPS has been studied in various populations and has been summarized comprehensively by Simons et al.[1] Fishbain et al[2] studied a cohort of 283 consecutive patients in a comprehensive pain center and found that 238 (84%) met the Simons and Travell criteria for MPS. Skootsky et al[3] reported that 30% of patients presenting with pain to the primary care general internal medicine practice at the University of California at Los Angeles Medical Care Center met the criteria for MPS, making this the single largest reason for patients with pain to present there for medical care. Gerwin[4] reported a prevalence of 93% for MPS and coexisting MPS and fibromyalgia in a study of 96 patients in a pain medicine center. More recently, in a study of older adults with low back pain (LBP) MPS was identified in 96% of symptomatic subjects versus 10% of controls.[5] Because most of these epidemiologic data are derived from studies carried out in specialized pain centers by clinicians with an interest in MPS, thereby suggesting both potential patient selection and rater bias, the prevalence of MPS in the general population remains unknown. However, the available research does suggest that MPS may be common in these clinically relevant patient populations studied.[2-5]

Although the International Association for the Study of Pain has included MPS in its 2005 *Core Curriculum for Professional Education in Pain*,[6] the diagnosis of MPS has met with notably less acceptance in other medical fields, including orthopaedic manual physical therapy. Perhaps due to the limited number of clinical experts in MPS,[7] the topic has received scant attention in the literature,[8] which has further decreased the penetration of this information into mainstream physical therapy and medicine. For example, a recent survey of chronic pain in Europe[9] did not even include MTrPs among the surveyed potential causes of chronic pain. This may have been related to the fact that in this survey, pain management specialists were involved in the care of only 2% of the patients.[9]

In contrast to other providers involved in greater numbers in this study, such as general practitioners and orthopaedists, perhaps pain management specialists do tend to consider the MPS construct, as evidenced by a survey of American Pain Society members, wherein 88.5% of respondents described MPS as a legitimate diagnosis and more than 80% concurred on diagnostic criteria.[10] Simons[11] further illustrated this seemingly limited relevance attached to MPS in mainstream medicine by indicating that between 1996 and 2002 only 0.5% of Medline-cited articles for low back pain even mentioned MTrPs.

Without a clinical gold standard diagnostic imaging or laboratory test for MTrPs,[8] clinicians need to rely solely on history and physical examination findings for the diagnosis of MPS. As Dommerholt et al have done in this book, the specific palpation techniques used have been described in great detail.[1,12,13] Simons et al[1] have proposed criteria for the identification of MTrPs (**Table 4-1**). With diagnosis to a great extent dependent on palpatory tests, establishing reliability of trigger point palpation is an even more important step toward establishing validity of the clinical construct of MTrPs. Adequate intra- and interrater reliability for the identification of MTrPs is justifiably considered the lowest threshold of proof required to satisfy construct validity of the MTrP concept. Therefore the goal of this chapter is to systematically review the research on reliability of trigger point palpation with the intent of providing a current best evidence synthesis with attention to implications for clinical practice and future research.

## TABLE 4-1   Recommended Criteria for Identification of MTrPs[1]

**Essential Criteria**

- Taut band palpable (where muscle is accessible)
- Exquisite spot tenderness of a nodule in a taut band
- Patient recognition of current pain complaint by pressure on the tender nodule (identifies an active trigger point)
- Painful limit to full stretch range of motion

**Confirmatory Observations**

- Visual or tactile identification of a local twitch response (LTR)
- Imaging of an LTR induced by needle penetration of tender nodule
- Pain or altered sensation (in the distribution expected from a trigger point in that muscle) on compression of tender nodule
- Electromyographic demonstration of spontaneous electrical activity characteristic of active loci in the tender nodule of a taut band

## Methods and Materials

A literature search was performed using the Medline via PubMed and CINAHL databases from their inception through June 2008. We combined the search terms "myofascial trigger point" and "reliability." We retrieved English-language studies that described reliability research into MTrP palpation of the spine and extremity muscles. Studies on the temporomandibular joint were excluded, as were studies on instrumented algometry. This literature-search strategy was expanded with a hand search of the reference lists of the articles retrieved and by contacting experts for additional references, if such existed.

Flawed studies and the resulting biased reliability statistics can provide the clinician with unwarranted confidence with regard to diagnosis. This review is a systematic review in that it uses the *Data Extraction and Quality Scoring Form for Reliability Studies of Spinal Palpation*. This methodological quality assessment tool was developed by Seffinger et al[14] and used in a systematic review of reliability studies of spinal palpatory tests. It collects information on study details with regard to subjects, examiners, study conditions, data analysis, and results. Scores are weighted, leading to a maximum score of 100. Both authors independently scored all papers retrieved and then determined a final score based on consensus.

With no established cutoff values and no research into the reliability of the methodological quality assessment tool used, we acknowledge that the assessment it provides is qualitative at best. Therefore, in addition to these scores we provide a narrative discussion of the biases in the reliability studies retrieved to allow for a current best evidence synthesis, taking into account potential methodological flaws not, or insufficiently, addressed in this methodological quality assessment tool.

## Results

The Medline search yielded nine references, of which three were retrieved.[15-17] The CINAHL search yielded five references, of which one was appropriate but a duplicate of the Medline-yielded references.[16] A hand search of the reference lists yielded an additional four references.[17-21] The expert search produced two more papers, for a total of nine original studies.[22,23] Of these studies, eight dealt with interrater reliability, whereas one studied intrarater reliability. **Table 4-2** provides the scores on the methodological quality assessment tool for all studies.

A synopsis of each paper is presented below in chronological order in the following format: rater details; training; MTrP diagnostic features tested; specific muscles tested; subject characteristics; methodology and process of study; data analysis and statistics used; results reported, including data on prevalence where provided; and author conclusions. No further data is provided on the rating scales used, because all studies used a dichotomous rating scale noting the presence or absence of diagnostic features.

TABLE 4-2 Methodological Quality Assessment Tool Scores[14]

| Criteria | Weight | Maximum score | Wolfe et al (1992) | Nice et al (1992) | Njoo et al (1994) | Lew et al (1997) | Gerwin et al I (1997) | Gerwin et al II (1997) | Hsieh et al (2000) | Sciotti et al (2001) | Al-Shenqiti (2005) | Bron et al (2007) |
|---|---|---|---|---|---|---|---|---|---|---|---|---|
| **Study subjects** | | | | | | | | | | | | |
| Study subjects adequately described | 1 | 8 | 7 | 5 | 7 | 5 | 3 | 7 | 7 | 6 | 5 | 7 |
| Inclusion/ exclusion criteria described | 1 | 2 | 1 | 1 | 2 | 2 | 2 | 2 | 2 | 2 | 2 | 2 |
| Subjects naïve/without vested interest | 1 | 2 | 0 | 0 | 0 | 0 | 0 | 0 | 0 | 0 | 0 | 0 |
| Number of subjects in study given | 1 | 4 | –2 | –2 | –2 | –2 | –2 | –2 | –2 | –2 | –2 | –2 |
| Dropouts described | 1 | 1 | 1 | 1 | 0 | 1 | 1 | 1 | 1 | 1 | 1 | 1 |
| Subjects not informed of findings | 1 | 1 | 0 | 0 | 0 | 0 | 0 | 0 | 0 | 0 | 0 | 0 |
| **Examiners** | | | | | | | | | | | | |
| Selection criteria for examiners described | 2 | 1 | 1 | 1 | 1 | 1 | 1 | 1 | 1 | 1 | 1 | 1 |
| Background of examiners described | 5 | 1 | 2 | 1 | 1 | 1 | 1 | 1 | 1 | 1 | 1 | 1 |

|  |  |  |  |  |  |  |  |  |  |  |  |
|---|---|---|---|---|---|---|---|---|---|---|---|
| Examiners blind to clinical presentation of subjects | 8 | 1 | 0 | 0 | 0 | 1 | 0 | 1 | 1 | 0 | 1 |
| Examiners blind to previous findings | 10 | 1 | 0 | 1 | 1 | 1 | 1 | 1 | 1 | 1 | 1 |
| **Study conditions** | | | | | | | | | | | |
| Consensus test procedures and training examiners | 4 | 2 | 2 | 2 | 1 | 0 | 2 | 2 | 2 | NA | 2 |
| Description of test/retest procedure and time interval | 3 | 1 | 1 | 1 | 1 | 1 | 1 | 1 | 0 | 1 | 1 |
| Study conditions described (e.g., facilities and setup) | 1 | 1 | 1 | 1 | 0 | 1 | 1 | 1 | 1 | 1 | 1 |
| Description of palpation test technique | 8 | 0 | 1 | 1 | 1 | 0 | 1 | 1 | 1 | 1 | 1 |
| Consensus test outcome | 5 | 1 | 1 | 1 | 1 | 1 | 1 | 1 | 1 | NA | 1 |
| **Data analysis** | | | | | | | | | | | |
| Appropriate statistical methods used | 10 | 1 | 1 | 1 | 1 | 1 | 1 | 1 | 1 | 1 | 1 |

*(continued)*

TABLE 4-2 Methodological Quality Assessment Tool Scores[14] (cont.)

| Criteria | Weight | Maximum score | Wolfe et al (1992) | Nice et al (1992) | Njoo et al (1994) | Lew et al (1997) | Gerwin et al I (1997) | Gerwin et al II (1997) | Hsieh et al (2000) | Sciotti et al (2001) | Al-Shenqiti (2005) | Bron et al (2007) |
|---|---|---|---|---|---|---|---|---|---|---|---|---|
| P value displayed | 8 | 1 | 1 | 0 | 0 | 0 | 1 | 1 | 0 | 0 | 0 | 0 |
| Precision of examiner agreement calculated and displayed as confidence interval | 7 | 1 | 0 | 0 | 1 | 0 | 0 | 0 | 0 | 0 | 0 | 0 |
| **Results** | | | | | | | | | | | | |
| Results displayed appropriately (e.g., figures, tables) | 1 | 1 | 0 | 1 | 1 | 1 | 0 | 1 | 1 | 1 | 1 | 1 |
| Results adequately described | 2 | 1 | 0 | 0 | 0 | 1 | 0 | 0 | 0 | 1 | 0 | 1 |
| Potential study biases identified | 4 | 1 | 0 | 1 | 1 | 1 | 1 | 1 | 1 | 1 | 1 | 1 |
| Unweighted total score | | 34 | 15 | 16 | 20 | 17 | 14 | 21 | 20 | 20 | 15/31 | 22 |
| Weighted total score | 100 | | 34 | 52 | 71 | 62 | 60 | 73 | 73 | 71 | 50/87 | 75 |

## Interrater Reliability Studies

*Wolfe et al (1992) study*

Wolfe et al[18] reported on a study, part of which established MTrP interrater reliability testing. Two physiatrists, one neurologist, and one internal medicine specialist, all considered MPS experts, were the raters. The initial study design intended to also include four rheumatologists as raters; however, these medical specialists could not become proficient in MTrP examination during the practice sessions, and therefore the design study was changed to include only the MPS experts. In addition, the researchers further altered the study by reducing the number of muscles tested to eight on only the right side of the body, because not all experts were able to assess the muscles in the allotted 15-minute examination period. A reported half-day training session preceded the actual study; however, much of this time was taken up with (unsuccessfully) attempting to train the rheumatologists in MTrP palpation (personal communication Dr. David Simons, November 2006). The clinicians tested for the presence or absence of a taut band, tender point, referred pain, recognized pain, and local twitch response (LTR). Operational definitions were taken from Travell and Simons.[12] An active MTrP was defined as having the diagnostic characteristics of spot tenderness, a taut band, an LTR, and referred pain recognized by the patient. In contrast, a latent MTrP only had spot tenderness, a taut band, and an LTR. The muscles tested were the levator scapulae, supraspinatus, anterior scalene, upper trapezius, infraspinatus, pectoralis major, the sternal section of sternocleidomastoid, and the iliocostalis and longissimus at T10–L1 area. Subjects were 23 females in three groups: seven subjects with fibromyalgia recruited from community-based rheumatology practices, including that of one of the participating rheumatologists; eight patients with MPS recruited from the practice of one of the MPS expert raters; and eight age- and sex-matched asymptomatic volunteers. Mean ages were 39.7, 32.6, and 34.2 years, respectively. Raters were blinded to subject diagnosis, and subjects were blinded to tester speciality. Eight subjects were examined in a 2- to 3-hour period and someone other than the raters documented the findings. Data were summed to obtain a total count for each characteristic tested, with missing data extrapolated by obtaining the means of all values for that subject and rater. The three diagnostic groups and raters were compared using a two-way analysis of variance. Tukey's multiple-comparison test was used for post-hoc analysis. Statistical significance was set at 0.05, and all tests were two-tailed.

Muscle tenderness was present in 75% of subjects in both patient groups. Taut bands were found in 50% of subjects in all groups, whereas an LTR was elicited in 30% of subjects in all groups. Referred pain sensations were noted in 45% of subjects in the patient groups. Examination produced pain recognized by the patient in 37.5% of sites examined in both patient groups. Latent MTrPs occurred in less than 3% of subjects in all groups, whereas active MTrPs occurred in 18% of subjects in both patient groups. Based on statistical analyses, the authors concluded that the MPS experts did not differ in their ability to identify referred pain, recognized pain, or latent MTrPs. In contrast, there were significant interrater differences for the MTrP count and identification of the taut band, the LTR, and active MTrPs. In fact the raters differed nearly twofold on MTrP count and identification of taut bands, greater than threefold on identification of the LTR, and more than fivefold on identification of active MTrPs.

However, when the criteria for MTrP identification were redefined as solely the presence of pain on palpation with the presence of referred pain recognized by the patient, the raters did not differ statistically with regard to MTrP identification. In the original study, use of the κ-statistic was avoided, reportedly due to the fact that subject findings might have been different at each examination because of previous examinations.

Simons and Skootsky[1] later analyzed the original data and reported the following interrater κ-values: taut band 0.29; spot tenderness 0.61; LTR 0.16; referred pain 0.40; and recognized pain 0.30. Overall, the reliability for MTrP identification was poor. Because latent MTrPs, taut bands, and LTR were equiprevalent in all groups, the authors questioned the pathological nature of such findings. The authors concluded that agreement on an MTrP definition was essential and that at the very least subsequent studies should specify the definition for research purposes. They also recommended that each definition must establish its own reliability and validity and suggested that specific training could lead to substantial increases in reliability.

## Nice et al (1992) study

The raters in the study by Nice et al[20] were 12 physiotherapists with 3–17 years of experience in treating patients with LBP. Three raters had had specialized training in MTrP examination. Seven raters examined patients for MTrPs routinely, of which two tested four to six and five examined one to three patients per week. A written description of Travell and Simons' 1983 assessment[13] for the iliocostalis lumborum and longissimus thoracis muscles was provided to each rater. A palpation practice session was completed until all the raters reported confidence in administering the palpation tests. Raters tested for MTrP presence or absence in the L1 iliocostalis lumborum and T10/11 and the L1 longissimus thoracis. Criteria for MTrP presence were onset or increase in pain in the expected reference zone for the muscle. Subjects were 50 patients with LBP (62% female; age 19–77; mean age of 39) recruited from the caseloads of the participating therapists with pain indicative of MTrP involvement in the muscles studied. The subjects were tested in random order by two raters chosen arbitrarily from the rater pool, excluding therapists involved in the patients' care. Each subject was positioned in side-lying position with hips and knees bent to 90°. Patients were included for data analysis if they presented with pain patterns as described by Travell and Simons. Of 235 MTrP examinations, 197 were deemed appropriate for data analysis. The authors used the κ statistic with standard error (SE), percentage agreement (PA), observed proportion of positive agreement ($P_{pos}$), and observed proportion of negative agreement ($P_{neg}$) for statistical analysis.

The authors calculated overall statistics as well as statistics for when only the correct technique was used. In addition, the authors provided statistics for when both correct technique was used and where patients reported pain immediately prior to examination. Data for all

TABLE 4-3   Interrater Reliability Statistics Nice et al[20] Study

| MTrP | n | κ (SE) | PA | $P_{pos}$ | $P_{neg}$ |
|------|---|--------|-----|-----------|-----------|
| **Overall interrater reliability** | | | | | |
| A | 67 | 0.29 (0.16) | 76 | 0.43 | 0.85 |
| B | 71 | 0.31 (0.16) | 79 | 0.52 | 0.87 |
| C | 59 | 0.38 (0.16) | 79 | 0.44 | 0.87 |
| **Interrater reliability with rater using correct technique** | | | | | |
| A | 37 | 0.35 (0.22) | 91 | 0.46 | 0.88 |
| B | 39 | 0.35 (0.22) | 82 | 0.46 | 0.89 |
| C | 36 | 0.46 (0.18) | 81 | 0.59 | 0.87 |
| **Interrater reliability with raters using correct technique and patient reporting pain immediately prior to examination** | | | | | |
| A | 23 | 0.25 (0.24) | 70 | 0.46 | 0.79 |
| B | 25 | 0.42 (0.23) | 80 | 0.56 | 0.87 |
| C | 20 | 0.38 (0.21) | 70 | 0.62 | 0.75 |

three scenarios are provided in **Table 4-3**. Separate analysis of the seven more experienced raters did not demonstrate an appreciable difference in reliability. The authors concluded that despite the high percentage agreement (76–79%), the low κ values (0.29–0.38) and $P_{pos}$ values (0.43–0.52) indicated consistently poor reliability for MTrP palpation and questioned the usefulness of examining for MTrPs in patients with LBP.

### Njoo and Van der Does (1994) study

Njoo and Van der Does[19] used one experienced general practitioner who had received additional training in a rheumatology university hospital and four last-year medical students trained by the experienced clinician over a 3-month period. During the study, a pool of three raters (the experienced clinician and two students) was always available. Prestudy training included performance, interpretation, and registration of the examinations, and practice application of 2 kg of force by the index finger was carried out using a balance for standardization of applied pressure. Characteristics defined and tested were absence or presence of spot tenderness, referred pain, taut band, LTR, limited range of motion, jump sign, and recognition of the patient's pain. The muscles tested were the bilateral quadratus lumborum and gluteus medius, as described by Travell and Simons.[13] Of 124 subjects, 61 were patients with nonspecific LBP (44.2% female; mean age 36.2) and 63 patients who had consulted their general practitioner for reasons other than low back pain and who also noted no low back pain at the time of consultation acted as controls (50.7% female; mean age 38.1). Subjects were recruited from general medical practices and health centers. The examination methodology included subjects completing a questionnaire and undergoing a physical (orthopaedic and neurologic) and MTrP examination. The first rater completed this part of the testing and then the second rater completed the MTrP examination blinded to the first rater's findings and to symptom status. The second rater tested for all characteristics, with exception of limited stretch range of motion. The reason provided for this exception was that including this characteristic would have entailed the subject moving around, which might have led to unblinding. Tables were used to give visual information on prevalence. Prevalence of MTrP characteristics varied greatly in patients in the quadratus lumborum (range 2–32) and in the gluteus medius (range 1–29); for the controls these ranges were 0–11 and 0–9, respectively. Reliability was expressed with κ-statistics with 95% confidence intervals (**Table 4-4**). The authors concluded that localized tenderness with recognition of the patient's complaint by palpation and presence of a jump sign had both good interrater reliability and discriminative value for distinction between patients with nonspecific LBP and controls. They also questioned the value of a palpable taut band as a prerequisite for MTrP diagnosis, because this finding occurred also without tenderness in the study subjects.

### Gerwin et al (1997) study

Gerwin et al[17] reported on a two-phase interrater reliability study. Phase I of the study included two physiatrists and two neurologists, all MPS experts. Prestudy training consisted of a discussion session the night before the study to ascertain the muscles to be studied and to review MTrP characteristics to be tested. Characteristics tested included tenderness, taut band, LTR, referred pain, reproduced pain, and presence or absence of an MTrP. The muscles tested bilaterally were the sternocleidomastoid, trapezius (upper and lower), anterior scalene, levator scapulae, infraspinatus, latissimus dorsi, teres minor,

TABLE 4-4    Interrater Reliability for Individual MTrP Characteristics[19]

| MTrP Symptom Tested | Quadratus Lumborum κ (95% CI) | Gluteus Medius κ (95% CI) |
|---|---|---|
| Localized tenderness | 0.73 (0.61–0.85) | 0.58 (0.43–0.74) |
| Referred pain | 0.36 (−0.04–0.76) | 0.46 (0.18–0.74) |
| Palpable band | 0.47 (0.28–0.68) | 0.51 (0.34–0.69) |
| Twitch response | 0.19 (−0.38–0.77) | −0.02 (−0.99–0.96) |
| Recognition of pain | 0.57 (0.38–0.78) | 0.58 (0.38–0.79) |
| Jump sign | 0.68 (0.53–0.83) | 0.71 (0.55–0.86) |

triceps, and extensor digitorum. No distinction was made with regard to active or latent trigger points. The subjects were 25 personnel at an army medical center (52% female; mean age 50). No exclusion criteria were set, because the study did not aim to relate MTrP presence to a specific diagnosis. Each subject was randomized and subjects were examined in 15-minute periods each in three groups of 8–10 subjects. Subjects were instructed to speak only in relation to their response to the examination (e.g., referred pain) and not to discuss symptom status. Statistical analysis was done with percentage agreement, a generalized version of Cohen's κ used to indicate pairwise agreement, called the $S_{av}$, and a test of significance to see if the $S_{av}$ value really differed from zero.

Phase I results were summarized with reliability being low across the characteristics and with no features approaching an $S_{av}$ of 0.5 except for tenderness of the left upper trapezius and left extensor digitorum muscles (0.52 and 0.55, respectively). The authors concluded from the phase I study a failure to demonstrate reliability for any of the features with exception of tenderness of the trapezius and extensor digitorum, as noted above.

Phase II used the same raters but included a much more in-depth 3-hour training session immediately prior to the study. Definitions of the MTrP characteristics were reviewed to achieve consensus among the four raters. Practical training included practice on a volunteer and the other raters, and consensus was achieved. The use of pincer and flat palpation depending on the muscle tested was discussed. The amount of pressure used was left at the discretion of the rater in that it needed to be sufficient to satisfy the examiner that the feature was present or absent. The LTR was confirmed either visually or by feel. A uniform process for subject's pain recognition and pain referral was agreed upon to exclude leading questions. The rating scale was dichotomous for the presence or absence of the same characteristics as phase I of the study, but raters also determined whether an active or latent MTrP was present. Point tenderness and a taut band with palpation reproducing the patient's recognized pain defined an active MTrP, whereas a latent MTrP was characterized only by a tender point and taut band. Referred pain and LTR were considered to confirm MTrP presence. Muscles tested bilaterally were the sternocleidomastoid, upper trapezius, infraspinatus, the axillary portion of the latissimus dorsi, and extensor digitorum. Ten subjects (70% female; mean age 42) were recruited from the practice of one of the raters and included both patients and asymptomatic friends or spouses of patients. Six subjects had cervical spondylosis or radiculopathy, one had piriformis syndrome, and three were pain-free. Subjects were randomized for examination sequence and were examined in a 15-minute period; they were instructed to speak only in relation to their response to the examination (e.g., referred pain) and not to discuss their symptom status. Statistical analysis was similar to phase I, but descriptive statistics on the presence and absence of the individual characteristics tested and the presence of active or latent MTrPs in each of the five tested muscles were added.

The number of MTrP features present varied from 23–80; the number absent ranged from 1–56. Phase II results demonstrated significant improvement over phase I, and reported $S_{av}$ values for the individual features were as follows: tenderness 0.48–1.0; taut band 0.40–0.46; LTR 0.11–0.57; referred pain 0.57–0.84; and patient-recognized pain

0.79–1.0. Due to almost complete agreement, $S_{av}$ was not applicable for tenderness and taut band in the sternocleidomastoid and tenderness and LTR in the extensor digitorum. Agreement for the presence or absence of an active or latent trigger point was 0.84 for the sternocleidomastoid, 0.66 for the upper trapezius, 0.65 for the infraspinatus, 0.79 for the latissimus, and 0.95 for the extensor digitorum.

The authors concluded based on their findings from phase II that four raters could agree on the MTrP features and on the presence or absence of latent and active MTrPs. They claimed that the study established reliability of the clinical signs of the MTrP. Furthermore, the diversity of the results between phase I and II was suggested to arise from study design. Whereas phase II included the same expert raters, the difference was the extent of the prestudy consensus and practical training process. The authors also noted that force required for palpation could not be standardized for all patients and that reliability seemed to differ across muscles.

### Lew et al (1997) study

Lew et al[22] used two experienced physical therapists-osteopaths considered MPS experts by their peers. These raters read Travell and Simons' 1983[12] Chapter 6 on the trapezius muscle, discussed the procedure, and agreed that their technique was similar to that of Travell and Simons. No hands-on palpation training was reported in the study. The raters established presence or absence of latent trigger points (both referring and nonreferring) in the upper trapezius. Criteria adopted in this study to confirm the presence of a latent MTrP were spot tenderness, taut band, and maximum local or referred pain. The study assessed the ability for the clinicians to identify the location of trigger points identified in the upper trapezius by transferring the MTrP position onto a quarter-size body chart by directing an assistant to mark the chart. Subjects were 58 asymptomatic volunteers (59% female, 41% male; mean age 28.7 and 28.9, respectively), who had not been treated for cervical, thoracic, or shoulder complaints in the prior 3 months. The subjects were randomized for testing and were examined at the rate of 15 per hour with 5 minutes between examination of one subject by the second of the two raters to allow for the reduction in palpatory erythema. The patient lay prone in the position suggested by Travell and Simons.[12] If the examiner suspected a taut band in the trapezius, verbal interaction was allowed and the clinician used subject feedback to locate the point of maximal tenderness and local or referred pain. At this stage, the examiner verbally directed an assistant to locate the position of the latent MTrP on a body chart using an "X." The quarter-size body chart had vertebrae, scapulae, and the borders of trapezius diagrammatically represented. The criteria used for agreement between the two examiners was a difference in location of less than 5.0 mm from the center of the Xs on the quarter-size life size chart (i.e., a 20-mm difference on the subjects). This criterion was based on an EMG study that claimed that MTrPs have a radius of 10 mm.[24]

Results were descriptively presented and percentage agreement on location of nonreferring and referring MTrPs was reported as 10% and 21%, respectively. There was discordance in the number of trigger points identified between the raters: 87 versus 174! The authors claimed from the data that κ could not be validly calculated, and therefore it was not reported. They also concluded that poor interrater reliability agreement existed for location of MTrPs in the upper trapezius and that the results suggested that MTrPs in the upper trapezius could not be reliably identified by palpation. The authors implied that prestudy training might not have been adequate to ensure a uniform approach to examination. The suggestion was made that prior to future studies "rigorous familiarization" training should be initiated to form consensus on practical application of tactile perception.

### Hsieh et al (2000) study

Hsieh et al[21] used four chiropractors and four physiatry residents, all considered nonexpert raters. The eight raters were split into trained and nontrained groups. The trained group consisted of two chiropractors with 3 and 5 years of licensure, a second-year physiatry resident with 3 years of licensure, and a third-year physiatry resident with 6 years of licensure. The nontrained group consisted of a senior chiropractic faculty member and a chiropractor, both with 15 years of licensure, and two second-year physiatry residents with 2 years of licensure. The trained group received three 2-hour lectures on MPS and MTrP localization, referencing Travell and Simons[12] textbook, and three 2-hour practical sessions on symptomatic and normal subjects. Standardization of the amount of palpatory pressure was practiced using an algometer with 3 kg/cm² for superficial and 7–8 kg/cm² for deep muscles. The untrained group was instructed to locate a taut band, LTR, or referred pain in the muscles tested. They were given a handout showing MTrP location but no other training. The clinicians were tested against an MPS expert clinician-researcher. Ten muscles (L1 iliocostalis, rectus femoris, lower portion of the rectus abdominis, tensor fasciae latae, the distal superficial quadratus lumborum, MTrP2 in the gluteus maximus, MTrP2 in the gluteus medius, the anterior portion of the gluteus minimus, MTrP1 in the piriformis, and MTrP1 in the soleus; numbering of trigger points was as provided in Travell and Simons[12]) were tested bilaterally for the presence or absence of a taut band, LTR, and any referred pain. Subjects were 26 patients with LBP (53.8% male; mean age 47.9) and 26 control subjects (57.7% male; mean age 42.5), who were recruited via 27 various media presentations. The patients were tested in groups of three to seven per session and were initially examined by the expert rater and then by two trained and two nontrained raters in a predetermined random order. The testers were blinded to the expert's findings, each other's findings, and to symptom status. Overall, stratified, and mean κ-coefficients (with SE) served as indicators of agreement.

Results reported for the palpation of the taut band, LTR, and referred pain yielded low κ values between expert and trained (0.215, 0.123, and 0.342, respectively) and between expert and untrained (0.050, 0.118, and 0.326, respectively). Interrater agreement for the nonexpert, trained examiners was 0.108, –0.001, and 0.435, respectively, and –0.019, 0.022, and 0.320, respectively, for the nonexpert, untrained examiners. The study concluded that for nonexpert physiatrists or chiropractors MTrP palpation was not reliable for detecting taut band and LTR and only marginal for referred pain after training. It was suggested that expertise in the form of extensive clinical experience might play a more important role in palpation of MTrP characteristics than training.

### Sciotti et al (2001) study

Sciotti et al[15] used four clinicians with 9–18 years of experience in MTrP diagnosis and management. Prestudy, the raters compiled a training manual and gathered relevant MTrP information and completed four 3-hour sessions of training and practical application testing on volunteer subjects. The right trapezius muscle was examined for the presence or absence of five characteristics: taut band, nodule, spot tenderness, jump sign, and LTR. To identify a latent MTrP, two of the following needed to be present: taut band, nodule, and/or spot tenderness. In addition to interrater reliability, clinical precision of palpatory location of the upper trapezius was measured by the 3D infrared OptoTRAK3020 camera system. Twenty asymptomatic subjects (60% female; age 20–40) were recruited from a local health clinic. Subjects were excluded if they had an existing clinical disorder and active MTrPs. Subjects were examined in randomized groups of four on any given day, and each clinician examined each subject individually in a dimly lit room to avoid identification of erythema from previous palpation. The order of the clinicians was randomized, and the right upper trapezius was palpated from medial to lateral. The subjects were able to interact with the clinicians on their response to the palpation, but they were prevented from discussing previous assessment findings. Upon MTrP identification an assistant placed a probe underneath the clinician's fingers over the site and the fingers were then removed from the site, at which time a 3D measurement was taken. Data were gathered and reported descriptively for the five tested features. The 3D precision of palpatory location was expressed with a generalizability coefficient and standard error of measurement (SEM).

Of the 20 subjects, 16 were identified as having an MTrP. Results revealed good agreement for palpation of a taut band, nodule, and spot tenderness. All raters were in complete agreement on 14 of these 16 subjects. The authors reported that palpation for the trapezius was reliable across the whole group of raters for identification of taut band, nodule, and spot tenderness features of the MTrP but very poor for the jump sign and the LTR. Based on a criterion reliability threshold of a generalizability coefficient ≥0.80, the use of only two raters was most reliable. This two-rater scenario yielded a precision of 3D location of the MTrP with a generalizability coefficient of 0.92, 0.86, and 0.83 and an SEM of 7.5, 7.6, and 6.5 mm in the medial-lateral, superior-inferior, and anterior-posterior directions, respectively. This accuracy of 3D location essentially approached the physical dimensions of the fingertips. Also, reliability was increased—not surprisingly—if the patient was inherently more tender to palpation.

### Bron et al (2007) study

Bron et al[23] used three physiotherapists working in a practice specializing in musculoskeletal disorders of neck, shoulder, and arm and with 2–21 years of experience in MTrP identification as raters. This study is included as Chapter 5 in this book. Prestudy, the raters completed 8 hours of training and consensus-building on palpation technique, position, amount of pressure, and MTrP localization. Three bilateral shoulder muscles, the infraspinatus (three MTrPs), posterior deltoid (one MTrP), and biceps brachii (two MTrPs) were examined for absence or presence of a nodule in a taut band, referred pain, LTR, and jump sign. The feature of recognized pain was omitted to maintain blinding of the raters to symptom status. The criteria for MTrP presence were a nodule in a taut band, referred pain, LTR, and a jump sign. Forty subjects were recruited from a physical therapy practice and consisted of 32 unilateral and bilateral patients with shoulder pain and referral diagnoses of rotator cuff disease, tendonitis, tendinopathy, subacromial impingement, or chronic subdeltoid–subacromial bursitis and eight control subjects. Raters were blinded to subject status, and the subjects were randomized for testing. The assessments were completed in 10 minutes, and muscles were tested in uniform positions in sitting (i.e., the infraspinatus with the arm by the side and the other two muscles with the forearms supported with slight elbow flexion). The subjects were instructed to inform the raters if they experienced referred pain but were prohibited from reporting if the pain was familiar, thus maintaining blinding to symptom status. Results were reported in proportion of observed agreement ($P_{obs}$) and κ values between pairs of raters for individual characteristics and for agreement on MTrP presence and also by calculating a prevalence index, the absolute value of the difference between the number of agreements on positive and negative findings divided by the total number of observations as an indicator of the effect of limited variation in the data set on κ values. The three rater-pairs were also compared for statistically significant differences using the Kruskal-Wallis test.

The authors summarized the results noting that $P_{obs}$ was ≥0.70 in five out of six trigger points for referred pain sensation (0.68–0.87) and the jump sign (0.63–0.93), yielding these as the most reliable features. Less reliable results were noted for nodule in a taut band (0.58–0.86) and the LTR (0.51–0.82). The reliability of the agreement on MTrP presence for the three infraspinatus MTrPs was 0.69, 0.76, and 0.78; for the anterior deltoid 0.66; and for the two MTrPs in the biceps brachii 0.59 and 0.63. The κ values were highly variable and affected by prevalence of findings. There were no statistically significant differences between the three rater-pairs with regard to the identification of absence of presence of MTrPs. The authors concluded that palpation of the shoulder muscles tested in this study was reliable among three blinded examiners, as demonstrated by acceptable agreement on the presence and absence of MTrPs. The findings were taken to imply that palpation is a potentially useful diagnostic tool in patients with shoulder pain but that reliability differs per muscle and even per MTrP in the same muscle.

## Intrarater Reliability

Al-Shenquiti and Oldham[16] published the only MTrP palpation intrarater reliability study. The rater was a physical therapist with 11 years of clinical experience and extensive training in MTrP examination. The MTrP characteristics tested were absence or presence of spot tenderness, taut band, jump sign, LTR, pain recognition by patient, and referred pain for the supraspinatus, infraspinatus, teres minor, and subscapularis. Subjects consisted of 58 patients (53% male; mean age 48.4) with a medical diagnosis of rotator cuff tendonitis of greater than 6 weeks' but less than or equal to 18 months' duration. The diagnosis required a painful resisted movement of at least one motion of abduction, internal, or external rotation with or without a painful arc. Full range of motion but impingement on end of range of passive flexion also served to include the patient. No asymptomatic controls were included in this study. After recording the patient's report of pain pattern, the rater performed a flat palpation of the four rotator cuff muscles for the six characteristics tested in each muscle in reported standardized positions in a period of approximately 8 minutes per subject. This was repeated 3 days later for each subject by the same rater blinded to the documented findings of the initial testing. Data were reported descriptively for MTrP presence at initial test using the criteria of spot tenderness, taut band, pain recognition, jump sign, and referred pain. The presence of MTrPs for each muscle on initial test was reported as 88%, 62%, 20.7%, and 5.2% for the supraspinatus, infraspinatus, teres minor, and subscapularis, respectively. Despite this fairly homogenous group, the κ-statistic was employed and reported for each muscle and characteristic. Results yielded κ values of 1.0 for spot tenderness, taut band, jump sign, and recognized pain for all four muscles, and the κ values for referred pain were reported as 0.85, 0.86, 0.88, and 0.79 for the supraspinatus, infraspinatus, teres minor, and subscapularis respectively. For the supraspinatus or subscapularis a κ for the LTR could not be calculated because there were no positives identified, but a κ = 0.75 was reported for the infraspinatus and κ = 1.0 for the teres minor based upon two positive findings. The authors concluded intrarater reliability of MTrP characteristics in the rotator cuff muscles of patients diagnosed with tendonitis was established for the presence of spot tenderness, taut band, jump sign, and recognized pain. The intrarater reliability for the LTR varied depending on the muscle tested. The study acknowledged that external validity might be limited due to rater expertise and that although the rater was blinded during the second test there was potential for subconscious recall of the initial assessment findings.

## Discussion

As we noted in the introduction, the goal of this chapter is to determine a current best evidence synthesis with regard to reliability of MTrP manual palpation. Crucial to this stated goal is an evaluation of the research validity of the retrieved research papers. Domholdt[25] defined research validity as the extent to which conclusions of a study are believable and useful. We will discuss three areas specific to these reliability studies on manual identification of MTrPs where research validity can be threatened: construct validity, external validity, and statistical conclusion validity. In addition to this narrative review, we will use the implications of the systematic review using the *Data Extraction and Quality Scoring Form for Reliability Studies of Spinal Palpation* criterion list to provide a current best evidence synthesis.

## Construct Validity

A construct is an artificial framework that is not directly observable. The main threat to construct validity in reliability research is the discrepancy between the construct as labeled and the construct as implemented.[25]

It is evident that absence of a uniform MTrP definition threatens construct validity of the studies. Although all interrater reliability studies referred to the work of Travell and Simons,[1,12,13] none have used the essential criteria proposed in Table 4-1 for MTrP identification. Njoo and Van der Does[19] and Hsieh et al[21] only studied individual MTrP characteristics. Nice et al[20] used the most simplistic MTrP definition as tenderness and reproduction of trigger–point-specific characteristic referred pain. These authors excluded 11% of responses based on referral outside of the patient-indicated area of LBP. As Gerwin et al[17] noted, this may have excluded points that did fulfil MTrP criteria from statistical analysis. All other studies either used two[15,23] or three[16-18] of the essential criteria with a variety of the additional confirmatory findings as proposed by Simons et al[1] added in to satisfy criteria for MTrP identification. Wolfe et al[18] did a secondary analysis of their data with definition of an MTrP based on palpatory tenderness and patient recognition of pain, which one can hardly consider specific findings unique to an MTrP. As Wolfe et al[18] noted, consensus on MTrP definition is required and in absence of that consensus it is required that various proposed definitions establish their specific reliability. When using MTrP palpation in a clinical situation, we need to verbalize which definition we adhere to, because this clearly determines reliability. A similar case can be made with regard to the operational definitions of the various MTrP characteristics in the studies discussed.

Another aspect of construct validity concerns training and experience. Are these studies testing solely MTrP palpation or are they studying MTrP palpation in combination with varying levels of training and clinical experience? **Table 4-5** qualitatively shows that reliability was supported only in those studies that used both expert raters and prestudy hands-on training.[15,17,23] This is also clearly illustrated by the difference in findings between phases I and II in the Gerwin et al[17] study. This again has clear implications for reliable use of MTrP palpation in clinical practice.

Another threat to construct validity is that of the MTrP being clearly localized. Although the integrated hypothesis clearly favors MTrP location near or at the motor endplate, theoretically MTrPs can form anywhere in the muscle belly, which is also confirmed by both our clinical observations. Limiting the palpatory examination to specific demarcated areas, as was done in the Nice et al[20] and Hsieh et al[21] studies limits, as also noted by Gerwin et al,[17] the likelihood of finding MTrPs and does not represent clinical reality.

Most articles studied presence or absence of referred pain;[16,19-21,23] however, only Nice et al[20] specified the exact referral pattern as defined by Travell and Simons.[13] Recent research[26] has cast doubt on at least one muscle referral pattern as proposed by these authors, which would seem to further question construct validity of the Nice et al[20] study.

Our narrative review revealed several—in our opinion fatal—flaws with regard to construct validity: insufficiently specific definition of an MTrP, assumptions with regard to a

TABLE 4-5    Effect of Level of Expertise and Prestudy Training on Reliability Findings

| Study | Expertise Level | Hands-On Pretraining | Reliability Conclusions |
|---|---|---|---|
| Wolfe et al[18] | Expert | None | Unsupported |
| Nice et al[20] | Expert, varied level | None | Unsupported |
| Njoo & Van der Does[19] | Expert and nonexpert | Yes | Partially supported |
| Gerwin et al[17] (Phase I) | Expert | None | Unsupported |
| Gerwin et al[17] (Phase II) | Expert | Yes | Supported |
| Lew et al[22] | Expert | None | Unsupported |
| Hsieh et al[21] | Expert and nonexpert | Yes | Unsupported |
| Sciotti et al[15] | Expert | Yes | Supported |
| Bron et al[23] | Expert | Yes | Supported |

fixed MTrP location, and the use of a nonvalidated referral pattern as the main diagnostic criterion. For these reasons, we omitted the Wolfe et al,[18] Nice et al,[20] and Hsieh et al[21] studies from consideration for our best evidence synthesis.

## External Validity

External validity deals with the degree to which study results can be generalized to different subjects (in this case raters, test subjects, muscles tested), settings, and times.[25]

Raters with various different professional backgrounds have been used in these studies, including medical students, general practitioners, and medical specialists,[17–19,21] physiotherapists,[16,20,22, 23] and chiropractors.[15–21] Again, looking at Table 4-5 we note adequate reliability reported in studies done by all three professions involved, but we also note that rather than professional background the level of expertise and prestudy training seem to determine study outcome. Expertise and prestudy training affect external as well as construct validity.

Four studies[15,17,18,22] identified latent MTrPs. Two of these studies[15,22] exclusively used asymptomatic subjects with latent upper trapezius MTrPs. Although one study[27] suggested that latent MTrPs may affect movement patterns, Wolfe et al[18] have questioned the clinical relevance of latent MTrPs. With regard to reliability, Nice et al[20] clearly showed greater reliability in subjects symptomatic at the time of evaluation. Not surprisingly, Sciotti et al[15] showed that reliability was directly related to the amount of palpatory tenderness: Greater tenderness yielded greater interrater reliability in locating the MTrP. Other studies have used symptomatic subjects with fibromyalgia,[18] MPS,[18] low back pain,[19-21] neck pain,[17] and shoulder pain,[23] allowing for careful extrapolation to these clinical populations only.

Various muscles have been used for palpation reliability testing, including upper extremity, neck, back, and buttock muscles. Gerwin et al[17] have stated that features of the MTrP examination should not be assumed to be generally reliable and that feature identification tends to vary from muscle to muscle.

Settings have included general medicine clinics,[17,19] specialist medicine clinics,[17,18] likely chiropractic college clinics,[15,21] generalist physiotherapy clinics,[16,20] and a specialist physiotherapy clinic.[23] Again, looking at Table 4-5, two of the studies that reported adequate reliability were done in specialist settings,[17,23] which together with the influence of a possible higher pain level in patients from such settings and its effect on reliability raises the possibility of selection bias.

Although we questioned the use of solely asymptomatic subjects and the possible selection bias resulting from specialty settings, none of these flaws seemed sufficient to exclude studies from further consideration.

## Statistical Conclusion Validity

Using inappropriate statistical tools for data analysis is a threat to statistical conclusion validity.[25] Reliability studies use indices of agreement to quantitatively express intra- or interrater agreement. Huijbregts[28] has provided an in-depth review of indices of agreement. For the purpose of this review it is sufficient to know that chance-corrected indices of agreement are preferable over non–chance-corrected indices. Examples of the former are variations of the $\kappa$-coefficient used by various studies reviewed here,[16,19,20,21,23] but this also includes the $S_{av}$ used by Gerwin et al[17] and the generalizability coefficient used by Sciotti et al.[15] The study by Njoo and Van der Does[19] was the only one to supply 95% confidence intervals, allowing us to also judge clinical relevance of the interrater reliability findings. **Table 4-6** provides consensus-based cutoff values for the clinical interpretation of $\kappa$ values. As did Seffinger et al,[14] we used a $\kappa$ value (and $S_{av}$- and G-coefficient values) of 0.40 as an indicator of acceptable reliability.

| TABLE 4-6 | Kappa ($\kappa$) Benchmark Values[28] |
|---|---|
| <40% | Poor to fair agreement |
| 40–60% | Moderate agreement |
| 60–80% | Substantial agreement |
| >80% | Excellent agreement |
| 100% | Perfect agreement |

The greatest limitation to κ statistics is that they do not provide an adequate representation of reliability in case of limited variation in the data set (i.e., a preponderance of agreement on negative or positive findings).[28] Various studies have provided descriptive or specific prevalence statistics. From the study description, it is clear that limited variation has played a role with regard to the identification of latent MTrPs in the Wolfe et al[18] study and with regard to identification of a taut band and tenderness in the sternocleidomastoid and identification of tenderness and an LTR in the extensor digitorum in phase II of the Gerwin et al[17] study. Nice et al[20] indicate that the low level of agreement on a positive finding negatively affected κ values in their study. Bron et al[23] were the only study to calculate a prevalence index that clearly showed an effect of low prevalence on κ values, and thereby made a sufficient case for their reliance of the non–chance-corrected statistic $P_{obs}$.

Three studies used tests of statistical significance. Wolfe et al[18] used this statistical test to compare raters for differences in summed findings for individual characteristics and identification of active and latent MTrPs, which provides no information on actual agreement. Bron et al[23] used a test of significance to compare rater pairs for differences in identification of absence or presence of MTrPs; again, this adds little in the sense of establishing reliability. Gerwin et al[17] used a test of significance to establish if $S_{av}$ values differed significantly from zero. Although this is determined to a great degree by sample size,[26] with the small sample used in phase II of this study this would seem to be a relevant test to support true reliability.

Although Sciotti et al[15] used appropriate statistics for the portion of their study that looked at reliability of 3D location of MTrPs, for the interrater reliability portion with regard to MTrP characteristics they only used descriptive statistics, and that did not provide sufficient data to allow the reader to calculate appropriate statistics.

We discarded the interrater reliability portion of the Sciotti et al[15] study with regard to MTrP characteristics, and the Lew et al[22] and the Wolfe et al[18] studies for failing to use appropriate indices of agreement to express reliability. In the Njoo and Van der Does[19] and the Gerwin et al[17] studies, interrater reliability for the LTR in the quadratus lumborum, gluteus medius, sternocleidomastoid, trapezius, and infraspinatus muscles and referred pain for the quadratus lumborum failed to meet the reliability cutoff value of κ = 0.40. Because raw data and information on the manner of calculation were insufficient, we also discarded the later analysis of the Wolfe et al data.[1]

## Methodological Quality Assessment

Table 4-2 provides scores on the methodological quality assessment tool used in this study. This tool systematically deflates all weighted total scores by 1 point: Unlike with some palpatory tests, subjects cannot be blinded to MTrP palpation findings, because their report of recognized and referred pain is part of the diagnostic criteria. However, due to the limited effect we found this to be acceptable. For the sole intrarater reliability studies, items related to rater consensus were obviously not relevant: This deflated the total score for the Al-Shenqiti and Oldham[16] study by an additional 13 points. Clearly, this tool is less suited for methodological quality assessment of intrarater studies.

What is evident from Table 4-2 is that there has been a clear improvement in methodological quality of interrater reliability studies from the first study by Wolfe et al[18] in 1992 to the most recent 2007 Bron et al[23] study. However, almost universal methodological flaws in need of attention in future studies include:

- Use of subjects not naïve to the palpatory test studied
- Lack of rater blinding to subject symptom status
- Lack of P values to show κ values differ significantly from zero (which, as we noted earlier, lends credence to reliability findings in the small sample sizes generally used in these studies)
- Lack of calculation of confidence intervals
- Insufficient description of study results

In the absence of cutoff values established by Seffinger et al, we decided to use an arbitrary value of 70 as an indication of sufficient methodological quality. In line with findings from the narrative review above this eliminated the Wolfe et al,[18] Nice et al,[20] Lew et al,[22] and the Gerwin et al (phase I) studies[17] from consideration.

## Best Evidence Synthesis

Based on our narrative and methodological assessment of study quality we feel confident in providing the following best evidence synthesis:

- Sufficient intrarater reliability has been established for identification of spot tenderness, taut band, jump sign, recognized pain, and referred pain for all four rotator cuff muscles and for the LTR in the infraspinatus and teres minor.[16]
- Sufficient interrater reliability has been established for identification of local tenderness, taut band, recognized pain, and jump signs for both the gluteus medius and the quadratus lumborum muscles, whereas identification of referred pain has sufficient interrater reliability for the gluteus medius only.[19]
- Sufficient interrater reliability has been established for identification of tenderness in the upper trapezius, infraspinatus, and the axillary portion of the latissimus dorsi; taut band in the upper trapezius, infraspinatus, the axillary portion of the latissimus dorsi, and extensor digitorum; referred and patient recognized pain and absence or presence of latent or active MTrPs in the sternocleidomastoid, upper trapezius, infraspinatus, the axillary portion of the latissimus dorsi, and extensor digitorum; and LTR in the latissimus.[17] Operational definition in this case for an active MTrP includes point tenderness and a taut band with palpation reproducing the patient's recognized pain, whereas a latent MTrP is characterized only by a tender point and taut band.

- If a latent MTrP is defined as needing to have two of the following characteristics present—taut band, nodule, and/or spot tenderness—accuracy of MTrP location in the upper trapezius is highly reliable between raters.[15]
- If the criteria for MTrP presence include a nodule in a taut band, referred pain, LTR, and a jump sign, MTrP identification in the posterior deltoid, biceps brachii, and infraspinatus is highly reliable between raters, with identification of referred pain and the jump sign as most reliable individual characteristics in these muscles.[23]

A caveat with these findings is that reliability seems dependent on a high level of rater expertise, intensive training and consensus discussion on technique and operational definitions, and possibly higher levels of patient-reported pain.

## Limitations

This chapter has not addressed the literature on MTrP palpation reliability in patients with temporomandibular joint dysfunction. We also excluded instrumented algometry studies, as we concentrated on manual palpation studies only; however, we acknowledge that algometry has obvious clinical utility and may augment reliability of manual palpatory techniques. Another limitation related to our literature selection is that we chose English-language articles only, and that we therefore may have missed research published in other languages.

Finally, the biggest limitation lies in our elimination of articles based on a narrative and systematic assessment of methodological quality. Identification of fatal flaws in the narrative portion of the assessment was based on our personal interpretation, although we hope we have defended our choices appropriately. The methodological quality assessment tool has itself not been evaluated for reliability and has no consensus-based cutoff score for sufficient methodological quality. However, the very limited variation noted after both authors independently scored all studies indicates sufficient reliability of this tool and the elimination by the tool of studies already eliminated by the narrative assessment of study quality hint at its validity.

# Conclusion

Reliability of manual palpatory tests for the diagnosis of MTrPs was investigated in nine separate studies over the period of 1992–2007. These studies show a clear improvement in methodological quality over time but suffer from using subjects not naïve to the test, lack of rater blinding, inadequate statistical analysis of the results, and inadequate presentation of the findings, all points that are relevant to further improving future studies in this area.

Critical analysis has shown reliability of various features of the MTrP manual diagnostic techniques in different muscles sufficient for confident, research-based clinical use, but even with these specific findings there is the caveat that reliability appears dependent on a high level of rater expertise, intensive training and consensus discussion on technique and operational definitions, and possibly higher levels of patient-reported pain.

# References

1. Simons DG, Travell JG, Simons LS. *Travell and Simons' Myofascial Pain and Dysfunction: The Trigger Point Manual.* 2nd ed. Vol. 1. Baltimore, MD: Williams & Wilkins; 1999.
2. Fishbain DA, et al. DSM-III diagnoses of patients with myofascial pain syndrome (fibrositis). *Arch Phys Med Rehabil* 1989;70:433–438.
3. Skootsky SA, Jaeger B, Oye RK. Prevalence of myofascial pain in general internal medicine practice. *West J Med* 1 989;151:157–160.
4. Gerwin R. A study of 96 subjects examined both for fibromyalgia and myofascial pain. *J Musculoskel Pain* 1995;3(suppl 1):121.
5. Weiner DK, et al. Chronic low back pain in older adults: Prevalence, reliability, and validity of physical examination findings. *J Am Geriatr Soc* 2006;54:11–20.
6. Charlton JE. *Core Curriculum for Professional Education in Pain.* Seattle, WA: International Association for the Study of Pain; 2005.
7. Simons DG. Myofascial pain syndrome: One term but two concepts: A new understanding. *J Musculoskel Pain* 1995;3(1):7–13.
8. Simons DG. Review of enigmatic MTrPs as a common cause of enigmatic musculoskeletal pain and dysfunction. *J Electromyogr Kinesiol* 2004;14:95–107.
9. Breivik H, et al. Survey of chronic pain in Europe: Prevalence, impact on daily life, and treatment. *Eur J Pain* 2006;10(4):287–333.
10. Harden RN, et al. Signs and symptoms of the myofascial pain syndrome: A national survey of pain management providers. *Clin J Pain* 2000;16:64–72.
11. Gerwin RD, Dommerholt J, Shah JP. An expansion of Simons' integrated hypothesis of trigger point formation. *Curr Pain Headache Rep* 2004;8:468–475.
12. Travell JG, Simons DG. *Myofascial Pain and Dysfunction: The Trigger Point Manual. Volume 1: The Upper Extremities.* Baltimore, MD: Williams & Wilkins; 1983.
13. Travell JG, Simons DG. *Myofascial Pain and Dysfunction: The Trigger Point Manual. Volume 2: The Lower Extremities.* Baltimore, MD: Williams & Wilkins; 1992.
14. Seffinger MA, et al. Reliability of spinal palpation for diagnosis of back and neck pain: A systematic review of the literature. *Spine* 2004;29:E14–E25.
15. Sciotti VM, et al. Clinical precision of myofascial trigger point location in the trapezius muscle. *Pain* 2001;93:259–266.
16. Al-Shenqiti AM, Oldham JA. Test–retest reliability of myofascial trigger point detection in patients with rotator cuff tendonitis. *Clin Rehabil* 2005;19:482–487.
17. Gerwin RD, et al. Interrater reliability in myofascial trigger point examination. *Pain* 1997; 69(1–2):65–73.
18. Wolfe F, et al. The fibromyalgia and myofascial pain syndromes: A preliminary study of tender points and trigger points in persons with fibromyalgia, myofascial pain syndrome and no disease. *J Rheumatol* 1992;19:944–951.
19. Njoo KH, Van der Does E. The occurrence and inter-rater reliability of myofascial trigger points in the quadratus lumborum and gluteus medius: A prospective study in nonspecific low back pain patients and controls in general practice. *Pain* 1994;58:317–323.
20. Nice DA, et al. Intertester reliability of judgments of the presence of trigger points in patients with low back pain. *Arch Phys Med Rehabil* 1992;73:893–898.

21. Hsieh CY, et al. Interexaminer reliability of the palpation of trigger points in the trunk and lower limb muscles. *Arch Phys Med Rehabil* 2000;81:258–264.
22. Lew PC, Lewis J, Story I. Inter-therapist reliability in locating latent myofascial trigger points using palpation. *Man Ther* 1997;2:87–90.
23. Bron C, et al. Interobserver reliability of palpation of myofascial trigger points in shoulder muscles. *J Manual Manipulative Ther* 2007;15:203–215.
24. Fricton JR, et al. Myofascial pain syndrome: Electromyographic changes associated with local twitch response. *Arch Phys Med Rehabil* 1985;66:314–317.
25. Domholdt E. *Physical Therapy Research: Principles and Applications.* Philadelphia, PA: WB Saunders Company; 1993.
26. Cornwall J, Harris AJ, Mercer SR. The lumbar multifidus muscle and patterns of pain. *Man Ther* 2006;11:40–45.
27. Lucas KR, Polus BI, Rich PS. Latent myofascial trigger points: Their effect on muscle activation and movement efficiency. *J Bodywork Movement Ther* 2004;8:160–166.
28. Huijbregts PA. Spinal motion palpation: A review of reliability studies. *J Manual Manipulative Ther* 2002;10:24–39.

Chapter 5

# Interrater Reliability of Palpation of Myofascial Trigger Points in Three Shoulder Muscles

*Carel Bron, PT, MT*

*Jo Franssen, PT*

*Michel Wensing, PhD*

*Rob A.B. Oostendorp, PhD, PT, MT*

## Introduction

Shoulder complaints are very common in modern industrial countries. Recent reviews[1-4] have indicated a 1-year prevalence ranging from 4.7–46.7%. These reviews have also reported a lifetime prevalence of 6.7–66.7%. This wide variation in reported prevalence can be explained by the different definitions used for shoulder complaints and by differences in the age and other characteristics of the various study populations. Because making a specific structure-based diagnosis for patients with shoulder complaints is considered to be difficult due to the lack of reliable tests for shoulder examination, current guidelines developed by the Dutch Society of General Practitioners have recommended instead using the term "shoulder complaints" as a working diagnosis.[5] Shoulder complaints have been defined in a similarly nonspecific manner as signs and symptoms of pain in the deltoid and upper arm region and stiffness and restricted movements of the shoulder, often accompanied by limitations in daily activities.[6]

Despite the absence of reliable diagnostic tests to implicate these structures, the prevailing assumption is that in nontraumatic shoulder complaints the anatomical structures in the subacromial space are primarily involved (i.e., the subacromial bursa, the rotator cuff tendons, and the tendon of the long head of the biceps muscle).[7-9] However, this

Courtesy of John M. Medeiros, PT, PhD, Managing Editor of the *Journal of Manual and Manipulative Therapy*.

assumption does not take into account that muscle tissue itself can also give rise to pain in the shoulder region.[10] In our clinical experience, myofascial trigger points (MTrPs) can lead to musculoskeletal pain in the shoulder and upper arm region and contribute to the burden of shoulder complaints.

The term *myofascial pain* was first introduced by Travell,[10] who described it as "the complex of sensory, motor, and autonomic symptoms caused by myofascial trigger points." An MTrP is a hyperirritable spot in skeletal muscle that is associated with a hypersensitive palpable nodule in a taut band. In addition, the spot is painful on compression and may produce characteristic referred pain, referred tenderness, motor dysfunction, and autonomic phenomena. Two different types of MTrPs have been described: active and latent. Active trigger points are associated with spontaneous complaints of pain. In contrast, latent trigger points do not cause spontaneous pain, but pain may be elicited with manual pressure or with needling of the trigger point. Despite not being spontaneously painful, latent MTrPs have been hypothesized to restrict range of motion[11] and to alter motor recruitment patterns.[12]

As noted, referred pain is a key characteristic of myofascial pain. Referred pain is felt remote from the site of origin.[13] The area of referred pain may be discontinuous from the site of local pain or it may be segmentally related to the lesion, both of which may pose a serious problem for the correct diagnosis and subsequent appropriate treatment of muscle-related pain. The theoretical model for this phenomenon of referred pain was first proposed by Ruch[14] and later modified by Mense[13,15] and Hoheisel.[16] Referred pain patterns originating in muscles have been documented using injection of hypertonic saline, electrical stimulation, or pressure on the most sensitive spot in the muscle.[17-21] In the clinical setting, palpation is the only method capable of diagnosing myofascial pain. Therefore, reliable MTrP palpation is the necessary prerequisite for considering myofascial pain as a valid diagnosis.[22] Published interrater studies have reported poor to good reliability for MTrP palpation.[23-29] The previous chapter by McEvoy and Huijbregts provides a comprehensive and systematic review of MTrP palpation reliability studies. However, only one of these studies included a muscle that could produce shoulder pain: Gerwin et al[27] reported a percent agreement (PA) of 83% for tenderness in the infraspinatus muscle ($\kappa = 0.48$), 83% ($\kappa = 0.40$) for the taut band, 59% ($\kappa = 0.17$) for the local twitch response, and 89% ($\kappa = 0.84$) for the referred pain.

In light of the near absence of data of the societal impact of shoulder complaints as noted earlier, and of the potential role of myofascial pain syndrome with regard to shoulder pain, the aim of this study was to determine the interrater reliability of MTrP palpation in three human shoulder muscles deemed by us to be clinically relevant: the infraspinatus, the anterior deltoid, and the biceps brachii muscles.

## Methods and Materials

### Subjects

Subjects were recruited from a consecutive sample of patients with unilateral or bilateral shoulder pain referred by their physician to a physical therapy private practice specializing in the management of persons with neck, shoulder, and upper extremity musculoskeletal disorders. To decrease limited variation within the data set and to control for rater bias, we also included asymptomatic subjects.

All subjects were unacquainted with and had not met the raters. Additional inclusion criteria for participation in the study were age between 18 and 75 years and the ability to read and understand the Dutch language. Exclusion criteria were known serious rheumatological, neurologic, orthopaedic, or internal diseases, such as adhesive capsulitis, rotator cuff tears, cervical radiculopathy, diabetes mellitus, recent shoulder or neck trauma, or shoulder/upper extremity complaints of uncertain origin, as diagnosed by the referring physicians. After reading a brief synopsis of the aim of the study and the test procedure, all subjects signed an informed consent form. The Committee on Research involving Human Subjects of the district Arnhem-Nijmegen approved the study design, the protocols, and the informed consent procedure.

## Raters and Observers

The raters were three physical therapists: rater A with 29, rater B with 28, and rater C with 16 years of clinical experience, respectively. All were employed at the private practice where this study was conducted. The raters had all specialized in the diagnosis and management of patients with musculoskeletal disorders of the neck, shoulder, and upper extremity; and they had 21, 16, and 2 years of experience, respectively, with regard to diagnosis and management of MTrPs.

The observers were three physical therapists who also had experience in treating patients with myofascial pain. Prior to the study, they were informed by the lead investigator (CB) about the study protocol, and they participated in the training sessions with the raters.

Both raters and observers participated in a total of 8 hours of training. During these sessions, they were able to practice their skills, to compare with each other, and to discuss palpation technique, subject positioning, the amount of pressure used by the examiners,[30] and the location of the MTrPs (**Figure 5-1**). Before proceeding with the study, they reached consensus about all aspects of the examination.

## Trigger Point Examination

Simons et al[31] documented 11 muscles in total that could refer pain to the frontal or lateral region of the shoulder and arm (**Table 5-1**). Based on our clinical observation that these muscles are frequently involved in patients with shoulder pain, we chose to study the infraspinatus, the anterior deltoid, and the biceps brachii. Without providing specific data on prevalence, Simons et al[31] reported that the infraspinatus is very often involved in shoulder pain. Hong[32] noted that the deltoid and the biceps brachii could give rise to satellite MTrPs of the infraspinatus muscle. Hsieh[33] provided evidence for the existence of a key–satellite relation between the infraspinatus muscle and the anterior deltoid muscle.

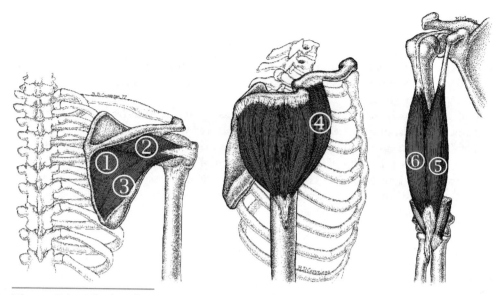

**Figure 5-1** The localization of trigger points in the infraspinatus muscle, biceps brachii, and the anterior deltoid muscles. The numbers correspond with the sequence of palpation during the test.

*Source:* Illustrations courtesy of Lifeart/Mediclip, Manual Medicine 1, Version 1.0a, Williams & Wilkins, 1997.

TABLE 5-1    Muscles with a Known Referred Pain Pattern to the Frontal or Lateral Region of the Shoulder and/or Arm[31]

Infraspinatus

Deltoid (anterior and middle part)

Biceps brachii

Supraspinatus

Coracobrachialis

Latissimus dorsi

Scalene

Pectoralis major

Pectoralis minor

Subclavius

Sternalis

A satellite trigger point may develop in the referral zone of a key MTrP located in the key muscle. It may also develop in an overloaded synergist that is substituting for the muscle that is harboring the key MTrP, in an antagonist countering the increased tension of the key muscle, or in a muscle that is linked apparently only neurogenically to the key MTrP. Sometimes this hierarchy is obvious, but it is not always evident. Key and satellite trigger points are related to each other; our clinical observations indicate that signs and symptoms related to satellite trigger points diminish when key MTrPs are treated appropriately.

Another reason for our choice of these specific muscles is that all three muscles studied here are part of the same functional unit, with all three muscles acting as synergists active during shoulder flexion. Although the infraspinatus muscle is traditionally known as an external rotator, this is only true for the anatomic (arm by the side) position. This muscle is one of the rotator cuff muscles that is active during flexion of the upper arm to provide stability of the glenohumeral joint during arm movements.[34,35]

Although MTrPs may be found anywhere in the muscle belly, we agreed to palpate for their presence only in close proximity to the motor endplate zones. The reason for this choice of location is that Simons et al[31] have suggested that the primary abnormality responsible for MTrP formation is associated with individual dysfunctional endplates in the endplate zone or motor point.

We bilaterally palpated these three muscles for MTrPs using four of the criteria proposed for the palpatory diagnosis of MTrPs:[31]

1.  Presence of a taut band with a nodule. The rater examined the subject by palpating the muscle perpendicular to the muscle fiber orientation with either a flat palpation (infraspinatus muscle and the anterior deltoid muscle) or a pincer palpation (biceps brachii muscle). When a taut band was identified, the rater palpated along the taut band to locate the nodule. The raters were asked to search for multiple MTrPs in each muscle. The palpatory findings were more important than the exact location of the MTrPs, as indicated by Simons et al.[31]

2.  Reported painful sensation during compression in an area consistent with the established referred pain pattern of the involved muscle. While compressing the palpable nodule in the taut band, the subject was asked if he or she felt any pain or any sensation (e.g., tingling or numbness) in an area remote from the compressed point. When the subjects reported referred sensation, they were asked to describe this area. The rater then decided whether this area was comparable to the established referred pain zone (**Figure 5-2**).

3.  Presence of a visible or palpable local twitch response (LTR) during snapping palpation. The rater rolled quickly the taut band under the fingertip, while examining the skin above the muscle fibers for this characteristic short and rapid movement.

4.  Presence of a general pain response during palpation, also known as a jump sign. While compressing the MTrP, the rater carefully examined the subject's reaction. A positive jump sign was defined as the subject withdrawing from palpation, wincing, or producing any pain-related vocalization.

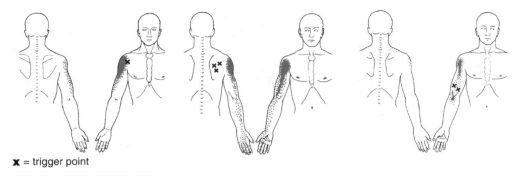

**x** = trigger point

**Figure 5-2** The localization of trigger points in the anterior deltoid, infraspinatus, and biceps brachii muscle and the referred pain patterns according to Simons et al.[31] Solid shading shows the essential referred pain zone, present in nearly all patients, while the stippling represents the spillover zone, present in some, but not all, patients.[31]

*Source:* Illustrations courtesy of Lifeart/Mediclip, Manual Medicine 1, Version 1.0a, Williams & Wilkins, 1997.

All four criteria were scored dichotomously:

- Yes if the rater was certain of presence of a parameter
- No if the rater was sure of the absence of a parameter or if the rater was unsure of presence or absence

Examination of the infraspinatus muscle was performed with the subjects seated with the arms hanging down by the side of the body. Examination of the anterior deltoid and biceps brachii muscles was performed with the forearms supported with slight elbow flexion (**Figure 5-3**).

The raters were blinded to subject status; that is, the subjects were not allowed to indicate whether they were symptomatic. They were instructed to inform the raters when they felt pain somewhere other than the palpation site or when they experienced a referred sensation. However, they were not allowed to tell the rater whether they felt a recognizable pain, because that would negate attempts at rater blinding.

In addition to scoring the separate criteria, the raters were asked to judge whether a trigger point was present or absent. Simons et al[31] suggested that minimal diagnostic criteria for an MTrP consist of a palpable nodule present in a palpable taut band. Simons et al also required that this produce the patient's recognizable pain upon compression, but we should note that in this study the subjects were not allowed to inform the examiners of their symptom status. Therefore, in this study the examiners decided that the MTrP was present when the palpable nodule in the taut band was present

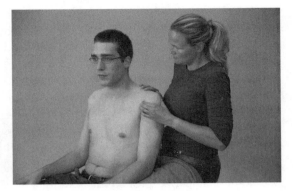

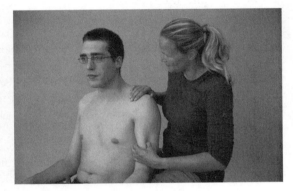

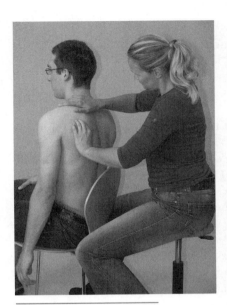

**Figure 5-3** Palpation technique for trigger point palpation of the infraspinatus muscle (left), anterior deltoid muscle (top right), and the biceps brachii muscle (bottom right), respectively.

together with at least one or more of the other clinical characteristics. In all other combinations, it was said that the MTrP was absent. As a result of this study design, no distinction was made between active and latent MTrPs, because the examiners were not allowed to inquire whether subjects recognized the pain from palpation. Therefore, examiners may have reported on both active and latent MTrPs in symptomatic and asymptomatic subjects.

## Methods

During two morning sessions separated by a 1-week interval, two different groups of 20 subjects each were examined. The raters completed the assessment of each of the four characteristics for the three bilateral muscles within a 10-minute period. Subjects were examined in groups of three, with each subject in a separate, private treatment room. Following the first assessment, the raters were randomly assigned to one of the two other rooms to assess another subject until all three raters had assessed all subjects. Upon completion of the assessment of the initial group of three subjects, three new subjects were assigned to the examination rooms, and the procedures were repeated. An observer was present in each room during all examinations to verify correct implementation of the testing procedures, but the observer did not interfere with the examination. According to the observers, all examinations were performed in an appropriate manner.

## Statistical Analysis

For the statistical analysis, we used the Statistical Package for the Social Sciences for Windows version 12.0.1 (SPSS Inc., Chicago, IL). Frequencies were calculated for the subject demographic information.

To express interrater reliability, we calculated both pairwise percentages of agreement (PA) and pairwise Cohen Kappa-values ($\kappa$). The PA value is defined as the ratio of the number of agreements to the total number of ratings made.[36] Using the terminology from the contingency matrix provided in **Table 5-2**, PA = $(a + d)/n$. Cohen's $\kappa$ is a coefficient of agreement beyond chance: $\kappa = PA - P_e/1 - P_e$. The agreement based on chance alone ($P_e$) is calculated by the sum of the multiplied marginal totals corresponding to each cell divided by the square of the total number of cases ($n$): $P_e = (f_1 g_1 + f_2 g_2)/n^2$.

The $\kappa$ value is widely used for dichotomous variables in interrater reliability studies, although there is no universally accepted value for good agreement.[37] Landis and Koch[38] proposed that a $\kappa$ value <0.00 be considered indicative of poor reliability and a value of 0.001–0.20 slight, 0.21–0.40 fair, 0.41–0.60 moderate, 0.61–0.80 substantial or good, and 0.81–1.00 almost perfect or very good reliability. In this study, we considered a PA value ≥70% indicative of interrater reliability acceptable for clinical use, because under ideal circumstances (i.e., equal prevalence of negative and positive findings), when using a dichotomous test, a PA value ≥70% leads to a $\kappa \geq 0.40$.

A major drawback to using $\kappa$ as an index of agreement is that this statistic is very sensitive to the prevalence of positive and negative findings. To quantify this effect on the $\kappa$

### TABLE 5-2    The Contingency Matrix

|  |  | Rater 1 | | |
|---|---|---|---|---|
|  |  | Positive | Negative | |
| Rater 2 | Positive | $a$ | $b$ | $g_1$ |
|  | Negative | $c$ | $d$ | $g_2$ |
| Total |  | $f_1$ | $f_2$ | $n$ |

values calculated, in this study we also determined the prevalence index ($P_i$), which is the absolute value of the difference between the number of agreements on positive findings (*a*) and agreements on negative findings (*d*) divided by the total number of observations (*n*): $P_i = |a - d|/n$.[39] If $P_i$ is high (closer to 1.0), chance agreement ($P_e$) is also high and κ is reduced accordingly. If the $P_i$ is closer to zero, chance agreement ($P_e$) is low and κ will increase. This means that the κ statistic is more useful as an index of agreement in case of a low $P_i$ than it is with higher $P_i$ values. **Table 5-3** provides examples of the influence of variations in $P_i$ on κ values. With κ values in this study strongly influenced by variations in prevalence as indicated by the wide range of $P_i$, we were forced to focus on the PA values for the interpretation of our findings.

TABLE 5-3a   Example of the Influence of a High Value of the Prevalence Index on the κ Value (Example Used: Trigger Point 3, Right Shoulder, Couple A/C, Palpation for a Nodule)[a]

|  |  | Observer 1 | | |
|---|---|---|---|---|
|  |  | Positive | Negative |  |
| Observer 2 | Positive | 35 | 2 | 37 |
|  | Negative | 2 | 1 | 3 |
| Total |  | 37 | 3 | 40 |

[a]In this case, the percentage of agreement is high (0.90), but because the prevalence index is also high (0.85), the κ value indicates only fair agreement (0.28).

TABLE 5-3b   Example of the Influence of a Low Value of the Prevalence Index on the κ Value (Example Used: Trigger Point 2, Right Shoulder, Couple B/C, Palpation of a Nodule)[a]

|  |  | Observer 1 | | |
|---|---|---|---|---|
|  |  | Positive | Negative |  |
| Observer 2 | Positive | 19 | 0 | 19 |
|  | Negative | 5 | 16 | 21 |
| Total |  | 24 | 16 | 40 |

[a]In this case, the percentage of agreement is high (0.85), but the prevalence index is low (0.08), so despite slightly lower percentage agreement than in Table 5-3a, the κ value (0.75) indicates good agreement.

To compare the three pairs of raters, we used the Kruskal-Wallis test, which is a non-parametric one-way analysis of variance. The test statistic $H$ will increase with increased variation. For graphical presentation, we used the box-and-whisker plot. To compare several data sets, this semigraphical way of summarizing data, which provides median value, lower and upper quartiles, and the extreme values, is considered simple and useful.[37]

## Results

### Patient Characteristics

Thirty-two subjects with unilateral or bilateral shoulder pain and eight subjects without shoulder pain were included in this study. The mean age of subjects was 40 (SD = 11.5; range 18 to 70). Of these 40 subjects, 24 (60%) were female and 16 (40%) were male. The study population had a gender and age profile similar to the patient population of the physical therapy practice where the study was conducted. Most of the subjects (53%) were not diagnosed with a specific medical diagnosis for their shoulder complaints, as suggested in the guidelines developed by the Dutch Society of General Practitioners.[5] **Table 5-4** provides physician referral diagnoses for the 32 patients involved in this study.

TABLE 5-4    Patient Diagnosis and Referral Information

| Referral Diagnosis | Number of Subjects | Percentage |
|---|---|---|
| No medical diagnosis | 17 | 53% |
| Calcifying tendonitis | 2 | 6% |
| Tendonitis/bursitis/tendinosis | 3 | 9% |
| Soft-tissue disorder | 7 | 22% |
| Degenerative changes in the acromioclavicular or glenohumeral joint | 2 | 6% |
| Subacromial impingement syndrome | 1 | 3% |
| Total | 32 | 100% |

The physician referred the patient to the practice without mentioning any medical diagnosis. This follows the Dutch guidelines for general practitioners.

## Pairwise Interrater Agreement

**Tables 5-5** through **5-8** present the data of the various clinical characteristics of the MTrP in the 80 shoulders of our 40 subjects (i.e., palpable nodule in a taut band, referred pain sensation, LTR, and the jump sign, respectively). The column PA provides the percentage agreement values for the three pairs of observers for both the left and right shoulder. The column κ shows the corresponding κ value; the third column shows the corresponding prevalence index ($P_i$).

Although we have insufficient information to calculate mean agreement values for all rater pairs, we can cautiously conclude that the rater pairs seemed to be demonstrating similar reliability. When comparing the pairwise PA values for the presence or absence of MTrPs, we found no significant difference between the rater pairs (Kruskal-Wallis one-way ANOVA on ranks, $H = 0.841$, $P > 0.05$; **Figure 5-4**).

TABLE 5-5    Percentage Agreement (PA), κ Coefficient, and Prevalence Index ($P_i$) for Palpation of a Nodule in a Taut Band in Six Localizations in Three Muscles (Left and Right)[a]

| | | Rater Pairs | | | | | | | | |
|---|---|---|---|---|---|---|---|---|---|---|
| | | A/B | | | A/C | | | B/C | | |
| MTrP | Side | PA | κ | $P_i$ | PA | κ | $P_i$ | PA | κ | $P_i$ |
| 1 | Left | 65 | 0.22 | 0.40 | 68 | 0.30 | 0.38 | 68 | 0.34 | 0.13 |
| | Right | 73 | 0.40 | 0.32 | 63 | 0.24 | 0.13 | 70 | 0.47 | 0.30 |
| 2 | Left | 70 | 0.35 | 0.30 | 80 | 0.60 | 0.10 | 65 | 0.30 | 0.20 |
| | Right | 73 | 0.44 | 0.18 | 70 | 0.43 | 0.05 | 88 | 0.75 | 0.08 |
| 3 | Left | 83 | 0.26 | 0.73 | 90 | 0.30 | 0.85 | 88 | 0.25 | 0.83 |
| | Right | 85 | 0.33 | 0.75 | 90 | 0.28 | 0.85 | 85 | 0.33 | 0.75 |
| 4 | Left | 63 | 0.34 | 0.03 | 70 | 0.40 | 0.20 | 63 | 0.25 | 0.18 |
| | Right | 75 | 0.50 | 0.15 | 63 | 0.26 | 0.13 | 68 | 0.35 | 0.03 |
| 5 | Left | 45 | 0.16 | 0.00 | 68 | 0.27 | 0.38 | 53 | 0.14 | 0.18 |
| | Right | 53 | 0.16 | 0.13 | 80 | 0.58 | 0.20 | 53 | 0.11 | 0.18 |
| 6 | Left | 53 | 0.22 | 0.03 | 73 | 0.25 | 0.53 | 45 | 0.15 | 0.05 |
| | Right | 53 | 0.22 | 0.03 | 75 | 0.44 | 0.35 | 58 | 0.24 | 0.13 |

[a]The numbers 1, 2, and 3 in the first column correspond with the localization in the infraspinatus muscle, 4 is localized in the anterior deltoid muscle, and 5 and 6 are localized in the biceps brachii muscle. In the second row, the three raters are mentioned as A, B, and C. The number of subjects is 40.

**TABLE 5-6** Percentage Agreement (PA), $\kappa$ Coefficient, and Prevalence Index ($P_i$) for Palpation of Referred Pain in Six Localizations in Three Muscles (Left and Right)

| | | Rater Pairs | | | | | | | | |
|---|---|---|---|---|---|---|---|---|---|---|
| | | A/B | | | A/C | | | B/C | | |
| MTrP | Side | PA | $\kappa$ | $P_i$ | PA% | $\kappa$ | $P_i$ | PA | $\kappa$ | $P_i$ |
| 1 | Left | 78 | 0.48 | 0.38 | 63 | 0.19 | 0.28 | 65 | 0.21 | 0.35 |
| | Right | 78 | 0.51 | 0.33 | 75 | 0.41 | 0.40 | 73 | 0.41 | 0.28 |
| 2 | Left | 88 | 0.38 | 0.78 | 88 | 0.55 | 0.68 | 80 | 0.23 | 0.70 |
| | Right | 80 | 0.25 | 0.70 | 85 | 0.33 | 0.75 | 85 | 0.53 | 0.6 |
| 3 | Left | 73 | 0.46 | 0.08 | 63 | 0.26 | 0.13 | 70 | 0.36 | 0.25 |
| | Right | 83 | 0.64 | 0.18 | 78 | 0.54 | 0.13 | 80 | 0.58 | 0.2 |
| 4 | Left | 78 | −0.13 | 0.78 | 85 | 0.31 | 0.75 | 78 | −0.13 | 0.78 |
| | Right | 88 | 0.55 | 0.68 | 80 | 0.25 | 0.70 | 88 | 0.22 | 0.83 |
| 5 | Left | 93 | 0.36 | 0.88 | 83 | 0.29 | 0.73 | 80 | 0.13 | 0.75 |
| | Right | 85 | 0.19 | 0.80 | 93 | 0.63 | 0.78 | 88 | −0.06 | 0.88 |
| 6 | Left | 90 | 0.45 | 0.80 | 75 | 0.25 | 0.60 | 70 | 0.03 | 0.65 |
| | Right | 88 | 0.38 | 0.78 | 75 | 0.15 | 0.65 | 78 | 0.20 | 0.68 |

**TABLE 5-7** Percentage Agreement (PA), $\kappa$ Coefficient, and Prevalence Index ($P_i$) for Palpation of a Local Twitch Response in Six Localizations in Three Muscles (Left and Right)

| | | Rater Pairs | | | | | | | | |
|---|---|---|---|---|---|---|---|---|---|---|
| | | A/B | | | A/C | | | B/C | | |
| MTrP | Side | PA | $\kappa$ | $P_i$ | PA | $\kappa$ | $P_i$ | PA | $\kappa$ | $P_i$ |
| 1 | Left | 80 | 0.09 | 0.75 | 73 | 0.21 | 0.58 | 78 | 0.36 | 0.58 |
| | Right | 85 | −0.04 | 0.85 | 75 | 0.05 | 0.75 | 75 | 0.15 | 0.65 |
| 2 | Left | 100 | n.c. | 1.00 | 73 | n.c. | 0.73 | 73 | n.c. | 0.73 |
| | Right | 95 | n.c. | 0.95 | 78 | n.c. | 0.78 | 78 | 0.11 | 0.73 |
| 3 | Left | 53 | 0.05 | 0.13 | 58 | 0.15 | 0.38 | 50 | 0.16 | 0.25 |
| | Right | 70 | 0.15 | 0.55 | 43 | 0.13 | 0.13 | 33 | 0.07 | 0.03 |
| 4 | Left | 73 | 0.04 | 0.68 | 63 | 0.14 | 0.38 | 65 | 0.11 | 0.55 |
| | Right | 65 | 0.21 | 0.35 | 60 | 0.20 | 0.20 | 60 | 0.20 | 0.15 |
| 5 | Left | 43 | 0.00 | 0.28 | 50 | 0.04 | 0.00 | 58 | 0.00 | 0.48 |
| | Right | 53 | 0.01 | 0.43 | 73 | 0.45 | 0.08 | 60 | 0.13 | 0.45 |
| 6 | Left | 53 | 0.17 | 0.28 | 68 | 0.32 | 0.28 | 50 | 0.16 | 0.25 |
| | Right | 60 | 0.23 | 0.35 | 63 | 0.25 | 0.08 | 58 | 0.21 | 0.33 |

TABLE 5-8    Percentage Agreement (PA), κ Coefficient, and Prevalence Index (P$_i$) for Palpation of the Jump Sign in Six Localizations in Three Muscles (Left and Right)

| | | Rater Pairs | | | | | | | | |
|---|---|---|---|---|---|---|---|---|---|---|
| | | A/B | | | A/C | | | B/C | | |
| MTrP | Side | PA | κ | P$_i$ | PA | κ | P$_i$ | PA | κ | P$_i$ |
| 1 | Left | 75 | 0.47 | 0.25 | 83 | 0.60 | 0.38 | 78 | 0.51 | 0.33 |
| | Right | 63 | 0.27 | 0.18 | 73 | 0.36 | 0.38 | 65 | 0.31 | 0.15 |
| 2 | Left | 70 | 0.07 | 0.60 | 68 | 0.12 | 0.53 | 88 | 0.68 | 0.53 |
| | Right | 68 | 0.02 | 0.63 | 75 | 0.19 | 0.65 | 93 | 0.58 | 0.43 |
| 3 | Left | 70 | 0.29 | 0.40 | 68 | 0.22 | 0.43 | 78 | 0.38 | 0.53 |
| | Right | 75 | 0.47 | 0.25 | 75 | 0.49 | 0.15 | 80 | 0.58 | 0.25 |
| 4 | Left | 78 | 0.56 | 0.18 | 65 | 0.31 | 0.15 | 73 | 0.36 | 0.38 |
| | Right | 78 | 0.54 | 0.18 | 78 | 0.48 | 0.43 | 70 | 0.34 | 0.40 |
| 5 | Left | 68 | 0.30 | 0.33 | 68 | 0.33 | 0.18 | 65 | 0.22 | 0.35 |
| | Right | 68 | 0.31 | 0.28 | 68 | 0.31 | 0.28 | 65 | 0.16 | 0.40 |
| 6 | Left | 68 | 0.35 | 0.28 | 70 | 0.40 | 0.05 | 63 | 0.28 | 0.18 |
| | Right | 70 | 0.37 | 0.25 | 83 | 0.64 | 0.18 | 73 | 0.41 | 0.28 |

## Palpable Nodule in a Taut Band

The PA value for the palpable nodule in a taut band in the muscle varied from 45% in the medial head of the biceps brachii muscle to 90% in the infraspinatus muscle. The PA tended to be higher in trigger point 3 (83–90%) than in point 1 (63–73%). In the anterior deltoid muscle, the PA varied from 63–75%. The PA for the biceps brachii varied from 45–75%. Only the rater pair A/C agreed in both points more than 70%. The κ value ranged from 0.11–0.75 (Table 5-5).

## Referred Pain Sensation

The agreement on the referred pain sensation elicited by pressure on the nodule reached a PA value ≥70% in all but three cases (range 63–93%). The scores for referred pain sensation were the lowest in the infraspinatus (trigger point 1). The κ value ranged from −0.13–0.64 (Table 5-6).

## Local Twitch Response

The LTR had only acceptable agreement for two locations in the infraspinatus. The lowest PA value was 33% in trigger point 3, which is the most central point in the infraspinatus

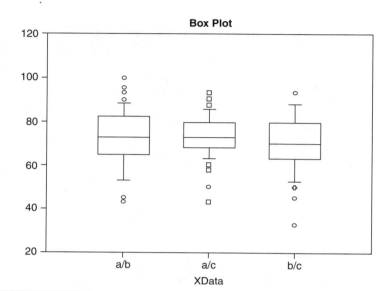

**Figure 5-4** This box-n-whisker plot shows the graphical expression [i.e., median, lower and upper quartile, minimum and the maximum value] of the dataset from the pairs of raters. This graphic shows only small differences (not statistically or clinically relevant differences) between the three pairs of observers.

muscle. All three raters were unable to elicit an LTR in trigger point 2 (also in the infraspinatus muscle) in almost any of the subjects. This led to an agreement of 100% in one case; in most cases it was not possible to calculate a κ value because of the absence of the LTR in all cases of one rater (Table 5-7).

## Jump Sign

The raters achieved the highest PA (93%) on the jump sign in the infraspinatus muscle and the lowest PA (63%) in the infraspinatus muscle and the biceps brachii muscle. The κ value ranged from 0.07–0.68 (Table 5-8).

## Overall Agreement

The percentage of agreement on MTrP presence or absence was acceptable for the infraspinatus muscle. In two out of three trigger point locations, PA values exceeded 70%. In the anterior deltoid muscle and in the biceps brachii muscle, the PA value was <70% (**Table 5-9**).

TABLE 5-9  Percentage Agreement (PA), κ Coefficient, and Prevalence Index (P$_i$) for Agreement on Presence or Absence of Myofascial Trigger Points[a]

| | Rater | | |
| | Pairs | PA | κ | P$_i$ |
|---|---|---|---|---|
| 1 Left | A/B | 75 | 0.50 | 0.05 |
| | A/C | 70 | 0.40 | 0.05 |
| | B/C | 70 | 0.40 | 0.05 |
| 1 Right | A/B | 65 | 0.33 | 0.00 |
| | A/C | 65 | 0.29 | 0.15 |
| | B/C | 70 | 0.41 | 0.05 |
| 2 Left | A/B | 78 | 0.38 | 0.53 |
| | A/C | 75 | 0.44 | 0.35 |
| | B/C | 73 | 0.38 | 0.38 |
| 2 Right | A/B | 70 | 0.19 | 0.55 |
| | A/C | 73 | 0.29 | 0.53 |
| | B/C | 88 | 0.72 | 0.33 |
| 3 Left | A/B | 73 | 0.18 | 0.58 |
| | A/C | 80 | 0.25 | 0.70 |
| | B/C | 83 | 0.29 | 0.73 |
| 3 Right | A/B | 73 | 0.30 | 0.48 |
| | A/C | 78 | 0.40 | 0.53 |
| | B/C | 85 | 0.48 | 0.65 |
| 4 Left | A/B | 63 | 0.31 | 0.13 |
| | A/C | 58 | 0.18 | 0.03 |
| | B/C | 65 | 0.25 | 0.30 |
| 4 Right | A/B | 80 | 0.60 | 0.00 |
| | A/C | 68 | 0.35 | 0.03 |
| | B/C | 63 | 0.25 | 0.08 |
| 5 Left | A/B | 53 | 0.22 | 0.13 |
| | A/C | 60 | 0.19 | 0.20 |
| | B/C | 58 | 0.18 | 0.28 |
| 5 Right | A/B | 58 | 0.15 | 0.28 |
| | A/C | 73 | 0.45 | 0.03 |
| | B/C | 55 | 0.12 | 0.25 |
| 6 Left | A/B | 58 | 0.28 | 0.08 |
| | A/C | 73 | 0.33 | 0.43 |
| | B/C | 50 | 0.20 | 0.00 |

*(continued)*

TABLE 5-9　Percentage Agreement (PA), κ Coefficient, and Prevalence Index ($P_i$) for Agreement on Presence or Absence of Myofascial Trigger Points[a] (cont.)

| | | Rater | | |
|---|---|---|---|---|
| | Pairs | PA | κ | $P_i$ |
| 6 Right | A/B | 60 | 0.27 | 0.15 |
| | A/C | 80 | 0.58 | 0.20 |
| | B/C | 60 | 0.27 | 0.15 |

[a]The numbers 1, 2, and 3 correspond with the localization in the infraspinatus muscle, 4 is localized in the anterior deltoid muscle, and 5 and 6 are localized in the biceps brachii muscle.

## Discussion

Palpation is the only method available for the clinical diagnosis of myofascial pain. Therefore, reliable MTrP palpation is the necessary prerequisite to considering myofascial pain as a valid diagnosis. This study indicated that referred pain was the most reliable criterion for palpatory diagnosis in all six MTrPs in all three muscles on both sides. Only in three of the 36 MTrP locations did the PA value not reach the predetermined value of 70%. This finding is consistent with the results of other interrater reliability studies of MTrP examination.[26,27] The nodule in the taut band, the LTR, and the jump sign were more reliable in the infraspinatus muscle than in the anterior deltoid and biceps brachii muscle. In general, the jump sign also proved a reliable palpatory characteristic in this study. This is in contrast to other studies, which may indicate that the raters in this study were more successful in standardizing the amount of pressure during the palpation. In general, the LTR was not a reliable characteristic although it did prove reliable for MTrP 1 and 2 in the infraspinatus on either side. Palpation of the nodule in the taut band had sufficient reliability for the diagnosis of MTrPs in the infraspinatus muscle, but less for diagnosis of MTrPs in the anterior deltoid and biceps brachii muscles. There was also a high level of agreement for the presence or absence of MTrPs in the infraspinatus muscle. This agreement was lower for the anterior deltoid and biceps brachii muscles.

　　Compared to various other commonly used physical examination tests, such as the assessment of intervertebral motion or muscle strength, whose established interrater reliability ranges from 41–97%,[40–43] the interrater agreement with regard to MTrP palpation in these three shoulder muscles seemed acceptable. However, the degree of agreement seemed to be strongly dependent on the muscle that was examined. Clinical experience suggests that some muscles are more accessible to palpation than others. There may even be differences within particular muscles. For trigger point 3 of the infraspinatus muscle, the raters achieved the highest agreement. Because MTrPs are often in close proximity to each other, raters did not always agree on which MTrP they were evaluating. For example, the raters may have had difficulty in distinguishing trigger points in the infraspinatus muscle, the teres minor muscle, and the posterior deltoid muscle. The area of referred pain may help in determining which muscle was palpated. However, recognition of pain elicited by palpation, as normally would occur in the clinical situation, was not determined in this study, because this could have endangered the blinding of the raters. Recognition of this characteristic pain by the patient may be an important aspect of reliable MTrP identification. For the biceps brachii muscle, the raters may have had difficulty distinguishing between the lateral and the medial head of the muscle. It is conceivable that such difficulties could contribute to the lower level of agreement noted for this muscle.

We realize that by collapsing rating categories in this study to *absent* or *present* and by not including a third category of indeterminate findings, we may have artificially inflated reliability findings. We decided to score dichotomously for the presence or absence of MTrPs and not include this indeterminate category, because the treatment choice would have been similar independent of a negative or indeterminate finding. When MTrPs are absent or when the physical therapist is unsure about the presence or absence of an MTrP, in the clinical situation no treatment will be directed to the MTrP.

We again note that in this study no distinction was made between active and latent MTrPs, because the examiners were not allowed to inquire whether subjects recognized the pain from palpation. Therefore, examiners may have reported on both active and latent MTrPs in symptomatic and asymptomatic subjects. This may affect external validity in this study in that its findings cannot be directly extrapolated to the clinical situation where patient report of recognition of pain is available and the distinction between active and latent trigger points therefore can be made.

In the interpretation of the study findings, we chose to emphasize PA over $\kappa$ values. PA values do not take into account the agreement that would be expected purely by chance. True agreement is the agreement beyond this expected agreement by chance, and $\kappa$ is a measure of true, chance-corrected agreement. However, as mentioned earlier, the $\kappa$ statistic is probably inappropriate for studies in which the positive and negative findings are not equally distributed.[39,44-46] In this study, even asymptomatic subjects had some (obviously latent) trigger points in the shoulder muscles. Subjects with unilateral shoulder pain often also may have latent or active trigger points in the contralateral shoulder.[47] Both may have contributed to the high prevalence of positive findings in this study. The resultant $P_i$ resulted in generally low $\kappa$ values despite high PA values, making the $\kappa$ statistic less appropriate for the statistical representation and subsequent interpretation of study findings.

Training would seem important to achieve sufficient agreement, even when raters have considerable clinical experience. McEvoy and Huijbregts also discussed this issue in more detail in the previous chapter. Prior to conducting this interrater reliability study, consensus about the standardization of manual palpation of MTrPs was achieved between raters. In this study, there was no statistically significant difference between the rater pairs, even though one rater had only 2 years of clinical experience with MTrP diagnosis and management. We recognize that this consensus training may impact external validity in that the results of this study may not apply to situations and clinicians where such training has not occurred. Future studies are needed to determine how many years of experience and what extent of prestudy consensus training is needed to achieve sufficient interrater reliability.

## Conclusion

In this study, three blinded raters were able to reach acceptable pairwise interrater agreement on the presence or absence of MTrPs, as described by Simons et al.[31] Referred pain was the most reliable feature in all six MTrPs in all three shoulder muscles on both sides. The nodule in the taut band, the LTR, and the jump sign were more reliable in the infraspinatus muscle than in the anterior deltoid and biceps muscle.

The results of this study support the idea that experienced raters can obtain acceptable agreement when diagnosing MTrPs by palpation in the three shoulder muscles studied. Allowing for patient report of pain recognition may provide for even better interrater reliability results. Interrater agreement seems dependent on the muscle, and even on the location of the trigger point within a muscle, and findings indicating acceptable interrater reliability cannot be generalized to all shoulder muscles. The distinction between active and latent trigger points should be considered in future studies, as should the effect of prestudy consensus training and clinical experience. However, in summary we conclude that this study provides preliminary evidence that MTrP palpation is a reliable and therefore potentially useful diagnostic tool in the diagnosis of myofascial pain in patients with nontraumatic shoulder pain.

## Acknowledgments

We would like to thank all subjects for participating in this study and our colleagues (B. Beersma, C. Ploos van Amstel, M. Onstenk, and B. de Valk) for their assistance as observers. The authors are grateful to Dr. Jan Dommerholt for his very helpful comments. We would also like to thank Dr. Peter Huijbregts for his extremely helpful contributions to this chapter.

## References

1. Bot SD, van der Waal JM, Terwee CB, van der Windt DA, Schellevis FG, Bouter LM, Dekker J. Incidence and prevalence of complaints of the neck and upper extremity in general practice. *Ann Rheum Dis* 2005;64:118–123.
2. Bongers PM: The cost of shoulder pain at work. *BMJ* 2001;322:64–65.
3. Luime JJ, Koes BW, Hendriksen IJ, Burdorf A, Verhagen AP, Miedema HS, Verhaar JA. Prevalence and incidence of shoulder pain in the general population: A systematic review. *Scand J Rheumatol* 2004;33:73–81.
4. Picavet HSJ, Gils HWV van, Schouten JSAG. *Klachten van het bewegingsapparaat in de Nederlandse bevolking: Prevalenties, consequenties en risicogroepen.* [Dutch: Musculoskeletal complaints in the Dutch population: Prevalence, consequences, and at risk groups] Bilthoven, The Netherlands: CBS; 2000.

5. De Winter AF. *Diagnosis and Classification of Shoulder Complaints*. Amsterdam, The Netherlands: VU University of Amsterdam; 1999.
6. Pope DP, Croft PR, Pritchard CM, Silman AJ. Prevalence of shoulder pain in the community: The influence of case definition. *Ann Rheum Dis* 1997;56:308–312.
7. Michener LA, McClure PW, Karduna AR. Anatomical and biomechanical mechanisms of subacromial impingement syndrome. *Clin Biomech* 2003;18:369–379.
8. Steinfeld R, Valente RM, Stuart MJ. A commonsense approach to shoulder problems. *Mayo Clin Proc* 1999;74:785–794.
9. Bang MD, Deyle GD. Comparison of supervised exercise with and without manual physical therapy for patients with shoulder impingement syndrome. *J Orthop Sports Phys Ther* 2000;30:126–137.
10. Travell JG, Simons DG. *Myofascial Pain and Dysfunction: The Trigger Point Manual*. Baltimore, MD: Williams & Wilkins, 1983.
11. Simons DG. Trigger points and limited motion. *J Orthop Sports Phys Ther* 2000;30:706–708.
12. Lucas KR, Polus BI, Rich PA. Latent myofascial trigger points: Their effects on muscle activation and movement efficiency. *J Bodywork Movement Ther* 2004;160–166.
13. Mense S, Russell IJ, Simons DG. *Muscle Pain: Understanding Its Nature, Diagnosis, and Treatment*. Philadelphia, PA: Lippincott Williams & Wilkins; 2001.
14. Ruch T. Visceral sensation and referred pain. In JF Fulton, ed. *Howell's Textbook of Physiology*. Philadelphia, PA: Saunders; 1949: 385–401.
15. Mense S. Neurologische grundlagen von muskelschmerz [German: Neurologic basis of muscle pain]. *Schmerz* 1999;13:3–17.
16. Hoheisel U, Koch K, Mense S. Functional reorganization in the rat dorsal horn during an experimental myositis. *Pain* 1994;59:111–118.
17. Kellgren JH. Observations on referred pain arising from muscle. *Clin Sci* 1938;3:175–190.
18. Graven-Nielsen T, Arendt-Nielsen L, Svensson P, Jensen TS. Quantification of local and referred muscle pain in humans after sequential i.m. injections of hypertonic saline. *Pain* 1997;69: 111–117.
19. Graven-Nielsen T, Mense S. The peripheral apparatus of muscle pain: Evidence from animal and human studies. *Clin J Pain* 2001;17:2–10.
20. Hwang M, Kang YK, Shin JY, Kim DH. Referred pain pattern of the abductor pollicis longus muscle. *Am J Phys Med Rehabil* 2005;84:593–597.
21. Hwang M, Kang YK, Kim DH. Referred pain pattern of the pronator quadratus muscle. *Pain* 1005;116:238–242.
22. Gerwin R, Shannon S. Interexaminer reliability and myofascial trigger points. *Arch Phys Med Rehabil* 2000;81:1257–1258.
23. Njoo KH, Van der Does E. The occurrence and inter-rater reliability of myofascial trigger points in the quadratus lumborum and gluteus medius: A prospective study in non-specific low back pain patients and controls in general practice. *Pain* 1994;58:317–323.
24. Nice DA, Riddle DL, Lamb RL, Mayhew TP, Rucker K. Intertester reliability of judgments of the presence of trigger points in patients with low back pain. *Arch Phys Med Rehabil* 1992;73:893–898.
25. Lew PC, Lewis J, Story I. Inter-therapist reliability in locating latent myofascial trigger points using palpation. *Man Ther* 1997;2:87–90.
26. Hsieh CY, Hong CZ, Adams AH, Platt KJ, Danielson CD, Hoehler FK, Tobis JS. Interexaminer reliability of the palpation of trigger points in the trunk and lower limb muscles. *Arch Phys Med Rehabil* 2000;81:258–264.
27. Gerwin RD, Shannon S, Hong CZ, Hubbard D, Gevirtz R: Interrater reliability in myofascial trigger point examination. *Pain* 1997;69:65–73.

28. Sciotti VM, Mittak VL, DiMarco L, Ford LM, Plezbert J, Santipadri E, Wigglesworth J, Ball K. Clinical precision of myofascial trigger point location in the trapezius muscle. *Pain* 2001;93: 259–266.

29. Wolfe F, Simons DG, Fricton J, Bennett RM, Goldenberg DL, Gerwin R, Hathaway D, McCain GA, Russell IJ, Sanders HO. The fibromyalgia and myofascial pain syndromes: A preliminary study of tender points and trigger points in persons with fibromyalgia, myofascial pain syndrome and no disease. *J Rheumatol* 1992;19:944–951.

30. Fischer AA. Pressure tolerance over muscles and bones in normal subjects. *Arch Phys Med Rehabil* 1986;67:406–409.

31. Simons DG, Travell JG, Simons LS, Travell JG. *Travell & Simons' Myofascial Pain and Dysfunction: The Trigger Point Manual*. Baltimore, MD: Williams & Wilkins; 1999.

32. Hong CZ. Considerations and recommendations regarding myofascial trigger point injection. *J Musculoskel Pain* 1994;2(1):29–59.

33. Hsieh Y-L, Kao MJ, Kuan TS, et al. Dry needling to a key myofascial trigger point may reduce the irritability of satellite MTrPs. *Am J Phys Med Rehabil* 2007;86(5):397–403.

34. Kronberg M. Muscle activity and coordination in the normal shoulder: An electromyographic study. *Clin Orthop* 1990;257:76–85.

35. Sugahara R. Electromyographic study on shoulder movements. *Rehab Med Jap* 1974;41–52.

36. Haas M. Statistical methodology for reliability studies. *J Manipulative Physiol Ther* 1991;14: 119–132.

37. Altman DG. *Practical Statistics for Medical Research*. Boca Raton, FL: Chapman & Hall; 1991.

38. Landis JR, Koch GG. The measurement of observer agreement for categorical data. *Biometrics* 1977;33:159–174.

38. Sim J, Wright CC. The kappa statistic in reliability studies: Use, interpretation, and sample size requirements. *Phys Ther* 2005;85:257–268.

39. Smedmark V, Wallin M, Arvidsson I. Inter-examiner reliability in assessing passive intervertebral motion of the cervical spine. *Man Ther* 2000;5:97–101.

40. Fjellner A, Bexander C, Faleij R, Strender LE. Interexaminer reliability in physical examination of the cervical spine. *J Manipulative Physiol Ther* 1999;22:511–516.

41. Pool JJ, Hoving JL, de Vet HC, van MH, Bouter LM. The interexaminer reproducibility of physical examination of the cervical spine. *J Manipulative Physiol Ther* 2004;27:84–90.

42. Pollard H, Lakay B, Tucker F, Watson B, Bablis P. Interexaminer reliability of the deltoid and psoas muscle test. *J Manipulative Physiol Ther* 2005;28:52–56.

43. Lantz CA, Nebenzahl E. Behavior and interpretation of the kappa statistic: Resolution of the two paradoxes. *J Clin Epidemiol* 1996;49:431–434.

44. Feinstein AR, Cicchetti DV. High agreement but low kappa. I. The problems of two paradoxes. *J Clin Epidemiol* 1990;43:543–549.

45. Cicchetti DV, Feinstein AR. High agreement but low kappa. II. Resolving the paradoxes. *J Clin Epidemiol* 1990;43:551–558.

46. Marcus DA, Scharff L, Mercer S, Turk DC. Musculoskeletal abnormalities in chronic headache: A controlled comparison of headache diagnostic groups. *Headache* 1999;39:21–27.

47. Audette JF, Wang F, Smith H. Bilateral activation of motor unit potentials with unilateral needle stimulation of active myofascial trigger points. *Am J Phys Med Rehabil* 2004;83:368–374.

# Chapter 6

# Contributions of Myofascial Trigger Points to Chronic Tension-Type Headache

*César Fernández-de-las-Peñas, PT, DO, PhD*

*Lars Arendt-Nielsen, DMSc, PhD*

*David G. Simons, BSc, MD, DSc (Hon), DSc (Hon)*

## Introduction

Headache is one of the most common problems seen in medical practice. Among the many types of headache disorders, tension-type headache (TTH), cervicogenic headache, and migraine are the most prevalent in adults. Population-based studies suggest 1-year prevalence rates of 38.3% for episodic TTH and 2.2% for chronic TTH.[1] Nillson reported the prevalence of cervicogenic headache in a Scandinavian population to be approximately 16%.[2] Other population-based studies estimated that 10–12% of adults have experienced migraine in the previous year.[3]

The International Headache Society has recently actualized the diagnostic criteria for TTH (**Table 6-1**) and migraine without aura (**Table 6-2**).[4] In addition, diagnostic criteria for cervicogenic headache (**Table 6-3**) have been also detailed in the literature.[5] Although some patients present with two types of headaches simultaneously (TTH with migraine features, cervicogenic headache with TTH characteristics, etc.), it seems that the pain quality and features of these headache disorders are distinctly different.

Differences in pain features and quality of headache disorders may implicate different structures as being responsible for nociceptive irritation of the trigeminal nucleus caudalis.[6] Because cervicogenic headache is characterized by unilateral nonlancinating pain, which is increased by head movement, maintained neck postures, or external pressure over the upper cervical joints,[5] joint dysfunctions in the upper cervical spine (C0–C2) should be implicated in the etiology of cervicogenic headache.[7] Likewise, the characteristic

Courtesy of John M. Medeiros, PT, PhD, Managing Editor of the *Journal of Manual and Manipulative Therapy*.

symptoms of TTH, including bilateral pressing or tightening pain, pressure or bandlike tightness, and/or increased tenderness on palpation of neck and shoulder muscles,[4] resemble the descriptions of referred pain originating in myofascial trigger points (MTrPs).[8] Finally, the pain quality of migraine is attributed to the activation of the trigeminovascular system,[9,10] provoked by the release of algogenic substances.[11,12]

In addition to different pain features, the effectiveness of spinal manipulation or mobilization directed at the upper cervical spine in cervicogenic headache,[13,14] but not in

---

**TABLE 6-1 International Headache Classification of Tension-Type Headache[4]**

The following criteria are a synthesis of the more common pain features and characteristics of the different TTH diagnoses.

Pain features and characteristics of headache attacks in TTH:

A. Headaches lasting from 30 minutes to 7 days

B. Headaches with at least two of the following pain characteristics:

    1. Bilateral location

    2. Pressing/tightening (nonpulsating) quality

    3. Mild or moderate intensity

    4. Not aggravated by routine physical activity such as walking or climbing stairs

C. Both of the following:

    1. No nausea or vomiting (anorexia may occur)

    2. No more than one of photophobia or phonophobia

D. Not attributed to other disorder[a]

In addition, TTH can be diagnosed as associated or not associated to pericranial tenderness (based on the data obtained with the total tenderness score).[b]

Finally, depending on the frequency of the headaches, patients can be diagnosed as:

a. **Infrequent episodic TTH**: At least 10 episodes occurring on <1 day per month on average (<12 days per year)

b. **Frequent episodic TTH**: At least 10 episodes occurring >1 but <15 days per month for at least 3 months (>12 but <180 days per year)

c. **Chronic TTH**: Headache occurring on >15 days per month, on average, for >3 months (>180 days per year)

[a]History and physical and neurologic examination do not suggest any of the disorders listed in groups 5–12, or history and/or physical and/or neurologic examination do suggest such disorders but it is ruled out by appropriate investigations, or such disorder is present but headache does not occur for the first time in close temporal relation to the disorder.
[b]Langemark M, Olesen J. Pericranial tenderness in tension headache. A blind controlled study. *Cephalalgia* 1987;7:249–255.

**TABLE 6-2  International Headache Classification of Migraine without Aura[4]**

Diagnostic criteria:

A.  At least five attacks fulfilling criteria B–D

B.  Headache attacks lasting 4–72 hours (untreated or unsuccessfully treated)

C.  Headaches with at least two of the following pain characteristics:

    1.  Unilateral location

    2.  Pulsating quality

    3.  Moderate or severe intensity

    4.  Aggravation by or causing avoidance of routine physical activity such as walking or climbing stairs

D.  During headache at least one of the following:

    1.  Nausea and/or vomiting

    2.  Photophobia and phonophobia

E.  Not attributed to other disorder[a]

[a]History and physical and neurologic examination do not suggest any of the disorders listed in groups 5–12, or history and/or physical and/or neurologic examination do suggest such disorders but it is ruled out by appropriate investigations, or such disorder is present but headache does not occur for the first time in close temporal relation to the disorder.

---

**TABLE 6-3  Major Diagnostic Criteria for Cervicogenic Headache[5]**

A.  Symptoms and signs of neck involvement:

    1.  Precipitation of comparable head pain by

        • Neck movement or sustained awkward head postures, and/or

        • External pressure over the upper cervical or occipital region on the symptomatic side

    2.  Restriction of range of motion in the neck

    3.  Ipsilateral neck, shoulder, or arm pain

B.  Confirmatory evidence by diagnostic blocks

C.  Unilaterality of head pain, without side shift

D.  Head pain characteristics:

    1.  Moderate-severe, nonthrobbing and nonlancinating pain

    2.  Episodes of varying duration

    3.  Fluctuating continuous pain

There are other characteristics, but of less importance.

TTH,[15,16] supports the hypothesis that upper cervical joint dysfunctions can be more relevant for the pathogenesis of cervicogenic headache than for TTH or migraine. The pain features (quality and distribution) of TTH suggest that MTrPs can be involved in its etiology. The present chapter discusses the scientific evidence supporting that hypothesis.

## Definition of Myofascial Trigger Points

Simons et al defined a myofacial trigger point (MTrP) as "a hyperirritable spot associated within a taut band of a skeletal muscle"; this spot is painful on compression and usually responds with a referred pain pattern distant from that spot (i.e., the MTrP).[17] From a clinical viewpoint, active MTrPs cause clinical symptoms, and their local and referred pain is responsible for patients' complaints. An active MTrP is distinguished from a latent one when referred pain elicited by pressure applied to the MTrP is recognized as a recent, familiar pain by the subject. In patients, this elicited pain corresponds to at least part of their clinical pain complaint. Both active and latent MTrPs can provoke motor dysfunctions (e.g., muscle weakness, muscle imbalance, altered recruitment pattern of the stabilizer muscles, or muscle inhibition[18]) in either the affected muscle or in functionally related muscles.[17] Furthermore, latent MTrPs may not be an immediate source of pain, but they can elicit referred pain with mechanical stimulation or muscle contraction. In addition, latent MTrPs may disturb normal patterns of motor recruitment and movement efficiency.[19]

The formation of MTrPs may result from a variety of factors, such as severe trauma, overuse, mechanical overload, or psychological stress.[8] Although the etiology of MTrPs is not completely known, recent studies have hypothesized that the pathogenesis of MTrPs results from injured or overloaded muscle fibers.[20] This could lead to endogenous (involuntary) shortening, loss of oxygen supply, loss of nutrient supply, and increased metabolic demand on local tissues.[21] The most credible etiological explanation of MTrPs is the integrated hypothesis, which suggests that abnormal depolarization of motor endplates and sustained muscular shortening give rise to a localized "ATP energy crisis" associated with sensory and autonomic reflex arcs that are sustained by central sensitization.[22] A recent study provides evidence of sympathetic facilitation of mechanical sensitization and facilitation of the local and referred pain reactions in MTrPs.[23]

## Referred Pain to the Head from Trigger Points in Neck, Head, and Shoulder Muscles

Animal[24] and human[25,26] studies clearly show the convergence of cervical and trigeminal afferents in the trigeminal nerve nucleus caudalis, constituting the anatomic basis for referred head pain from neck and shoulder MTrPs. Because nociceptive somatic afferents from muscles of different upper cervical roots, particularly C1–C3, and the trigeminal nerve converge on the same relay neurons, it is assumed that the message to supraspinal structures can be misinterpreted and localized as pain in other structures distant from the site of painful stimulus (referred pain). Dorsal horn neurons that receive afferents from muscles frequently receive input from other deep structures and from the skin.[27,28] This extensive convergent input to dorsal horn neurons may account for the often diffuse and poorly localized nature of deep pain sensation in humans, particularly when pain is intense. In addition, animal studies[29] have demonstrated spinal-level spread of the pain message from one dorsal horn cell to another that is initiated by strong input from muscle nociceptors[30] and that can be interpreted as a likely contributing cause of the referred pain originating at MTrPs.[31]

Simons et al[17] described the referred pain patterns from different MTrPs in several head and neck muscles that have the potential to refer pain to the head. In addition, other authors have illustrated and described similar, but not equal, referred pain patterns.[32,33] Further, our research group has also compiled similar referred pain patterns from several headache patients. In the present chapter, we will show the referred pain patterns as described by Simons et al and our own patterns:

a. Referred pain elicited by upper trapezius muscle MTrPs spreads ipsilaterally from the posterior-lateral region of the neck, behind the ear, and to the temporal region (**Figure 6-1**).

b. MTrPs located in the sternocleidomastoid muscle refer pain to the occiput, the frontotemporal area, the retroauricular area, the forehead, and the cheek (**Figure 6-2**).

c. Temporalis muscle MTrP referred pain is located into the temporoparietal region and perceived inside the head (**Figure 6-3**).

d. Referred pain from suboccipital muscle MTrPs spreads to the side of the head over the occipital, temporal, and frontal bones and is usually perceived as bilateral headache (**Figure 6-4**).

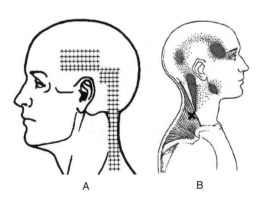

A           B

**Figure 6-1**  Referred pain from the upper trapezius muscle.

*Source:* Figure 6.1B illustration courtesy of Lifeart/Mediclip, Manual Medicine 1, Version 1.0a, Williams & Wilkins, 1997.

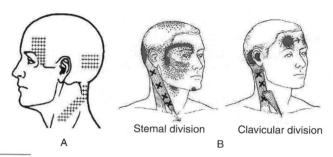

**Figure 6-2**   Referred pain from the sternocleidomastoid muscle.

*Source:* Figure 6.2 B illustration courtesy of Lifeart/Mediclip, Manual Medicine 1, Version 1.0a, Williams & Wilkins, 1997.

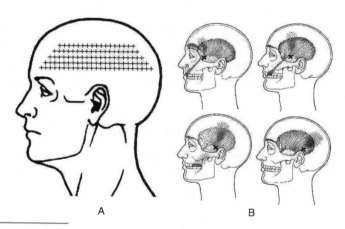

**Figure 6-3**   Referred pain from the temporalis muscle.

*Source:* Figure 6.3 B illustration courtesy of Lifeart/Mediclip, Manual Medicine 1, Version 1.0a, Williams & Wilkins, 1997.

e.   Splenius capitis muscle MTrPs refer pain to the vertex of the head, whereas splenius cervicis muscle MTrPs refer pain to the side of the head and behind the eyes (**Figure 6-5**).

f.   MTrPs located into the semispinalis cervicis muscle refer pain to the occiput bone, and those located into the semispinalis capitis muscle refer pain to the temporal region and behind the eyes (**Figure 6-6**).

Although referred pain patterns have highly clinical value for our patients, clinicians should take into account that these patterns can be slightly different between subjects.

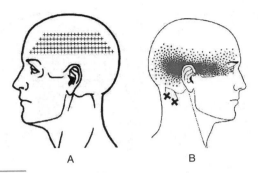

**Figure 6-4** Referred pain from the suboccipital muscles.

*Source:* Figure 6.4 B illustration courtesy of Lifeart/Mediclip, Manual Medicine 1, Version 1.0a, Williams & Wilkins, 1997.

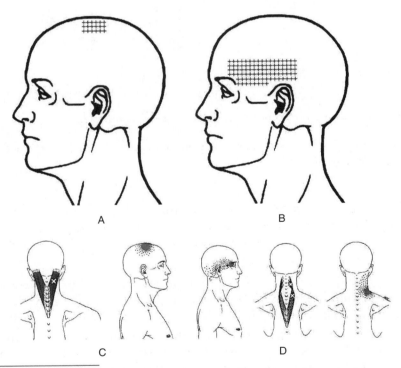

**Figure 6-5** Referred pain from the splenius capitis and cervicis muscle.

*Source:* Figure 6.5 C & D illustrations courtesy of Lifeart/Mediclip, Manual Medicine 1, Version 1.0a, Williams & Wilkins, 1997.

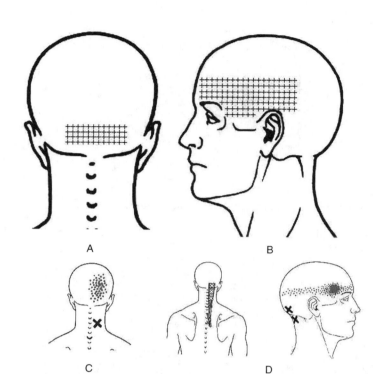

A          B

C          D

**Figure 6-6**  Referred pain from the semispinalis cervicis muscle.

*Source:* Figure 6.6 C & D illustrations courtesy of Lifeart/Mediclip, Manual Medicine 1, Version 1.0a, Williams & Wilkins, 1997.

In addition, we should recognize that these patterns have been described based on a small number of patients, so further studies with greater sample sizes are required.

Several pain models have described upper trapezius and temporalis muscle referred pain patterns:

a.  Referred pain elicited by the infusion of hypertonic saline into the upper trapezius muscle spreads ipsilaterally to the posterior-lateral region of the neck and to the temporal region in both healthy subjects[34] and headache patients.[35]

b.  The infusion of hypertonic saline into the temporalis muscles elicits referred pain to both the trigeminal territory (anterior part of the muscle) and to the cervical innervated dermatome (posterior part of the muscle).[36]

In addition, the referred pain patterns elicited by manual exploration of MTrPs in the upper trapezius[37] and the temporalis muscles[38] have been clinically confirmed in chronic

TTH patients, demonstrating that referred pain from these muscles is contributing to pain perception in chronic tension-type headache (CTTH).

## Clinical Evidence of Trigger Points in Chronic Tension-Type Headache

Recent studies demonstrate clinical evidence of the presence of MTrPs in certain neck and shoulder muscles in CTTH and unilateral migraine. Marcus et al[39] found in a nonblinded study that TTH subjects had a greater number of either active or latent MTrPs than healthy subjects. However, these authors did not specify in which muscles the MTrPs were observed more frequently.

We recently demonstrated, in blinded controlled studies, that CTTH was associated with active MTrPs in the suboccipital muscles[40] and in the upper trapezius, sternocleido-mastoid, and temporalis muscles.[41] Suboccipital muscle MTrPs were found in all 20 of our CTTH patients (100%), of which 13 (65%) elicited a referred pain that reproduced the same head pain as during headache attacks (i.e., active MTrPs).[40] In a second study with a sample of 25 patients with CTTH, MTrPs in the temporalis muscles were found in 20 of 25 (80%) on the right and 15 of 25 (60%) on the left side. MTrPs in the upper trapezius muscle were found in 19 of 25 (76%) on the right and 14 of 25 (56%) on the left side, whereas MTrPs into the sternocleidomastoid muscle were found in 16 of 25 (64%) on the right side and 12 of 25 (48%) on the left.[41] From all of these MTrPs, more than half elicited a referred pain pattern recognized by the patients as their usual headache, consistent with active MTrPs. In our studies, control subjects showed latent, but not active, MTrPs, as has been previously described.[42] We also demonstrated that those CTTH patients with active MTrPs had greater headache intensity and frequency than those with latent MTrPs[40,41] (**Table 6-4**).

We have demonstrated that unilateral migraine subjects showed a significantly greater number of active MTrPs ($P < 0.001$), but not latent MTrPs, than healthy controls.[43] In a sample of 20 patients with strictly unilateral migraine, MTrPs in the upper trapezius (10 latent and 6 active) and in the sternocleidomastoid (6 latent and 10 active) muscles were the most prevalent on the symptomatic side of the headache attacks. Active MTrPs were mostly located ipsilateral to migraine headaches, as compared to the nonsympto-matic side ($P < 0.01$).[43] Recently, Calandre et al[44] found that 73 out of 98 (73%) patients with migraine without aura showed MTrPs in the anterior temporal and suboccipital regions, as compared to 9 out of 32 (29%) healthy subjects ($P < 0.001$).

Referred pain from two extraocular muscle MTrPs (i.e., the superior oblique[45] and lateral rectus[46] muscles) has recently been described in CTTH. The superior oblique muscle referred pain is perceived as an internal and deep pain located at the retro-orbital region. This referred pain can extend to the supraorbital region and sometimes to the ipsilateral forehead (**Figure 6-7**). The lateral rectus muscle referred pain is also perceived as a deep ache located at the supraorbital region or the ipsilateral forehead (Figure 6-7).

TABLE 6-4 Headache Intensity, Frequency, and Duration Depending on the Type of Myofascial Trigger Point in Each Muscle within Our Chronic Tension-Type Headache Patients[a] (adapted from 40, 41)

| | | Headache Intensity (VAS)[b] | Headache Frequency (days/week) | Headache Duration (hours/day) |
|---|---|---|---|---|
| Right upper trapezius (n = 25) | Active MTrPs (n = 9) | 5.6 (1.7)[c] | 5.1 (1.1) | 8.9 (4.2)[c] |
| | Latent MTrPs (n = 10) | 4.5 (1.6) | 4.6 (1.2) | 6.7 (5.4) |
| Left upper trapezius (n = 25) | Active MTrPs (n = 6) | 5.6 (1.6) | 5.5 (1.9) | 9.2 (4.6) |
| | Latent MTrPs (n = 8) | 5.4 (1.2) | 4.8 (1.8) | 9.8 (5.1) |
| Right sternocleidomastoid (n = 25) | Active MTrPs (n = 6) | 6.1 (1.9) | 5.2 (1.8) | 9.6 (5.1) |
| | Latent MTrPs (n = 6) | 5.5 (2) | 5.3 (2.3) | 9.4 (5.7) |
| Left sternocleidomastoid (n = 25) | Active MTrPs (n = 5) | 6.4 (2.5)[c] | 5.6 (1.8) | 10.8 (5.1)[c] |
| | Latent MTrPs (n = 11) | 4.5 (1.2) | 4.9 (2.4) | 7.5 (4.8) |
| Right temporalis (n = 25) | Active MTrPs (n = 9) | 5.5 (1.8) | 5.2 (2.1) | 11.6 (1.9)[c] |
| | Latent MTrPs (n = 11) | 5.2 (1.9) | 5.4 (1.8) | 7.2 (2.9) |
| Left temporalis (n = 25) | Active MTrPs (n = 8) | 5.7 (1.4)[c] | 5.1 (1.7) | 9.4 (4.7) |
| | Latent MTrPs (n = 7) | 4.3 (1.6) | 4.4 (2.3) | 8.4 (5.5) |
| Suboccipital muscles[a] (n = 20) | Active MTrPs (n = 13) | 6 (3.15–9) | 6 (4–7) | 8.7 (3–12) |
| | Latent MTrPs (n = 7) | 4.6 (2.2–7) | 4.9 (4–6) | 9.8 (4–13) |

[a]Values are expressed as means (standard deviations) for all muscles, except for the suboccipital muscles, which is mean (min-max).
[b]VAS = Visual Analogue Scale (0–10)
[c]Significant in comparison with the latent MTrPs subgroup (unpaired students' t-test, $P < 0.05$).

Further, referred pain from MTrPs in the superior oblique muscle has also been found in unilateral migraine patients.[47] In addition, MTrPs in the superior oblique muscle are located bilaterally in TTH[44] but unilaterally on the symptomatic side in migraine patients.[47] Further, in a sample of 15 patients with episodic TTH, nine (60%) reported referred pain with manual exploration of the superior oblique muscle.[45] Because visual stress can be involved in MTrP perpetuation, particularly MTrPs in the upper trapezius muscle,[48] manual exploration of MTrPs in the extraocular muscles should be performed in patients with chronic headaches.

Referred pain from MTrPs located in other muscles (e.g., masseter, lateral pterygoid, scalenes, and levator scapulae) can also contribute to the pain distribution seen in chronic TTH (**Figure 6-8**).

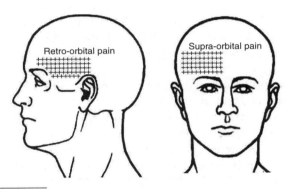

**Figure 6-7**    Referred pain from the superior oblique and lateral rectus muscles.

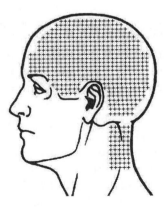

**Figure 6-8**    Composite pain pattern of tension type headache.

## Are Trigger Points Consequences of Central Sensitization?

Although scientific evidence suggests a close relationship between MTrPs in certain head and neck muscles, CTTH,[37,40,41,45] and migraine headache,[43,47] the data reported to date do not establish a cause-and-effect relationship between MTrPs and these chronic headaches.

Bendtsen[49] postulated that hyperalgesia in CTTH subjects may be due to an increased sensitivity (hyperexcitability) in the central nervous system provoked by nociceptive stimuli from peripheral structures. Central sensitization may be also involved in the generation of muscle referred pain from MTrPs.[50] Different studies have found that the area of the referred pain correlated with the intensity of the muscle pain in patients with fibromyalgia and whiplash-associated disorders.[51,52] Secondary hyperalgesia surrounding a painful area is related to central sensitization, which may account for muscle-referred pain. In that way, muscle-referred pain may also correlate with the phenomena of secondary hyperalgesia and tenderness seen in CTTH patients.[50] In addition, peripheral and central sensitization and decreased descending inhibition induced by long-term nociceptive stimuli from trigger points may also be involved in referred pain to the trigeminal region from active MTrPs.[53]

Active MTrPs have also been found in other chronic conditions, including mechanical neck pain,[54] osteoarthritis,[55] and lateral epicondylalgia.[56] Because active MTrPs are related to several chronic conditions accounting for sensitization of central pathways, clinicians should be aware that untreated MTrPs can cause chronic pain and that they should be treated as soon and as effectively as possible to avoid such occurrence.

If the central sensitization were causing the MTrPs, active MTrPs would not be expected in patients suffering from the episodic form of TTH, in which central sensitization has not been demonstrated.[49] Because there is a lesser degree of central sensitization in episodic TTH,[49] one would expect fewer active and more latent MTrPs in episodic TTH patients than in chronic TTH patients. Clinical studies have demonstrated that active MTrPs in the suboccipital, temporalis, upper trapezius, and sternocleidomastoid muscles are present to similar degrees in both episodic TTH[57,58] and chronic TTH patients[40,41] (**Table 6-5**). This seems to indicate that active MTrPs are not the consequence of central sensitization, because they are also present in the episodic form of TTH. However, without actual research-based knowledge, we cannot confirm, but only hypothesize, that active MTrPs can be a causative factor for sensitization of central pathways.

One clinical phenomenon that is observed by many clinicians and that has been reported in one research paper[59] is the fact that the degree of chronicity is strongly correlated with the number of treatments required to inactivate MTrPs. With increased duration of symptoms, there is increased central sensitization (hyperexcitability of the central nervous system, which is characterized by increased tenderness, hyperalgesia, or allodynia, and decreased pressure pain sensitivity levels), and one of the few available clinical treatments to normalize this sensitization is to do repeated treatment as often as necessary to

**TABLE 6-5** Percentage of Subjects with Myofascial Trigger Points (Active or Latent) in Chronic and Episodic Tension-Type Headache (adapted from 40, 41, 57, 58)

| | Suboccipital Muscles | Upper Trapezius Muscle | | Sternocleidomastoid Muscle | | Temporalis Muscle | |
|---|---|---|---|---|---|---|---|
| | | Left Side | Right Side | Left Side | Right Side | Left Side | Right Side |
| **Subjects with Chronic Tension-Type Headache** | | | | | | | |
| Active MTrPs | 65% | 24% | 36% | 20% | 24% | 32% | 36% |
| Latent MTrPs | 35% | 32% | 40% | 44% | 24% | 28% | 44% |
| **Subjects with Episodic Tension-Type Headache** | | | | | | | |
| Active MTrPs | 60% | 33% | 14% | 20% | 14% | 40% | 46% |
| Latent MTrPs | 40% | 40% | 40% | 14% | 46% | 33% | 27% |

MTrP = Myofascial trigger point/n (number of subjects).
Suboccipital muscle MTrPs in CTTH are based on a sample of n = 20; whereas in ETTH on a sample of n = 10.
Upper trapezius, sternocleidomastoid, and temporalis muscle MTrPs in CTTH are based on a sample of n = 25; whereas in ETTH on a sample of n = 15.

maintain the patient nearly pain-free. One should eliminate the MTrP source of chronic pain that is contributing to the sensitization. In the authors' clinical practice, with recent onset of pain one or two treatments generally suffice. With greater chronicity, the period of pain relief following a treatment is not shortened as much as it would be in acute cases, and consequently it takes more treatments to normalize this state of central sensitization and eliminate the return of spontaneous central pain.

## How Might Trigger Points Contribute to Chronic Tension-Type Headache?

The current pain model for CTTH states that the main problem is central sensitization due to prolonged nociceptive inputs from pericranial tissues, and that this mechanism is of major importance for the conversion of episodic into chronic TTH.[49,60] Olesen[61] proposed that headache might be due to an excess of nociceptive inputs from peripheral structures. According to his model, perceived headache intensity would be the sum of nociceptive inputs from cranial and extracranial tissues converging on the neurons of the trigeminal nucleus caudalis. Convergence of the nociceptive afferents from the receptive fields of cervical roots C1–C3, which include the upper trapezius, sternocleidomastoid, and suboccipital muscles, and those of the trigeminal nerve, which include the temporalis and the superior oblique muscles, occurs in the nucleus caudalis.[62] This fits nicely with the concept that nociceptive input from MTrPs in these muscles makes a major contribution to CTTH.

Higher levels of algogenic substances (i.e., bradykinin, calcitonin gene-related peptide, substance P, tumor necrosis factor-$\alpha$, interleukin-1$\beta$, serotonin, and norepinephrine) have been found in active but not in latent MTrPs,[63] and not in tender points.[64] This nociceptive input originated from MTrPs in head and neck muscles could produce afferent activity. That would result in temporal and spatial summation of neuron signals, and it might be one of the reasons for the central sensitization seen in CTTH.[49] In these patients, the persistent nociceptive input from TrPs may lead to sensitization of nociceptive second-order neurons at the level of the spinal dorsal/trigeminal nucleus.

Based on new available data,[40,41,43,45,57,58] it seems that TTH can be partly caused by referred pain from MTrPs in the posterior cervical, head (including extraocular), and shoulder muscles, mediated through the spinal cord and the brainstem trigeminal nucleus caudalis, rather than only tenderness of the pericranial muscles themselves. However, blinded controlled studies of treatment results are required to determine if MTrPs are the cause of the headache.

An MTrP role in headache does not negate the importance of other physical (e.g., malalignment of upper cervical vertebrae[65] or forward head posture[66]) or psychological (e.g., anxiety or depression) factors in exacerbating and sustaining CTTH. These same factors are known to aggravate and promote MTrP activity. Many elements traditionally deemed important in the genesis of CTTH may result from imperfect strategies devised to cope with MTrP-induced head pain.

Finally, because an association between MTrPs and TTH has been confirmed, a therapeutic approach based on MTrP management in TTH and migraine headaches should be explored in future studies. Although some evidence indicates that inactivation of MTrPs can relieve head pain from patients with migraine,[67] there is a need for high-quality randomized controlled trials that assess the effectiveness of different manual therapy approaches and new developments such as frequency-specific microcurrent,[68] shockwave therapy,[69] or high-power ultrasound[70] that are directed at treating MTrPs[71] in TTH and migraine headaches.

## Conclusion

Scientific evidence suggests that referred pain elicited by myofascial trigger points (MTrPs) from the upper trapezius, sternocleidomastoid, suboccipital, and extraocular muscles contributes to pain perception in chronic tension-type headache. The release of algogenic substances from MTrPs may cause nociceptive input to the trigeminal nerve nucleus caudalis, and it may cause sensitization, as seen in CTTH. More research is needed to further define the role of MTrPs in the etiology and/or maintenance of chronic headaches.

## Acknowledgments

We would like to thank Dr. Robert D. Gerwin, Johns Hopkins University, and Dr. Hong-You Ge, Aalborg University, for their kind encouragement and support.

## References

1. Schwartz BS, Stewart WF, Simon D, Lipton RB. Epidemiology of tension-type headache. *JAMA* 1998;279:381–383.
2. Nillson N. The prevalence of cervicogenic headache in a random population sample of 20- to 59-year-olds. *Spine* 1995;20:1884–1888.
3. Stewart WF, Lipton RB, Celentano DD, Reed ML. Prevalence of migraine headache in the United States: Relation to age, income, race and other sociodemographic factors. *JAMA* 1992;267:64–69.
4. IHS: Headache Classification Subcommittee of the International Headache Society. The International Classification of Headache Disorders, 2nd ed. *Cephalalgia* 2004;24(suppl 1):9–160.
5. Sjaastad O, Fredriksen T A, Pfaffenrath V. Cervicogenic headache: Diagnostic criteria. *Headache* 1998;38:442–445.
6. Nillson N. Evidence that tension-type headache and cervicogenic headache are distinct disorders. *J Manipulative Physiol Ther* 2000;23:288–289.
7. Jull GA, Niere R. The cervical spine and headache. In: Ferguson L, Gerwin R, eds. *Grieve's Modern Manual Therapy of the Vertebral Column*. Edinburgh: Churchill Livingstone; 2004:291–311.
8. Gerwin R. Headache. In: *Clinical Mastery in the Treatment of Myofascial Pain*. Philadelphia, PA: Lippincott Williams & Wilkins; 2005:1–24.
9. Goadsby PJ, Lipton RB, Ferrari MD. Migraine: Current understanding and treatment. *N Engl J Med* 2002;346:257–270.

10. Edvinsson L. Aspects on the patho-physiology of migraine and cluster headache. *Pharmacol Toxicol* 2001;89:65–73.
11. Fusco M, D'Andrea G, Miccichè F, Stecca A, Bernardini D, Leon Cananzi A. Neurogenic inflammation in primary headaches. *Neurol Sci* 2003;24(suppl):S61–S64.
12. Durham L. Calcitonin gene-related peptide (CGRP) and migraine. *Headache* 2006;46(suppl 1): S3–S8.
13. Fernández-de-las-Peñas C, Alonso-Blanco C, Cuadrado ML, Pareja JA. Spinal manipulative therapy in the management of cervicogenic headache. *Headache* 2005;45:1260–1263.
14. Bronfort G, Assendelft JJ, Evans R, Haas M, Bouter L. Efficacy of spinal manipulation for chronic headache: A systematic review. *J Manipulative Physiol Ther* 2001;24:457–466.
15. Fernández-de-las-Peñas C, Alonso-Blanco C, Cuadrado ML, Miangolarra JC, Barriga FJ, Pareja JA. Are manual therapies effective in reducing pain from tension-type headache? A systematic review. *Clin J Pain* 2006;22:278–285.
16. Astin JA, Ernst E. The effectiveness of spinal manipulation for the treatment of headache disorders: A systematic review of randomized clinical trials. *Cephalalgia* 2002;22:617–623.
17. Simons DG, Travell J, Simons LS. *Travell & Simons' Myofascial Pain and Dysfunction: The Trigger Point Manual.* Vol. 1. 2nd ed. Baltimore: Williams & Wilkins; 1999.
18. Headley B. The use of biofeedback in pain management. *Orthop Phys Ther Pract* 1993;2:29–40.
19. Lucas KR, Polus BI, Rich PA. Latent myofascial trigger points: Their effects on muscle activation and movement efficiency. *J Bodywork Movement Ther* 2004;8:160–166.
20. Gerwin RD, Dommerholt D, Shah JP. An expansion of Simons' integrated hypothesis of trigger point formation. *Curr Pain Headache Rep* 2004;8:468–475.
21. Simons DG. Review of enigmatic MTrPs as a common cause of enigmatic musculoskeletal pain and dysfunction. *J Electromyogr Kinesiol* 2004;14:95107.
22. McPartland JM, Simons DG. Myofascial trigger points: Translating molecular theory into manual therapy. *J Manual Manipulative Ther* 2006;14:232–239.
23. Ge HY, Fernández-de-las-Peñas C, Arendt-Nielsen L. Sympathetic facilitation of hyperalgesia evoked from myofascial tender and trigger points in patients with unilateral shoulder pain. *Clin Neurophysiol* 2006;117:1545–1550.
24. Bartsch T, Goadsby PJ. Stimulation of the greater occipital nerve induces increased central excitability of dural afferent input. *Brain* 2002;125:1496–1509.
25. Piovesan EJ, Kowacs PA, Oshinsky ML. Convergence of cervical and trigeminal sensory afferents. *Curr Pain Headache Rep* 2003;7:377–383.
26. Ge HY, Wang K, Madeleine P, Svensson P, Sessle BJ, Arendt-Nielsen L. Simultaneous modulation of the exteroceptive suppression periods in the trapezius and temporalis muscles by experimental muscle pain. *Clin Neurophysiol* 2004;115:1399–1408.
27. Schaible HG, Schmidt RF, Willis WD. Convergent inputs from articular, cutaneous and muscle receptors onto ascending tract cells in the cat spinal cord. *Exp Brain Res* 1987;66:479–488.
28. Hoheisel U, Mense S. Response behaviour of cat dorsal horn neurons receiving input from skeletal muscle and other deep somatic tissues. *J Physiol* 1990;426:265–280.
29. Hoheisel U, Mense S, Simons DG, Yu XM. Appearance of new receptive fields in rat dorsal horn neurons following noxious stimulation of skeletal muscle: A model for referred muscle pain? *Neurosci Lett* 1993;153:9–12.
30. Mense S. Referral of muscle pain: New aspects. *Am Pain Soc J* 1994;3:1–9.
31. Simons DG. Neuro-physiological basis of pain caused by trigger points. *Am Pain Soc J* 1994;3:17–19.
32. Wright E F: Referred craniofacial pain patterns in patients with temporomandibular disorder. *JADA* 2000;131:1307–1315.

33. Dejung B, Gröbli C, Colla F, Weissman R. *Triggerpunkt-Therapie* (Trigger Point Therapy). Bern, Switzerland: Verlag Hans Huber; 2003.

34. Ge HY, Arendt-Nielsen L, Farina D, Madeleine P. Gender-specific differences in electromyographic changes and perceived pain induced by experimental muscle pain during sustained contractions of the upper trapezius muscle. *Muscle Nerve* 2005;32:726–733.

35. Mørk H, Ashina M, Bendtsen J, Olesen J, Jensen R. Induction of prolonged tenderness in patients with tension-type headache by means of a new experimental model of myofascial pain. *Eur J Neurol* 2003;10:249–256.

36. Schmidt-Hansen PT, Svensson P, Jensen TS, Graven-Nielsen T, Bach FW. Patterns of experimentally induced pain in peri-cranial muscles *Cephalalgia* 2006;26:568–577.

37. Fernández-de-las-Peñas C, Ge HY, Arendt-Nielsen L, Cuadrado ML, Pareja JA. Referred pain from trapezius muscle trigger point shares similar characteristics with chronic tension-type headache. *Eur J Pain* 2007;11:475–482.

38. Fernández-de-las-Peñas C, Ge HY, Cuadrado ML, Madeleine P, Pareja JA, Arendt-Nielsen L. Bilateral pressure pain sensitivity mapping of the temporalis muscle in chronic tension-type headache. *Headache* 2008;48:1067–1075.

39. Marcus DA, Scharff L, Mercer S, Turk DC. Musculoskeletal abnormalities in chronic headache: A controlled comparison of headache diagnostic groups. *Headache* 1999;39:21–27.

40. Fernández-de-las-Peñas C, Alonso-Blanco C, Cuadrado ML, Gerwin RD, Pareja JA. Trigger points in the suboccipital muscles and forward head posture in tension-type headache. *Headache* 2006;46:454–460.

41. Fernández-de-las-Peñas C, Alonso-Blanco C, Cuadrado ML, Gerwin RD, Pareja JA. Myofascial trigger points and their relationship with headache clinical parameters in chronic tension-type headache. *Headache* 2006;46:1264–1272.

42. Chaiamnuay P, Darmawan J, Muirden KD, Assawatanabodee P. Epidemiology of rheumatic disease in rural Thailand: A WHOILAR COPCORD study. Community Oriented Programme for the Control of the Rheumatic Disease. *J Rheumatol* 1998;25:1382–1387.

43. Fernández-de-las-Peñas C, Cuadrado ML, Pareja JA. Myofascial trigger points, neck mobility and forward head posture in unilateral migraine. *Cephalalgia* 2006;26:1061–1070.

44. Calandre EP, Hidalgo J, García-Leiva JM, Rico-Villademoros F. Trigger point evaluation in migraine patients: An indication of peripheral sensitization linked to migraine predisposition? *Eur J Neurol* 2006;13:244–249.

45. Fernández-de-las-Peñas C, Cuadrado ML, Gerwin RD, Pareja JA. Referred pain from the trochlear region in tension-type headache: A myofascial trigger point from the superior oblique muscle. *Headache* 2005;45:731–737.

46. Fernández-de-las-Peñas C, Cuadrado ML, Gerwin RD, Pareja JA. Referred pain from the lateral rectus muscle in subjects with chronic tension-type headache (abstract). *Headache* 2006;46:880.

47. Fernández-de-las-Peñas C, Cuadrado ML, Gerwin RD, Pareja JA. Myofascial disorders in the trochlear region in unilateral migraine: A possible initiating or perpetuating factor. *Clin J Pain* 2006;22:548–553.

48. Treaster D, Marras WS, Burr D, Sheedy JE, Hart D. Myofascial trigger point development from visual and postural stressors during computer work. *J Electromyogr Kinesiol* 2006;16:115–124.

49. Bendtsen L. Central sensitization in tension-type headache: Possible patho-physiological mechanisms. *Cephalalgia* 2000;29:486–508.

50. Arendt-Nielsen L, Svensson P. Referred muscle pain: Basic and clinical findings. *Clin J Pain* 2001;17:11–19.

51. Graven-Nielsen T, Arendt-Nielsen L, Svensson P, Jensen T. Quantification of local and referred muscle pain in humans after sequential intra-muscular injections of hypertonic saline. *Pain* 1997;69:111–117.

52. Arendt-Nielsen L, Graven-Nielsen T. Central sensitization in fibromyalgia and other muscu-loskeletal disorders. *Curr Pain Headache Rep* 2003;7:355–361.

53. Arendt-Nielsen L, Laursen RJ, Drewes A. Referred pain as an indicator for neural plasticity. *Prog Brain Res* 2000;129:343–356.

54. Fernández-de-las-Peñas C, Alonso-Blanco C, Miangolarra JC. Myofascial trigger points in subjects presenting with mechanical neck pain: A blinded, controlled study. *Man Ther* 2007;12:29–33.

55. Bajaj P, Graven-Nielsen T, Arendt-Nielsen L. Osteoarthritis and its association with muscle hyperalgesia: An experimental controlled study. *Pain* 2001;93:107–114.

56. Fernández-Carnero J, Fernández-de-Las-Peñas C, de la Llave-Rincón AI, Ge HY, Arendt-Nielsen L. Prevalence of and referred pain from myofascial trigger points in the forearm muscles in patients with lateral epicondylalgia. *Clin J Pain* 2007;23:353–360.

57. Fernández-de-las-Peñas C, Alonso-Blanco C, Cuadrado ML, Pareja JA. Myofascial trigger points in the suboccipital muscles in episodic tension-type headache. *Man Ther* 2006;11:225–230.

58. Fernández-de-las-Peñas C, Cuadrado ML, Pareja JA. Myofascial trigger points, neck mobility and forward head posture in episodic tension-type headache. *Headache* 2007;47:662–672.

59. Hong CZ, Simons DG. Response to treatment for pectoralis minor myofascial pain syndrome after whiplash. *J Musculoskel Pain* 1993;1(1):89–131.

60. Buchgreitz, AC, Lyngberg L, Bendtsen R, Jensen R. Frequency of headache is related to sensiti-zation: A population study. *Pain* 2006;123:19–27.

61. Olesen J. Clinical and patho-physiological observations in migraine and tension-type headache explained by integration of vascular, supraspinal and myofascial inputs. *Pain* 1991;46:125–132.

62. Bogduk N. The anatomical basis for cervicogenic headache *J Manipulative Physiol Ther* 1992;15:67–70.

63. Shah JP, Phillips TM, Danoff JV, Gerber LH. An *in vitro* microanalytical technique for measuring the local biochemical milieu of human skeletal muscle. *J Appl Physiol* 2005;99:1977–1984.

64. Ashina M, Stallknecht B, Bendtsen L, Pedersen JF, Schifter S, Galbo H, Olesen J. Tender points are not sites of ongoing inflammation: *In vivo* evidence in patients with chronic tension-type headache. *Cephalalgia* 2003;3:109–116.

65. Bogduk N. Cervicogenic headache: Anatomic basis and pathophysiologic mechanisms. *Curr Pain Headache Rep* 2001;5:382–386.

66. Fernández-de-las-Peñas C, Alonso-Blanco C, Cuadrado ML, Pareja JA. Forward head posture and neck mobility in chronic tension-type headache: A blinded, controlled study. *Cephalalgia* 2006;26:314–319.

67. Calandre EP, Hidalgo J, García-Leiva JM, Rico-Villademoros F. Effectiveness of prophylactic trigger point inactivation in chronic migraine and chronic daily headache with migraine fea-tures (abstract). *Cephalalgia* 2003;23:713.

68. McMakin C. Micro-current therapy: A novel treatment method for chronic low back myofascial pain. *J Bodywork Movement Ther* 2004;8:143–153.

69. Kraus M, Reinhart E, Krause H, Reuther J. Low energy extra-corporeal shockwave therapy (ESWT) for treatment of myogelosis of the masseter muscle (German). *Mund Kiefer Gesichtschir* 1999;3:20–23.

70. Majlesi J, Unalan H. High-power pain threshold ultrasound technique in the treatment of active myofascial trigger points: A randomized, double-blind, case-control study. *Arch Phys Med Rehabil* 2004;85:833–836.

71. Fernández-de-las-Peñas C, Sohrbeck-Campo M, Fernández-Carnero J, Miangolarra-Page JC. Manual therapies in the myofascial trigger point treatment: A systematic review. *J Bodywork Movement Ther* 2005;9:27–34.

Part 3

# Management

# Chapter 7

# Effectiveness of Noninvasive Treatments for Active Myofascial Trigger Point Pain: A Systematic Review

*Luke D. Rickards, B.App.Sc, M.Osteo*

## Introduction

Musculoskeletal pain is among the leading reasons for visits to physicians and physical therapists.[1,2] It has been reported that between 30–85% of patients complaining of regional muscular pain meet the diagnostic criteria for myofascial pain syndrome (MPS).[3-6] If these estimates are valid, then MPS constitutes a considerable burden to patients and society.[4] Simons, Travell, and Simons[7] have defined MPS as a condition caused by hyperirritable foci, called myofascial trigger points (MTrPs), within taut bands of skeletal muscle. MTrPs are painful upon compression and may give rise to characteristic patterns of referred pain, tenderness, autonomic symptoms, and restricted range of motion.[7]

Simons, Travell, and Simons[7] described the following clinical diagnostic features for MTrPs:

- Taut muscle band containing a discrete nodule
- Focal tenderness
- Consistent and reproducible pattern of referred pain
- Local twitch response cause by snapping palpation
- Spontaneous exclamation of pain by the patient ("jump sign") as a result of mechanical pressure

MTrPs are classified as active or latent, depending on the presence of a characteristic pattern of pain referral. Active MTrPs refer pain at rest, with muscular activity, and upon direct palpation. In contrast, latent MTrPs remain nonpainful and only refer pain when steady direct pressure is applied.[7]

Trigger points may arise in any muscle group. However, the most common sites are the muscles involved in maintaining posture: the levator scapulae, upper trapezius, sternocleidomastoid, scalenes, erector spinae, quadratus lumborum, and gluteal muscles.[7] Patients described as having active MTrPs usually report regional, persistent pain that often results in a decreased range of motion. Associated signs, such as joint swelling and neurologic deficits, are usually absent on physical examination, and the pain does not follow a dermatomal or nerve root distribution.[7]

The etiology of MPS and MTrP formation is believed to be multifactorial, with postural stresses, inefficient biomechanics, repetitive overuse, direct trauma, and psychological stress the most frequently stated causes.[3,7-12] However, MTrPs present a complex of clinical and research findings that defy a simplistic explanation, and no substantiated scientific theory exists that explains the precise physiological nature of these clinical entities.[3,6,9,13-16] Several theories describing MTrP pathogenesis have been proposed, including Simons' "integrated hypothesis," which incorporates the local myofascial tissues, the central nervous system, and biomechanical factors, and endeavors to account for the major clinical characteristics of MTrPs.[7,14] Gerwin et al[17]—as discussed by Dommerholt et al in a previous chapter in this text—have expanded upon this integrated hypothesis, but further research is still required.[4,9,17] The lack of substantiating data relating to MTrP pathophysiology has made the objective diagnosis and management of MPS a clinical challenge.[3,14,18,19]

Despite this lack of knowledge with regard to their exact etiology, clinicians in many health-care disciplines routinely identify and treat MTrPs. However, at present there are no accepted biochemical, electromyographic, or diagnostic imaging criteria recognized as the definitive diagnostic gold standard.[4,9,14,20] The detection of MTrPs remains solely dependent on manual palpation skills and patient feedback.[20,21] This has raised many concerns regarding the nonsubstantive manner in which MTrPs are diagnosed.[4,20] Furthermore, no reliable list of physical diagnostic criteria for MTrPs currently exists.[4,6,9,14] The four criteria most commonly used by researchers to diagnose the presence of an MTrP are: tender spot in a taut band of skeletal muscle, patient pain recognition, predicted pain referral pattern, and local twitch response.[4] The tender spot in a taut band is considered the most reliable of the MTrP features. Reproduction of patient-recognized pain denotes an MTrP as active or latent. Referred pain patterns and the local twitch response are less reliable and have been considered confirmatory signs.[22,23] More information on the reliability of trigger point palpation can be found in Chapter 4.

Most relevant for the purposes of this systematic review is that the evidence from diagnostic reliability studies is varied and inconsistent.[4] Researchers have yet to demonstrate that the clinical features of MTrPs are reproducible among different examiners, thereby establishing the reliability of the physical examination in the diagnosis of MPS.[9,16,22] Gerwin et al[22] have demonstrated that the interrater reliability varies not only for the different MTrP features, but also for the identification of these features among different muscles. An implication of this finding is that researchers investigating MPS or MTrPs need to properly operationally define the MTrP for the purposes of their study. The criteria by which an MTrP is identified, or by which the diagnosis of MPS is made, need to be clearly stated in order to ensure the validity of the data.[22]

Although various treatment methods are considered to be effective in the resolution of MTrP symptomatology, the mechanisms underlying the claimed efficacy of these MTrP treatments are also poorly understood.[5,9] This has given rise to a multitude of interventions used in the treatment of MPS.[16] In a preliminary search of the current literature, the following interventions were used in various studies examining or reviewing the treatment of active MTrPs: transcutaneous electrical nerve stimulation (TENS), electrical muscle stimulation (EMS),[24] ischemic compression, myofascial release therapy, stretch with coolant spray, interferential current,[25] stretch, ultrasound, direct dry needling,[26] trigger point injection (with various solutions and medications),[27] neuroreflexotherapy,[28] deep pressure soft-tissue massage, hydrocollator superficial heat,[18] exercise, yoga,[19] acupuncture, ice massage,[8] magnetic stimulation,[29] laser therapy,[30] botulinum toxin, topical anesthetic preparation,[31] passive rhythmic release, active rhythmic release,[14] counterstrain, high-velocity low-amplitude thrust,[32] sulfur mud baths,[33] biofeedback, and clinical psychophysiology.[34] Such a variety of therapies, each requiring different skills, levels of training, and licensing, leaves clinicians with a dilemma when deciding the best course of treatment for their patient.

Cummings and White[1] have conducted a systematic literature review examining the effectiveness of various needling therapies in the treatment of MTrP pain. The review compared "wet" and "dry" needling methods and direct and indirect needling methods. The results suggested that needling appeared to be an effective treatment for MTrP pain, as marked improvements were recorded in all groups that received this intervention. The effect was shown to be due to the therapeutic effect of the needle itself or perhaps to the placebo effect of needling rather than the injection of saline or drugs. The review concluded that further controlled trials are needed to investigate whether needling has an effect beyond placebo in treating MTrP pain. Because there was no difference in effectiveness between wet and dry needling, the reviewers recommended dry needling techniques, because they are safer and more comfortable for the patient. Dommerholt et al discuss needling therapies in more detail in another chapter of this text.

With the effectiveness of the most common invasive interventions for MTrP pain addressed by Cummings and White,[1] the aim of this chapter is to review the evidence for the effectiveness of noninvasive interventions in the treatment of patients with a diagnosis of MPS resulting from active MTrPs.

## Materials and Methods

### Literature Search Strategy

A systematic literature search was performed using the Medline, PubMed, CINAHL, EMBASE, PEDro, and CENTRAL/CCTR electronic databases. The search terms were: key term—"trigger point" OR "trigger points"; indexing terms—"randomized controlled trial" OR "controlled clinical trial." The key terms were searched for in the title, abstract, and keywords. Searching was done from the inception date of the databases up to November 2007 to identify published randomized controlled trials examining noninvasive interventions in the treatment of MPS arising from MTrPs. In addition, reference lists of retrieved studies were scanned to identify additional relevant trials. Hand searching of the 1999 edition of *Simons, Travell, and Simons' Myofascial Pain and Dysfunction: The Trigger Point Manual*[7] was also performed.

## Study Selection

### Types of Studies

Randomized controlled studies or quasi-randomized studies examining the effectiveness of noninvasive treatment interventions for active MTrP pain were included. Studies examining the treatment outcomes of various interventions and those comparing different interventions were reviewed. The treatment group had to be compared with a known placebo, no treatment, or other treatment interventions. Studies comparing invasive and noninvasive treatments were included if the active noninvasive treatment groups were compared to a placebo or to a no-treatment control group. Trials in which allocation to the treatment or control group was not concealed from the outcome assessor were excluded.

### Types of Participants

Studies of men and/or women with the diagnosis MPS were included if the presence of active MTrPs had been identified. A clear definition of the criteria for determining the diagnosis of active MTrP pain was required. The minimum criteria for diagnosis were the presence of a taut band and spot tenderness on palpation. Studies examining the treatment of latent MTrPs were not included, because there is insufficient evidence to suggest that these are clinically relevant entities in patients complaining of muscle pain symptoms.

### Types of Intervention

Studies were included where the intervention involved one or more types of noninvasive method aimed at the treatment of active MTrP pain. Interventions were required to be clearly described.

### Types of Outcome Measures

Studies that stated the use of subjective pain-based outcome measures were included in the review. At least one patient-rated outcome measure, such as pain intensity, frequency, duration, or improvement, was required from individual patients before and after administration of the study treatments. These measures included visual analogue scores for pain intensity or pain relief, categorical scores for pain intensity or pain relief, and global ratings of treatment effectiveness as made by the study subjects. The review excluded studies using pain threshold algometry as the sole outcome measure, because changes in this measure do not guarantee clinically relevant reductions in subjective pain symptoms.[35] Studies that did not include subjective measures of either pain intensity or pain relief as part of the overall assessment of effectiveness, both before and after treatment, were excluded.

## Methodological Quality Assessment

Data on population, inclusion and exclusion criteria, study design, randomization, interventions used, blinding, description of dropouts, outcome measures, statistical analysis, results, and conclusions were extracted for each study.

The included studies were assessed for internal validity and methodological quality with an assessment tool used by Bronfort et al[36] in a review of noninvasive treatments for headache. This evaluation list contains 20 methodological items, of which 14 have been classified as internal validity items and six as descriptive information items (**Table 7-1**). The validity score (VS) is given as a percentage of the score of validity items, from a maximum of 14. The cutoff VS for high- versus low-quality studies was set in this review at 50.

## Levels of Evidence

The following levels of evidence determined the results of the analysis:

- *Significant evidence:* consistent findings in multiple high-quality (VS >50) randomized controlled trials
- *Moderate evidence:* consistent findings in multiple low-quality trials (VS <50) and/or a single relevant high-quality randomized controlled trial
- *Limited evidence:* a single low-quality randomized trial
- *Unclear evidence:* inconsistent or conflicting results in multiple randomized trials
- *No evidence:* no studies identified
- *Evidence of adverse effect:* trials with lasting negative changes

# Results

## Literature Search Results

The searches revealed 50 potentially relevant trials, 24[35,37-59] of which were subsequently excluded (see **Table 7-2**). Twenty-six studies met the inclusion criteria for this review.

The included trials could be divided into five categories based on the type of intervention studied:

- Laser therapies—seven trials
- Electrotherapies—five trials
- Ultrasound—five trials
- Magnet therapies—three trials
- Physical/manual therapies—six trials

## TABLE 7-1 Methodological Evaluation Scores

| | Smania et al (2003) | Altan et al (2003) | Brown et al (2002) | Hanten et al (2000) | Esenyel et al (2000) | Hou et al (2002) | Gam et al (1998) | Lee et al (1997) | Ardic et al (2002) | Hsueh et al (1997) | Gur et al (2004) | Tanrikut et al (2003) | Ilbuldu et al (2004) |
|---|---|---|---|---|---|---|---|---|---|---|---|---|---|
| **Internal Validity Items** | | | | | | | | | | | | | |
| Group comparability | + | + | + | + | − | − | p | − | + | + | + | p | + |
| Randomization procedure | p | − | − | p | − | − | p | − | − | − | p | + | − |
| Outcome measure | + | + | + | + | + | + | + | + | + | + | + | + | + |
| Patient blinding | + | − | p | na | na | na | p | p | + | p | p | p | − |
| Treatment provider blinding | p | − | + | na | na | na | + | − | − | − | − | na | − |
| Unbiased outcomes assessment | + | + | + | p | − | p | + | + | − | + | + | − | + |
| Attention bias | + | p | + | p | p | − | − | − | + | + | + | − | p |
| A priori hypothesis | + | + | + | + | + | + | + | + | + | + | + | − | + |
| Appropriate statistical tests | + | + | + | + | − | + | + | p | + | p | − | − | + |
| Adequate statistical power | − | − | + | − | − | + | + | − | − | − | + | + | + |
| Dropouts analysis | − | p | + | na | − | na | + | na | − | na | p | p | − |
| Missing data analysis | − | − | + | na | − | na | p | na | − | na | − | p | − |
| Intention-to-treat analysis | − | − | p | na | − | na | − | na | − | na | − | − | − |
| p-level adjustments | + | − | p | na | + | + | − | − | − | − | p | − | p |
| Total validity score (%) | 64 | 42 | 82 | 68 | 29 | 61 | 71 | 36 | 28 | 60 | 64 | 28 | 39 |
| **Descriptive Information Items** | | | | | | | | | | | | | |
| Defined inclusion and exclusion criteria | + | + | + | + | + | + | + | + | + | + | + | + | p |
| Adequate follow-up period | p | p | − | − | p | − | + | − | + | − | + | − | + |
| Defined intervention protocol | + | + | + | + | p | + | + | + | + | + | + | + | p |
| Comparison to existing treatments | p | + | + | + | − | + | p | + | p | + | + | p | p |
| Confidence intervals | + | + | + | + | − | + | + | p | + | + | + | − | p |
| Appropriate conclusions | + | + | + | + | + | + | + | p | + | + | + | + | p |

*Note:* + = yes; − = no; p = unclear; na = not applicable

| Internal Validity Items | Edwards et al (2003) | Ceccherelli et al (1989) | Snyder-Mackler et al (1989) | Hakguder et al (2003) | Graff-Radford et al (1989) | Smania et al (2005) | Chatchawan et al (2005) | Farina et al (2004) | Fernandez et al (2006) |
|---|---|---|---|---|---|---|---|---|---|
| Group comparability | + | - | - | + | - | + | + | + | + |
| Randomization procedure | p | - | p | p | - | p | p | p | p |
| Outcome measure | + | + | + | + | + | + | + | + | + |
| Patient blinding | na | p | p | - | p | p | na | p | na |
| Treatment provider blinding | - | p | p | - | p | + | na | + | na |
| Unbiased outcomes assessment | - | p | p | + | + | + | + | + | + |
| Attention bias | - | + | p | - | p | + | p | + | + |
| A priori hypothesis | + | + | + | + | + | + | + | + | + |
| Appropriate statistical tests | + | + | + | + | + | + | + | + | + |
| Adequate statistical power | - | - | - | - | - | - | + | - | - |
| Dropouts analysis | na | na | na | na | na | p | na | - | na |
| Missing data analysis | na | na | na | na | na | - | na | - | na |
| Intention-to-treat analysis | na | na | na | na | na | p | + | - | na |
| p-level adjustments | - | + | p | - | + | + | p | p | na |
| Total validity score (%) | 41 | 59 | 54 | 50 | 59 | 71 | 85 | 61 | 72 |
| **Descriptive Information Items** | | | | | | | | | |
| Defined inclusion and exclusion criteria | + | p | - | + | - | + | + | + | |
| Adequate follow-up period | p | p | - | p | - | p | p | + | + |
| Defined intervention protocol | + | + | + | p | + | + | + | + | - |
| Comparison to existing treatments | p | - | p | + | + | + | p | p | + |
| Confidence intervals | + | + | + | + | + | + | + | + | + |
| Appropriate conclusions | + | + | + | + | + | + | p | + | + |

*Note:* + = yes; - = no; p = unclear; na = not applicable

(continued)

TABLE 7-1   Methodological Evaluation Scores (cont.)

| Internal Validity Items | Majlesi et al (2004) | Dundar et al (2007) | Gemmel et al (2007) | Esenyel et al (2007) |
|---|---|---|---|---|
| Group comparability | + | + | + | p |
| Randomization procedure | – | p | p | – |
| Outcome measure | + | + | + | + |
| Patient blinding | p | p | na | na |
| Treatment provider blinding | na | – | na | na |
| Unbiased outcomes assessment | + | + | + | – |
| Attention bias | p | + | + | p |
| A priori hypothesis | + | + | + | + |
| Appropriate statistical tests | + | + | + | + |
| Adequate statistical power | – | – | – | – |
| Dropouts analysis | – | na | na | – |
| Missing data analysis | – | na | na | – |
| Intention-to-treat analysis | – | na | na | – |
| p-level adjustments | – | p | p | p |
| **Total validity score (%)** | 46 | 68 | 77 | 33 |
| **Descriptive Information Items** | | | | |
| Defined inclusion and exclusion criteria | + | + | + | + |
| Adequate follow-up period | p | p | – | p |
| Defined intervention protocol | + | + | + | + |
| Comparison to existing treatments | p | + | p | p |
| Confidence intervals | p | + | + | p |
| Appropriate conclusions | p | + | + | + |

Note: + = yes; – = no; p = unclear; na = not applicable

Some overlap of interventions occurred between categories. The methodological quality scores and extracted characteristics of the included trials are reported in **Tables 7-3** through **7-7**. In many cases, even relatively high-quality trials (VS >50) had limitations that may have affected the interpretation of study results. Studies with lower validity scores are acknowledged as having substantial limitations.

**TABLE 7-2  Excluded Papers Describing Noninvasive Therapies for Myofascial Trigger Point (MTrP) Pain**

| Study | Reason for Exclusion |
| --- | --- |
| Airaksinen et al[37] | No criteria for diagnosis of MTrP. |
| Airaksinen et al[38] | No patient-rated outcome measures used. |
| Airaksinen et al[39] | No patient-rated outcome measures used; no MTrP criteria. |
| Ceylan et al[40] | No patient-rated outcome measures used. |
| Chee & Walton[41] | No outcome measures apparent. |
| Curl & Emmerson[42] | Not randomized or blinded. |
| Dardzinski et al[43] | Not randomized or blinded. |
| Fryer & Hodgson[44] | Treatment of latent MTrPs. |
| Hanten et al[45] | No patient-rated outcome measures used. |
| Hong et al[46] | No patient-rated outcome measures used. |
| Jaeger & Reeves[35] | Not randomized or blinded. |
| Lewith & Machin[47] | No criteria for diagnosis of MTrP. |
| Lundeberg[48] | Not specific to MTrP pain. |
| McCray & Patton[49] | No criteria for diagnosis of MTrP; not limited to MTrP pain. |
| Melzack[50] | Not limited to MTrP pain. |
| Nilsson[51] | Not specific to MTrP pain. |
| Pratzel et al[52] | Not specific to MTrP pain. |
| Ruiz-Saez et al[53] | Treatment of latent MTrPs. |
| Schnider et al[54] | Noninvasive therapy compared to invasive therapy only. |
| Srbely & Dickey[55] | No patient-rated outcome measures used. |
| Simunovic[56] | Not randomized. |
| Simunovic et al[57] | Not specific to MTrP pain. |
| Snyder-Mackler et al[58] | MTrPs diagnosed by skin resistance only. |
| Yagci et al[59] | No criteria for diagnosis of MTrP. |

Of the 26 included trials, 23 assessed the treatment of MTrPs in the neck and/or upper trapezius region. In one of these trials,[30] MTrPs in the lower back were also treated. Although Graff-Radford et al[60] report diagnosing MTrPs in the temporalis and masseter muscles, it is unclear if these points were treated. Of the remaining three trials, Brown et al[61] assessed the treatment of MTrPs on the abdomen for chronic pelvic pain, Chatchawan et al[62] assessed

**TABLE 7-3  Laser Therapies for Trigger Points**

| Study | VS | Diagnosis | n | Intervention/Control | Outcome Measures | FU | Result |
|---|---|---|---|---|---|---|---|
| Dundar et al[69] | 68 | MPS in the neck | 64 | A: Ga-As-Al LLLT + stretching exercise<br>B: Placebo Ga-As-Al LLLT + exercise & stretching | Pain VAS<br>Range of motion<br>Neck disability index (NDI) | 4w | A equal to B ($P$ >.05); significant improvement in both groups attributed to exercise/stretching |
| Gur et al[65] | 64 | Chronic MPS in the neck | 60 | A: Ga-As LLLT<br>B: Placebo Ga-As LLLT | Neck pain and disability scale<br>VAS, Beck depression inventory, Nottingham health profile, n TrP | 10w | A superior to B; ($P$ <.01) on all measures |
| Snyder-Mackler et al[30] | 54 | MPS in the neck or lower back | 24 | A: He-Ne cold laser<br>B: Placebo He-Ne cold laser | Pain VAS<br>Skin resistance (dermometer) | 1d | A superior to B; pain ($P$ <.005).<br>No correlation between pain and skin resistance |
| Ceccherelli et al[67] | 59 | MPS in the neck | 27 | A: Ga-As LLLT<br>B: Placebo Ga-As LLLT | Pain VAS<br>McGill pain questionnaire (MPQ) | 3m | A superior to B; MPQ ($P$ <.008), pain ($P$ <.001) |

| Study | VS | n | Condition | Interventions | Outcome measures | FU | Results |
|---|---|---|---|---|---|---|---|
| Hakguder et al[68] | 50 | 62 | MPS the neck or upper back | A: Ga-As-Al LLLT and stretching<br>B: Stretching | Pain VAS<br>Pain threshold algometry<br>Thermographic asymmetry and difference | 3w | A superior to B; pain (P <.001), pain threshold (P <.001), thermography—asym. (P <.001)/diff (P <.01) |
| Ilbuldu et al[64] | 39 | 60 | Trigger points in upper trapezius muscle | A: He-Ne laser<br>B: Dry needling<br>C: Placebo He-Ne laser<br>All groups: trapezius and pectoralis stretches | Pain VAS (rest and activity)<br>Pain threshold algometry<br>Cervical range of motion<br>Nottingham health profile (NHP) | 6m | A superior to B and C post-treatment: pain (P <.001), ROM (P <.001), NHP—pain (P <.001)/phys activity (P <.05)<br>A equal to B and C at 6m FU |
| Altan et al[66] | 42 | 53 | MPS in the neck | A: Ga-As LLLT + exercise and stretching<br>B: Placebo Ga-As LLLT + exercise and stretching | Pain VAS<br>Pain threshold algometry<br>Cervical lateral flexion range | 3m | A equal to B; significant improvement in both groups attributed to exercise/stretching |

Note: VS = validity score; FU = follow up; n = number treated; MPS = myofascial pain syndrome; LLLT = low level laser therapy; VAS = visual analogue scale

TABLE 7-4 Electrotherapies for Trigger Points

| Study | VS | Diagnosis | n | Intervention/Control | Outcome Measures | FU | Result |
|---|---|---|---|---|---|---|---|
| Graff-Radford et al[60] | 59 | Chronic MPS in the back, neck, or head | 60 | A: TENS mode A<br>B: TENS mode B<br>C: TENS mode C<br>D: TENS mode D<br>E: Placebo TENS | Pain VAS<br>Pain threshold algometry | 5min | B superior to C and D<br>C & D superior to A & E; pain (P <.001) (B = 100 Hz, 250 µsec)<br>Pain threshold—all groups equal |
| Farina et al[73] | 61 | Trigger point pain in upper trapezius on one side | 40 | A: FREMS<br>B: TENS | NDPVAS<br>Pain threshold algometry<br>Cervical range of motion (ROM)<br>MTrP characteristics | 3m | Significant effect of FREMS at 3m; NDPVAS (P <.001)<br>Significant effect of TENS at 1m; NDPVAS (P <.001)<br>No sig. diff between groups |
| Hsueh et al[24] | 60 | Trigger point pain in upper trapezius on one side | 60 | A: Placebo electrotherapy<br>B: TENS<br>C: EMS | Pain VAS<br>Pain threshold algometry<br>Cervical range of motion (ROM) | 5min | B superior to A and C; pain and threshold (P <.05)<br>C superior to B & C; ROM (P <.05) |
| Ardic et al[71] | 28 | Trigger point pain in upper trapezius on one side | 40 | A: TENS and trapezius stretching<br>B: EMS and trapezius stretching<br>C: Trapezius stretching | Pain VAS<br>Pain threshold algometry<br>Cervical range of motion (ROM) | 3m | A equal to B, A and B superior to C; pain and threshold (P <.01)<br>A superior to B immediately after treatment (P <.01) |
| Tanrikut et al[74] | 28 | MPS in the neck or upper back | 45 | A: HVGS and exercise<br>B: Placebo HVGS and exercise<br>C: Exercise | Pain VAS<br>Analgesic use<br>Patient global assessment | 15d | A superior to B and C; pain (P <.05), global (P <.05)<br>A equal to B & C; analgesic use |

Note: EMS = electrical muscle stimulation; TENS = transcutaneous electrical nerve stimulation; HVGS = high voltage galvanic stimulation; FREMS = frequency modulated neural stimulation

TABLE 7-5   **Magnet Therapies for Trigger Points**

| Study | VS | Diagnosis | n | Intervention/Control | Outcome Measures | FU | Result |
|-------|-----|-----------|-----|----------------------|------------------|-----|--------|
| Brown et al[61] | 82 | Chronic pelvic pain with presence of trigger points | 33 | A: Active 500g magnets<br>B: Placebo magnets | McGill pain questionnaire<br>Pain disability index (PDI)<br>Clinical global impressions (CGI) | 1m | A superior to B; PDI ($P$ <.05), CGI-severity ($P$ <.05), CGI-improvement ($P$ <.01)<br>Blinding possibly compromised ($P$ <.05) |
| Smania et al[78] | 71 | Trigger point pain in upper trapezius | 53 | A: rMS<br>B: TENS<br>C: Placebo US with gel | Pain disability NPDVAS<br>Pain threshold algometry<br>MTrP characteristics<br>Cervical range of motion (ROM) | 3m | A superior to B; pain ($P$ <.001), pain threshold ($P$ <.001), MTrP characteristics ($P$ <.001)<br>B superior C immediately after treatment; pain ($P$ <.001) |
| Smania et al[29] | 64 | Trigger point pain in upper trapezius | 18 | A: rMS<br>B: Placebo rMS | Pain VAS<br>Pain disability NPDVAS<br>Pain threshold algometry<br>Cervical range of motion (ROM) | 1m | A superior to B; pain ($P$ <.022), pain disability ($P$ <.016), pain threshold ($P$ <.016)<br>A equal to B; ROM ($P$ <.066) |

*Note:* rMS = repetitive magnetic stimulation

TABLE 7-6  Ultrasound Therapies for Trigger Points

| Study | VS | Diagnosis | n | Intervention/Control | Outcome Measures | FU | Result |
|---|---|---|---|---|---|---|---|
| Gam et al[75] | 71 | Chronic MPS in the neck or shoulder | 67 | A: US, massage and exercise<br>B: Placebo US, massage and exercise<br>C: Control | Pain VAS<br>MTrP characteristics<br>Daily analgesic use | 6m | A equal to B equal to C; Analgesic use and VAS; A & B superior to C; MTrP characteristics |
| Maljesi & Unalan[76] | 46 | Trigger point pain in upper trapezius on one side | 72 | A: HPPT-US<br>B: Conventional US | Pain VAS<br>Cervical range of motion | 4w | A superior to B; pain ($P <.05$)<br>A equal to B; ROM ($P >.05$) |
| Esenyel et al[77] | 33 | Trigger point pain in upper trapezius on one side | 90 | A: Botox<br>B: Lidocaine<br>C: US<br>D: HPPT-US<br>E: Stretches<br>A, B, C, and D: + Stretches | Pain VAS | 1m | Significant change in all groups ($P <.005$)<br>C equal to D equal to E |
| Lee et al[70] | 36 | Trigger point pain in upper trapezius | 26 | A: Placebo US<br>B: US<br>C: Electrotherapy<br>D: US and electrotherapy | Pain VAS<br>Pain threshold algometry<br>Cervical range of motion | 5min | C superior to A; pain ($P <.05$).<br>D superior to A,B,C; ROM ($P <.05$) |
| Esenyel et al[26] | 29 | Trigger point pain in upper trapezius on one side | 102 | A: US and neck stretches<br>B: TrP injection and neck stretches<br>C: Neck stretches | Pain VAS<br>Pain threshold algometry<br>Cervical range of motion<br>Beck depression inventory<br>Taylor manifest anxiety sc | 3m | A and B superior to C, pain ($P <.001$) pain threshold ($P <.001$), ROM ($P <.05$)<br>A equal to B Anxiety > depression in MPS<br>Correlation between depression/anxiety and pain duration but not intensity |

Note: US = ultrasound; HPPT-US = high power pain threshold ultrasound;

TABLE 7-7    Physical and Manual Therapies for Trigger Points

| Study | VS | Diagnosis | n | Intervention/Control | Outcome Measures | FU | Result |
|---|---|---|---|---|---|---|---|
| Chatchawan et al[62] | 85 | Back pain with at least one MTrP in the upper or lower torso | 180 | A: Traditional Thai massage + stretches; B: Swedish massage + stretches | Pain VAS; Oswestry Disability Index; Pain threshold algometry; Thoracolumbar ROM | 1m | VAS and ODI reduced by half (P <.05) in both groups. No sig. dif. between groups |
| Gemmel et al[81] | 77 | Trigger point pain in upper trapezius | 45 | A: IC; B: TPPR; C: Placebo US | Pain VAS; Pain threshold algometry; Cervical ROM | 5min | A equal to B equal to C (P >.05) |
| Fernández-de-las-Peñas et al[80] | 72 | Trigger point pain in upper trapezius | 40 | A: IC; B: TFM | Pain VAS; Pain threshold algometry | 2min | Significant effect of A and B on VAS (P <.05); A equal to B (P <.05); VAS |
| Hanten et al[79] | 68 | MPS in the neck or upper back | 40 | A: Home program—IC followed by sustained stretching; B: Active range of motion exercises | Pain VAS; Pain threshold algometry; Percentage of time in pain | 3d | A superior to B; pain (P = .043) pain threshold (P = .000); A equal to B for time in pain |
| Hou et al[25] | 61 | Trigger point pain in upper trapezius | 119 | A: HtP & AROM; B: A + IC; C: A + IC and TENS; D: A + SwS; E: A + SwS and TENS; F: A + IFC and MFR | Pain VAS; Pain tolerance; Pain threshold algometry; Cervical range of motion | 5min | C, D, and F superior to A; pain (P <.05); D, E, and F superior to A; ROM (P <.05); B, C, D, E, F equal; F; largest VAS↓ |
| Edwards & Knowles[63] | 41 | MPS, region unspecified | 40 | A: Superficial dry needling and stretching; B: Stretching; C: No treatment control | Short form MPQ; Pain threshold algometry | 3w | A superior to C; MPQ (P <.05); B equal to C |

*Note:* IC = ischemic compression; TPPR = trigger point pressure release; TFM = transverse friction massage; HtP = hot pack; AROM = active range of motion exercise; SwS = stretch with spray; IFC = interferential current; MFR = myofascial release the treatment of MTrPs in the upper and lower back, and Edwards and Knowles[63] did not specify the region of treatment.

## Data Synthesis

### Laser Therapies

Two types of low-level laser therapies (LLLT) were used by trials included in this review: helium–neon (He–Ne)[30,64] and infrared lasers with a diode of gallium–arsenide (Ga–As)[65-67] or gallium–arsenide–aluminium (Ga–As–Al).[68,69] In five of the seven trials, a statistically significant difference was found between the treatment group and the control group following treatment. Two trials[65,67] reported that a statistically significant effect persisted at a 3-month follow-up. Hakguder et al[68] reported significant reductions in pain intensity with laser and stretching. Ilbuldu et al[64] measured outcomes at 6 months and found no difference between the treatment and placebo groups.

Altan et al[66] reported conflicting results, attributing the statistically significant effect in both the treatment and placebo groups to a concurrent program of exercise and stretching. Dundar et al[69] compared laser to placebo laser and reported no statistically significant difference between groups, also attributing the significant change in both the treatment and placebo groups to a concurrent program of exercise and stretching.

### Electrotherapies

Five trials studied electrotherapies directly and in three other trials (Hou et al[25], Lee et al[70], Smania et al[72]) electrotherapies were used as part of a mixed-intervention protocol. Five types of electrotherapies were studied: transcutaneous electrical nerve stimulation (TENS), electrical muscle stimulation (EMS), high-voltage galvanic stimulation (HVGS), frequency-modulated neural stimulation (FREMS), and interferential current (IFC).

Six of these eight trials used TENS. Hsueh et al[24] and Ardic et al[71] compared TENS to EMS, and in both studies TENS was superior to EMS in reducing pain. Hou et al[25] reported a significant reduction in pain intensity when TENS or IFC was used in combination with other physical therapy modalities and/or manual techniques. Graff-Radford et al[60] compared four different modes of TENS and reported a superior effect on pain levels with 100 Hz, 250 µsec stimulation. However, it is difficult to base any solid conclusions of long-term treatment effectiveness on these results, because in all but one trial (Ardic et al[71], which had a very low VS) the final outcome assessment was immediately post-treatment. Therefore, no evidence of medium- or long-term effectiveness is available. Smania et al[72] compared TENS to placebo ultrasound as part of a study examining repetitive magnetic stimulation and also found that TENS had an immediate effect; however, this did not persist at 1 month.

Farina et al[73] compared TENS with FREMS. Although both treatments showed significant effect on pain scores and MTrP characteristics at 1 month, there was no difference between groups. The effect persisted at the final follow-up of 3 months for the FREMS group but not the TENS group.

Lee et al[70] compared ultrasound to placebo ultrasound, combined-current electrotherapy, and ultrasound plus combined-current electrotherapy and found that only electrotherapy had a significant effect on pain intensity.

Tanrikut et al[74] reported a significant reduction in pain intensity at 15 days (but not in analgesic usage) after the application of HVGS; however, the internal validity of this trial was poor.

## Ultrasound

In two of the five trials using ultrasound (US), which included one very high-quality paper (Gam et al[75]), US was reported to have no significant effect on pain. Esenyel et al[26] reported a superior effect; however, this study was of very poor quality and attention bias was a significant limitation. Lee et al[70] reported no significant difference between US and placebo US.

Maljesi and Unalan[76] compared high-power pain-threshold ultrasound (HPPT-US) to conventional US and reported a statistically significant reduction in pain intensity in the HPPT-US group. However, the validity score of this trial was also low. Esenyel et al[77] compared ultrasound (HPPT-US) with stretching to conventional US with stretching and stretching alone and reported that pain intensity improved in all three groups; however, there was no significant difference noted between the groups.

## Magnet Therapies

The three trials examining magnet therapies for MTrPs were of high quality. Brown et al[61] reported a superior effect over placebo using magnets taped to MTrPs on the abdomen for the treatment of chronic pelvic pain. Although this study had a high VS, patient blinding was shown to be compromised.

Smania et al[29] reported that repetitive magnetic stimulation technique (rMS) was superior to placebo in reducing pain from MTrPs in the upper trapezius muscle; however, this was a very small study with only nine patients in each group. In a later study, Smania et al[78] repeated the rMS treatment with a larger population and found statistically significant changes in outcomes up to 3 months following treatment when compared with TENS and placebo US.

## Physical/Manual Therapies

Hou et al[25] studied various combinations of exercise, manual therapy, stretching, and modalities. In this study, all groups that received some form of electrotherapy modality had a superior effect on pain intensity when compared to the control group. The combination of hot pack, range of motion exercise, IFC, and myofascial release showed the largest reduction in pain. However, the final follow-up in this trial was only 5 minutes post-treatment.

Hanten et al[79] studied the effects of a home program of self-applied ischemic compression followed by stretching compared to active range of motion exercises and found a statistically significant difference in pain intensity for the home program group, but no difference in total time in pain. The follow-up in this trial was only 3 days. Edwards and Knowles[63] reported no difference in pain scores between a stretching group and a no-treatment control group after 3 weeks; however, this trial was of poor methodological quality.

Chatchawan et al[62] compared Thai massage plus stretches with Swedish massage plus stretches. This was a very well-conducted study, although no control was used. Both groups showed significant reductions in pain and disability measures; however, there was no difference between groups.

Fernández-de-las-Peñas et al[80] compared ischemic compression with transverse friction massage and found a significant reduction in pain intensity for both groups but no difference between groups. However, no conclusion regarding medium- to long-term effectiveness can be drawn, because the only outcomes measurement was immediately post-treatment. Gemmel et al[81] compared ischemic compression with trigger point pressure release and reported small but equal reductions in both groups.

Gam et al[75] also used massage and exercise in both the US treatment and placebo US groups and made comparisons with a no-treatment control group. No significant difference in pain intensity or analgesic use was measured between any of the groups at any time. However, significant reduction in the MTrP characteristics and prevalence was noted for both groups that received massage and exercise. Esenyel et al[77] used stretching with two active US groups and stretching alone and reported significant but equal reductions in pain intensity across the three groups.

Altan et al[66] and Dundar et al[69] compared laser and an isometric exercise and stretching protocol to placebo laser and the exercise protocol. Both studies found equal improvement in the active laser and placebo laser groups, which was attributed to the exercise with stretching.

# Discussion

## Summary of Findings

The results of this review highlight a considerable discrepancy between the vast range of noninvasive treatment modalities proposed as effective for MTrPs and those in fact supported by the literature. Most modalities have not been subjected to clinical trial, and therefore no evidence of effectiveness (or lack thereof) is available. Of those that have been studied, the evidence for effectiveness must be considered at best preliminary due to the paucity of clinical trials to date. In addition, it is important to remember that most of the current evidence on the noninvasive treatment of MTrPs is limited to the upper trapezius and cervical region.

### Laser Therapies

This review has found unclear evidence that laser therapy is effective as a short-term intervention for reducing pain intensity in MTrP pain of the neck and upper back.

Conflicting results between the studies need to be resolved. Hakguder et al[68] suggested that inadequate dosages may be the principal factor involved in the inconsistency among reports of LLLT efficacy. However, Gur et al[65] found good results with a lower dosage than was used by Hakguder et al.[68] In contrast, Dundar et al[69] used a higher dose than Hakguder et al[68] yet reported no difference between the active and placebo groups. Further studies are necessary to establish long-term effectiveness, the most effective type of laser, the optimum dosage, wavelength, and other parameters, and duration and frequency of treatment.

*Electrotherapies*
TENS appears to have an immediate effect with regard to decreasing pain intensity in MTrP pain of the neck and upper back. However, the data is insufficient to determine the effectiveness for TENS beyond the immediate post-treatment effect. There is limited evidence for the use of FREMS, HVGS, EMS, and IFC for MTrP pain. This conclusion reflects the results of a Cochrane review that found the current evidence for electrotherapies for neck disorders lacking, limited, or conflicting.[84]

*Ultrasound*
Moderate evidence derived from one high-quality and two lower-quality studies indicated that conventional ultrasound is no more effective than placebo or no treatment for MTrP pain in the neck and upper back. Robertson and Baker[85] also supported this conclusion. Further research is needed to evaluate the effectiveness of high-power pain-threshold ultrasound, because results from the two existing trials were conflicting.

*Magnet Therapies*
Although the three trials investigating magnet therapy were generally of good quality, each had a number of significant methodological flaws. Further research is necessary to support the findings of these trials. Contraindications of magnet therapies and minor adverse effects reported in one of the studies must also be considered. The contraindications reported for magnet therapy include cardiovascular disease, hypertension, coagulopathy, ulcer, recent severe hemorrhage, renal insufficiency, severe hepatic disease, neoplasia, epilepsy, cutaneous pathology, pain of central origin, patients with metallic implants (clips, cardiac valves, pacemakers), and pregnancy.[78] Brown et al[61] reported minor adverse events in half of the study participants. These included skin irritation, bruising, and erythema.

*Physical/Manual Therapies*
Due to the heterogeneity of trials investigating physical and manual therapies, the current evidence did not exceed the moderate level. Further, most of these trials examined multimodal treatment programs, so the presence of positive effects cannot be solely attributed to a particular physical or manual therapy intervention. Several studies reported that exercise and stretching appeared to be the effective therapy when included in treatment groups comparing active to placebo modalities.

The higher-quality trials[25,62,75,79-81] examining manual techniques suggested that such approaches may be effective. However, no conclusions regarding medium- to long-term effectiveness could be drawn. Additionally, effectiveness beyond placebo is neither supported nor refuted. Larger high-quality trials with longer follow-up periods are needed to support the findings of these studies. Fernández-de-las-Peñas et al[86] have performed a similar review of the evidence for manual therapies in the treatment of MTrPs. Their review also concluded that although a number of studies demonstrated statistically significant reductions in pain scores and pressure pain threshold, the current evidence neither supported nor refuted effectiveness beyond placebo.

## Methodological Limitations

When interpreting the results of randomized controlled trials, a distinction must be made between statistically versus clinically significant results.[36,82] Inappropriate conclusions about treatment efficacy are commonly drawn based solely on the presence or absence of between-group statistical differences.[36,83] However, statistically significant results cannot automatically be interpreted as clinically relevant.[82,83] To inform decisions about the management of individual patients, it may be more appropriate to consider available treatment options that have shown a meaningful clinical effect.[36] However, little is known about what is considered by patients to be a minimal clinically important change in myofascial pain-related outcome measures.[83]

Heterogeneity of study populations increases the effect size required for statistical significance. The trials included in this review have reported a large range in the baseline means for pain intensity measured by VAS. In the 24 trials that used this measure, the mean baseline VAS ranged from 2.6[79] to 8.4.[76] Some trials reported a difference of more than 4 VAS points between participants in the same study group. These findings suggest that heterogeneity of the patients included in the studies affects not only the potential for finding statistical significance, but also the external validity of study findings.

## Underlying Theoretical Considerations

The clinical uncertainties surrounding MTrP diagnosis present several challenges to the interpretation of clinical treatment trials. In the absence of an accurate diagnosis, the results of any epidemiologic, pathophysiological, or clinical investigation will be misleading.[4] For example, the trials examined in this review may have included a significant proportion of false positives, thus leading to an apparent failure of effective treatments. Until reliable diagnostic criteria have been established, research studies must present greater transparency as to how a case of MPS is defined.[4] Further, Sciotti et al[16] have pointed out that the routine ability to obtain precise location dimensions of MTrPs with actual visualization, such as 3D measurement techniques, is essential to the establishment of reliable data on pathogenesis, clinical diagnosis, and treatment. Until this is achieved and implemented in clinical trials assessing treatments for MTrP pain, reliable evidence of treatment effectiveness will remain elusive.

Although this review included only trials that were explicit with regard to the diagnostic characteristics of MTrPs, it is significant that only three of the 26 trials that met this inclusion criterion documented changes in these diagnostic characteristics as part of the outcomes assessment. Each of these trials used an index described by Gam et al.[75] The index involves rating the presence of tenderness and increased local muscle consistency on palpation using a score from 0–3 with 0 = increased consistency but where palpation produces no pain; 1 = increased consistency but the patient indicates pain only after being asked; 2 = increased consistency and the patient spontaneously expresses pain; and 3 = increased consistency and the patient withdraws from the palpation (jump sign). The number of MTrPs is recorded, and an index score is calculated as the sum of the scores for all MTrPs present at each treatment session. It should be noted that the reliability and validity of this index have not been established. The three trials[74,75,78] all reported statistically significant reductions in the taut band and spot tenderness as measured using this index. Gerwin[87] has suggested that with appropriate treatment the taut band will significantly reduce or disappear within 1 minute, along with the associated symptoms. However, Gam et al[75] have demonstrated that a significant reduction in both the prevalence and intensity of MTrP characteristics with massage and exercise was not accompanied by a reduction in pain intensity or analgesic use. Without more extensive substantiating evidence that changes in the clinical characteristics of the MTrP occur following treatment and that a reduction in subjective symptoms correlates with resolution of MTP findings, it is unclear whether treatments for MPS effectively address the entity by which diagnosis is made or if positive outcomes are due to other factors.

The mechanisms underlying the efficacy of the various treatments for MPS are poorly understood,[5,9] and the multitude of proposed treatments reflects the deficiency in understanding the precise pathophysiology of MTrPs. If treatments directed at MTrP entities specifically address the proposed pathophysiology, then the heterogeneous outcome of common treatments for pain arising from MTPs should be viewed as a challenge to that assertion. In addition to the possibility of placebo mechanisms, the common feature of treatments that appear to have some evidence of effectiveness is the application of direct stimulation at the hyperalgesic foci.[9] The proposed mechanisms for these treatments include direct mechanical disruption of muscle contraction knots,[5] reactive hyperaemic response,[7] equalization of sarcomere length,[88] central opioid release,[89] and supraspinal pain control mechanisms.[90] Research on therapeutic mechanisms is notoriously difficult due to the complexity of interactions between multiple local and systemic systems.[9] Improved understanding of the pathophysiology of the MPS clinical presentation may aid both our understanding of the effects of treatments for MPS and the development of appropriate and effective MTrP treatment strategies.

Although it is commonly argued that long-term relief of MTrP pain is critically dependent on the alleviation or correction of all contributing or perpetuating factors,[6,7,9,12,79,87,91] none of the trials included in this review carefully addressed or even controlled for such factors. Simons, Travell, and Simons[7] suggested mechanical stress and ergonomic issues, such as poor posture or muscle overuse/injury, nutritional inadequacies, metabolic or endocrine disorders, allergies, impaired sleep, psychological factors, chronic infection, radiculopathy, and chronic visceral disease as perpetuating factors for MTrP pain. However, many of these factors are controllable. In a cohort study of 25 patients with chronic myofascial head and neck pain, Graff-Radford et al[92] examined the use of a structured interdisciplinary format of physical and cognitive-behavioral therapies aimed at reducing factors that perpetuate MPS. The results immediately following treatment and at 3, 6, and 12 months post treatment showed highly reliable reductions in self-reported pain and medication intake when compared to pretreatment scores. However, no randomized controlled trials have addressed the duration of pain relief associated with management of contributing and perpetuating factors.[79]

In a study investigating factors that may influence the outcome of trigger point injection therapy, Hopwood and Abram[93] found that an increased risk of treatment failure was associated with unemployment due to pain at the start of treatment, no relief from analgesic medication, constant pain, high levels of pain-at-its-worst and pain-at-its-least, prolonged duration of pain, change in social activity, lower levels of coping ability, and alcohol use. They concluded that several factors should be considered in treating patients with MPS with trigger point injections. The study is consistent with the evidence that MPS is a multidimensional phenomenon and that a plethora of factors may influence treatment outcome.[94] This view was supported in a recent review of MPS,[95] suggesting that the pathogenesis of myofascial pain likely has a central mechanism with peripheral clinical manifestations.

Also relevant from an underlying theoretical perspective is that MTrPs have been identified with nearly every painful musculoskeletal condition.[12] Further, the symptoms produced by MTrPs have been said to mimic other common musculoskeletal disorders, such as radiculopathy, fibromyalgia, and articular or somatic dysfunctions.[4,14,88] Because it is unlikely that MTrPs represent the underlying pathophysiology for nearly all musculoskeletal pain disorders, an alternative explanation is the possibility that MTrP findings are a clinical epiphenomenon of musculoskeletal pathology and pain, the manifestation of which could be explained via peripheral and central sensitization mechanisms. Graven-Nielson and Arendt-Nielsen[94] have suggested that the number of MTrPs may be a manifestation of the degree of central sensitization. This was supported by their recent finding that a significantly higher number of MTrPs were found in the lower limb muscles in patients suffering from knee osteoarthritis compared with controls.[96] Niddam et al[90] have noted that the focal hyperalgesia found in MPS may in part be induced by central sensitization and changes in descending inhibitory or facilitatory mechanisms. This has important repercussions for the clinical management of MPS presentations, further suggesting that therapy should involve enhancing central inhibition with pharmacological or behavioral and psychological techniques in addition to reducing peripheral inputs with physical therapies.[92]

In a recent histological study examining MTrPs, the preliminary results of a novel microanalytical technique for assaying soft tissue using a microdialysis needle revealed significant differences in the levels of pH, substance P, CGRP, bradykinin, norepinephrine,

TNF, and IL-1 in those subjects with an active MTrP, compared with subjects with a latent MTrP and normal subjects.[97] Simons[98] has claimed that the results of this study strongly substantiate the integrated hypothesis as a valid explanation for the pain associated with MTrPs, providing a credible etiology for MTrPs. However, the authors of the study stated that the significance of the data in relation to an etiology of MTrP pain is unclear and that the study does not indicate that the assayed metabolites cause MTrPs.[97] In fact, the differences between the active and control groups were apparent from the time of needle insertion, suggesting the presence of confounding factors, including the possibility that introduction of the needle itself affected the data. Considering that the same metabolites are responsible for peripheral and central sensitization processes following a nociceptive event[99] and are also implicated in neuropathological pain mechanisms,[100] the proposed correlation with theories describing MTrP pathogenesis should be regarded with caution.

As a final critical note, Quintner and Cohen[101] have criticized the MTrP construct as the result of circular reasoning, and they have suggested that the emphasis on the primacy of the MTrP phenomenon has directed attention away from the possibility of nonmuscular explanations for the origin of the MPS clinical presentation. They have proposed that because the characteristics of the MPS presentation are indistinguishable from peripheral neural pain, a primary neuropathological cause involving sensitization of the nervi nervorum is a more likely explanation. Quintner and Cohen[101] suggested that there are sound anatomic and physiological grounds to indicate that the phenomenon of the MTrP, on which the theory of MPS depends, is better understood as a region of secondary hyperalgesia of peripheral nerve origin. This was supported by Butler,[102] who suggested that the concept of ectopic impulse generation or abnormal impulse generating sites (AIGS) and accompanying sensitization processes in peripheral and cutaneous sensory nerves compel reconsideration of the myofascial trigger point hypothesis. Although McPartland[32] has stated that it is in fact the pathological mechanisms of the MTrP that cause the development of peripheral nerve sensitization and AIGS, interestingly Butler[102] was cited as the source. Further research is needed to examine these hypotheses.

## Limitations

Publication bias was a limitation in this review. Optimally, reviews should include all trials, including unpublished research, regardless of language.[103] Due to resource and language constraints, only English-language publications were included in the review, and no effort was made to identify unpublished trials other than those held in the CENTRAL database. However, it is also recognized that unpublished data can be a source of bias.[104]

The methodological quality of the included trials is usually assessed by two or more reviewers.[105] Unfortunately, only one reviewer conducted the methodological quality assessment. Assessment was also unblinded. Although there is some evidence that blinded assessments of the quality of trials may be more reliable than assessments that are not blinded,[106] blinding can be difficult to achieve, is time consuming, and may not substantially alter the results of a review.[107]

In addition, the reliability of different methodological scoring systems may be a source of ambiguity. Conclusions with regard to the weight of evidence are dependent on the choice of methodological quality scoring system and on the exact definition of the evidence classification system used.[36,108] Therefore, as suggested by Bronfort et al[36] the commonly used methodological assessment tool, a 5-point scoring system developed by Jadad et al,[106] was initially used in addition to the 20-item scale described above. The Jadad system addresses randomization, double-blinding, and description of dropouts, all of which may be important sources of bias if addressed inadequately. However, the correlation between the total scores of the two scoring systems was low. The explanation for this is the proportionally high weight placed on the importance of blinding both the patient and the therapist in the Jadad scale compared to the 20-item scale. Complete blinding for many physical treatments (e.g., exercise and manual therapies) is difficult or impossible to achieve.[109] Consequently, the validity scores derived from the Jadad scale were excluded from the data analysis.

A conciliatory approach presuming that MTrP diagnosis is reliable was taken in order to review the current outcome data and examine other issues raised in the current literature on MPS. However, the absence of accurate and reliable diagnostic criteria for MPS signifies a possibility that some of the content in the sources used in this review may be misleading. Where this is the case, the related data and conclusions of this review will be flawed.

## Conclusion

### Implications for Clinical Practice

The evidence for effectiveness of the different noninvasive interventions for MTrP pain rests on only small groups of separate trials or in some cases on an individual trial. Even where trials were generally of good quality, the presence of significant methodological flaws must be acknowledged. Thus, the strength of evidence is limited in most cases. A few of the treatments studied may be effective. However, it is not known whether they actually address the proposed pathological entity or other pathological processes. Greater attention should be given to the possibility that a diagnosis of MPS may lack validity and that chronic musculoskeletal pain is a multidimensional problem that requires a structured multimodal approach to treatment.

Considering the current evidence of effectiveness from this review together with other factors that affect clinical decision making, such as the cost of modalities, practitioner training, potential side effects, contraindications, and cost-effectiveness, it is recommended that clinicians consider neck exercises, stretching, and self-administered manual release as the first choice of noninvasive MTrP-specific therapy for patients presenting with MPS of the upper trapezius and neck. In addition, dry needling of MTrPs can be considered an option by clinicians with appropriate training in this technique.

## Implications for Research

Further high-quality trials are needed to establish a firmer basis for considering these treatments as viable options. The clinical effectiveness of the commonly used therapies for which there is some evidence of effect needs to be researched further. Trials should document the diagnostic criteria and precise location of MTrPs, and changes in the diagnostic characteristics of MPS should be included in the outcomes measurement. Where possible, future research should control for contributing and perpetuating factors. Greater attention should also be paid to randomization procedures and to ensuring adequate statistical power, because these were consistently weak throughout the included trials. To better inform decisions about patient management, trials should evaluate and document not only the differences between group means, but also the distribution of clinical values or outcomes within each treatment group.[36]

## Acknowledgment

This chapter was largely based on a paper published earlier in the *International Journal of Osteopathic Medicine* 2006;9(4):120–136.

## References

1. Cummings TM, White AR. Needling therapies in the management of myofascial trigger point pain: A systematic review. *Arch Phys Med Rehabil* 2001;82:986–992.
2. Kraft GH. Myofascial pain update. *Phys Med Rehabil Clin N Am* 1997;8:1–21.
3. Wheeler AH. Myofascial pain disorders: Theory to therapy. *Drugs* 2004;64:45–62.
4. Tough EA, White AR, Richards S, Campbell J. Variability of criteria used to diagnose myofascial trigger point pain syndrome: Evidence from a review of the literature. *Clin J Pain* 2007;23:278–286.
5. Cummings M. Regional myofascial pain: Diagnosis and management. *Best Pract Res Clin Rheumatol* 2007;21:367–387.
6. Bennett R. Myofascial pain syndromes and their evaluation. *Best Pract Res Clin Rheumatol* 2007;21:427–445.
7. Simons DG, Travell JG, Simons LS. *Travell & Simons' Myofascial Pain and Dysfunction: The Trigger Point Manual*. Vol 1. 2nd ed. Baltimore, MD: Lippincott Williams & Wilkins; 1999.
8. Daniels JM, Ishael T, Wesley RM. Managing myofascial pain syndrome: Sorting through the diagnosis and honing treatment. *Phys Sports Med* 2003;31:39–45.
9. Huguenin LK. Myofascial trigger points: The current evidence. *Phys Ther Sport* 2004;5:2–12.
10. Fernández-de-las-Peñas C, Campo MS, Fernández-Carnero J, Miangolarra-Page JC. Manual therapies in myofascial trigger point treatment: A systematic review. *J Bodywork Movement Ther* 2005;9:27–34.
11. Treaster D, Marras WS, Burr D, Sheedy JE, Hart D. Myofascial trigger point development from visual and postural stressors during computer work. *J Electrophys Kinesiol* 2006;16:115–124.
12. Dommerholt J, Bron C, Franssen J. Myofascial trigger points: An evidence-informed review. *J Manual Manipulative Ther* 2006;14:203–221.

13. Rivner MH. The neurophysiology of myofascial pain syndrome. *Curr Pain Headache Rep* 2001;5:432–440.
14. Simons DG. Review of enigmatic MTrPs as a common cause of enigmatic musculoskeletal pain and dysfunction. *J Electrophys Kinesiol* 2004;14:95–107.
15. Alvarez DJ, Rockwell PJ. Trigger points: Diagnosis and management. *Am Fam Phys* 2002;65:653–661.
16. Sciotti VM, Mittak VL, DiMarco L, Ford LM, Plezbert J, Santipadri E, Wigglesworth J, Ball K. Clinical precision of myofascial trigger point location in the trapezius muscle. *Pain* 2001;93: 259–266.
17. Gerwin RD, Dommerholt J, Shah JP. An expansion of Simon's integrated hypothesis of trigger point formation. *Curr Pain Headache Rep* 2004;8:468–475.
18. Hong C. Current research on myofascial trigger points: Pathophysiological studies. *J Musculoskel Pain* 1999;7:21–29.
19. Hong C. New trends in myofascial pain syndrome. *Chinese Medical Journal (Taipei)* 2002;65:501–512.
20. Sciotti VM, Mittak VL, DiMarco L, et al. Clinical precision of myofascial trigger point location in the trapezius muscle. *Pain* 2001;93:259–266.
21. Ward RC. *Foundations for Osteopathic Medicine.* Baltimore, MD: Lippincott, Williams & Wilkins; 1997:915.
22. Gerwin RD, Shannon S, Hong CZ, Hubbard D, Gevirtz R. Interrater reliability in myofascial trigger point examination. *Pain* 1997;69:65–73.
23. Al-Shenqiti AM, Oldham JA. Test–retest reliability of myofascial trigger point detection in patients with rotator cuff tendonitis. *Clin Rehabil* 2004;19:482–487.
24. Hsueh TC, Cheng PT, Kuan TS, Hong CZ. The immediate effectiveness of electrical nerve stimulation and electrical muscle stimulation on myofascial trigger points. *Am J Phys Med Rehabil* 1997;76:471–476.
25. Hou CR, Tsai LC, Cheng KF, Chung KC, Hong CZ. Immediate effects of various physical therapeutic modalities on cervical myofascial pain and trigger-point sensitivity. *Arch Phys Med Rehabil* 2002;83:1406–1414.
26. Esenyel M, Caglar N, Aldemir T. Treatment of myofascial pain. *Arch Phys Med Rehabil* 2000;79:48–52.
27. Greenwald R. Trigger point injections: A review of the literature. *Am J Pain Management* 2000;10:79–81.
28. Kovacs FM, Abraira V, Pozo F, et al. Local and remote sustained trigger point therapy for exacerbations of chronic low back pain. *Spine* 1997;22:786–797.
29. Smania N, Corato E, Fiaschi A, Pietropoli P, Aglioti SM, Tinazzi M. Therapeutic effects of peripheral repetitive magnetic stimulation on myofascial pain syndrome. *Clin Neurophysiol* 2003;114:350–358.
30. Snyder-Mackler L, Barry AJ, Perkins AI, Soucek MD. Effects of helium-neon laser irradiation on skin resistance and pain in patients with trigger points in the neck or back. *Phys Ther* 1989;69:336–341.
31. Jenson MG. Reviewing approaches to trigger point decompression. *Physician Assistant* 2002;26:37–41.
32. McPartland JM. Travell trigger points: Molecular and osteopathic perspectives. *J Am Osteopath Assoc* 2004;104:244–249.
33. Pratzel HG, Eigner UM, Weinert D, et al. The analgesic efficacy of sulfur mud baths in treating rheumatic diseases of the soft tissues: A study using the double-blind control method. *Vopr Kurortol Fizioter Lech Fiz Kult* 1992;May:37–41.

34. Sorrell MR, Flanagan W. Treatment of chronic resistant myofascial pain using a multidisciplinary protocol [The Myofascial Pain Program]. *J Musculoskel Pain* 2003;11:5–9.
35. Jaeger B, Reeves JL. Quantification of changes in myofascial trigger point sensitivity with the pressure algometer following passive stretch. *Pain* 1986;27:203–210.
36. Bronfort G, Nilsson N, Haas M, Evans R, Goldsmith CH, Assendelft WJJ, Bouter LM. Non-invasive physical treatments for chronic/recurrent headache (Cochrane Review). In: *The Cochrane Library*, Issue 3, 2004.
37. Airaksinen O, Pontinen PJ. Effects of the electrical stimulation of myofascial trigger points with tension headache. *Acupunct Electrother Res* 1992;17:285–290.
38. Airaksinen O, Kolari PJ, Rantanen P, Pontinen PJ. Effects of laser irradiation at the treated and non-treated trigger points. *Acupunct Electrother Res* 1988;13:238–239.
39. Airaksinen O, Rantanen P, Pertti K, Pontinen PJ. Effects of the infrared laser therapy at treated and non-treated trigger points. *Acupunct Electrother Res* 1989;14:9–14.
40. Ceylan Y, Hizmetli S, Silig Y. The effects of infrared laser and medical treatments on pain and serotonin degradation products in patients with myofascial pain syndrome. A controlled trial. *Rheumatol Internat* 2004;24:260–263.
41. Chee EK, Walton H. Treatment of trigger points with microamperage transcutaneous electrical nerve stimulation (TENS)—(the Electro-Acuscope 80). *J Manipulative Physiol Ther* 1986;9:131–134.
42. Curl DD, Emmerson GW. A preliminary study using infrared thermography to examine the effect of low voltage stimulation in treating trigger points. *American Chiropractor* 1987;66–67.
43. Dardzinski JA, Ostrov BE, Hamann LS. Myofascial pain unresponsive to standard treatment. Successful use of a strain and counterstrain technique with physical therapy. *J Clin Rheumatol* 2000;6:169–174.
44. Fryer G, Hodgson L. The effect of manual pressure release on myofascial trigger points in the upper trapezius muscle. *J Bodywork Movement Ther* 2005;9:248–255.
45. Hanten WP, Barrett M, Gillespie-Plesko M, Jump KA, Olson SL. Effects of active head retraction with retraction/extension and occipital release on the pressure pain threshold of cervical and scapular trigger points. *Physiother Theory Pract* 1997;13:285–291.
46. Hong CZ, Chen YC, Pon CH, Yu JJ. Immediate effects of various physical medicine modalities on pain threshold of an active myofascial trigger point. *J Musculoskel Pain* 1993;1:37–53.
47. Lewith GT, Machin D. A randomised trial to evaluate the effect of infrared stimulation of local trigger points, versus placebo, on the pain caused by cervical osteoarthrosis. *Acupunct Electrother Res* 1981;6:277–284.
48. Lundeberg TC. Vibratory stimulation for the alleviation of chronic pain. *Acta Physiol Scand* 1983;523(suppl);S1–S51.
49. McCray RE, Patton NJ. Pain relief at trigger points: A comparison of moist heat and shortwave diathermy. *J Orthop Sports Phys Ther* 1984;5:175–78.
50. Melzack R. Prolonged relief of pain by brief, intense transcutaneous somatic stimulation. *Pain* 1975;1:357–373.
51. Nilsson N. A randomized controlled trial of the effect of spinal manipulation in the treatment of cervicogenic headache. *J Manipulative Physiol Ther* 1995;18:435–440.
52. Pratzel HG, Tent G, Weinert D. Analgesic effect of thiosulfate bath treatment in tendomyopathy. *Physikalische Medizin Rehabilitationsmedizin Kurortmedizin* 1995;5:11–14.
53. Ruiz-Sáez M, Fernández-de-las-Peñas C, Blanco CR, Martínez-Segura R, García-León R. Changes in pressure pain sensitivity in latent myofascial trigger points in the upper trapezius muscle after a cervical spine manipulation in pain-free subjects. *J Manipulative Physiol Ther* 2007;30:578–583.

54. Schnider P, Moraru E, Vigl M, et al. Physical therapy and adjunctive botulinum toxin type A in the treatment of cervical headache: A double-blind, randomised, placebo-controlled study. *J Headache Pain* 2002;3:93–99.

55. Srbely JZ, Dickey JP. Randomized controlled study of the antinociceptive effect of ultrasound on trigger point sensitivity: Novel application in myofascial therapy? *Clin Rehabil* 2007;21: 411–417.

56. Simunovic Z. Low level laser therapy with trigger points technique: A clinical study on 243 patients. *J Clin Laser Med Surg* 1996;14:163–167.

57. Simunovic Z, Trobonjaca T, Trobonjaca Z. Treatment of medial and lateral epicondylitis—tennis and golfer's elbow—with low level laser therapy: A multicenter double blind, placebo-controlled clinical study on 324 patients. *J Clin Laser Med Surg* 1998;16:145–151.

58. Snyder-Mackler L, Bork C, Bourbon B, Trumbore D. Effect of helium-neon laser on musculoskeletal trigger points. *Phys Ther* 1986;66:1087–1090.

59. Yagci N, Uygur F, Bek N. Comparison of connective tissue massage and spray-and-stretch technique in the treatment of chronic cervical myofascial pain syndrome. *The Pain Clinic* 2004;16:469–474.

60. Graff-Radford SB, Reeves JL, Baker RL, Chiu D. Effects of transcutaneous electrical nerve stimulation on myofascial pain and trigger point sensitivity. *Pain* 1989;37:1–5.

61. Brown CS, Ling FW, Wan JY, Pilla AA. Efficacy of static magnetic field therapy in chronic pelvic pain: A double-blind pilot study. *Am J Obstet Gynaecol* 2002;187:1581–1587.

62. Chatchawan U, Thinkhamrop B, Kharmwan S, Knowles J, Eungpinichpong W. Effectiveness of traditional Thai massage versus Swedish massage among patients with back pain associated with myofascial trigger points. *J Bodywork Movement Ther* 2009;9:298–309.

63. Edwards J, Knowles N. Superficial dry needling and active stretching in the treatment of myofascial pain: A randomised controlled trial. *Acupunct Med* 2003;21(3):80–86.

64. Ilbuldu E, Cakmak A, Disci R, Aydin R. Comparison of laser, dry needling, and placebo laser treatments in myofascial pain syndrome. *Photomedicine Laser Surgery* 2004;22:306–311.

65. Gur A, Sarac AJ, Cevik R, Altindag O, Sarac S. Efficacy of 904 nm gallium arsenide low level laser therapy in the management of chronic myofascial pain in the neck: A double-blind and randomize-controlled trial. *Lasers Surg Med* 2004;35:229–235.

66. Altan L, Bingol U, Aykac M, Yurtkuran M. Investigation of the effect of Ga-As laser therapy on cervical myofascial pain syndrome. *Rheumatol Internat* 2003;25:23–27.

67. Ceccherelli F, Altafini L, Lo Castro G, Avila A, Ambrosio F, Giron GP. Diode laser in cervical myofascial pain: A double-blind study versus placebo. *Clin J Pain* 1989;5:301–304.

68. Hakguder A, Birtane M, Gurcan S, Kokino S, Turan FN. Efficacy of low level laser therapy in myofascial pain syndrome: An algometric and thermographic evaluation. *Lasers Surg Med* 2003;33:339–343.

69. Dundar U, Evcik D, Samli F, Pusak, Kavuncu V. The effect of gallium arsenide aluminium laser therapy in the management of cervical myofascial pain syndrome: A double blind, placebo-controlled study. *Clin Rheumatol* 2007;26:930–934.

70. Lee JC, Lin DT, Hong C. The effectiveness of simultaneous thermotherapy with ultrasound and electrotherapy with combined AC and DC current on the immediate pain relief of myofascial trigger points. *J Musculoskel Pain* 1997;5:81–90.

71. Ardic F, Sarhus M, Topuz O. Comparison of two different techniques of electrotherapy on myofascial pain. *J Back Musculoskel Rehabil* 2002;16:11–16.

72. Smania N, Corato E, Fiaschi A, Pietropoli P, Aglioti SM, Tinazzi M. Repetitive magnetic stimulation: A novel approach for myofascial pain syndrome. *J Neurol* 2005;252:307–314.

73. Farina S, Casarotto M, Benelle M, Tinazzi M, Fiaschi A, Goldoni M, Smainia, N. A randomised controlled study on the effect of two different treatments (FREMS and TENS) in myofascial pain syndrome. *Europa Medicophysica* 2004;40:293–301.

74. Tanrikut A, Ozaras N, Ali Kaptan H, Guven Z, Kayhan O. High voltage galvanic stimulation in myofascial pain syndrome. *J Musculoskel Pain* 2003;11:11–15.

75. Gam AN, Warming S, Larsen LH, et al. Treatment of myofascial trigger-points with ultrasound combined with massage and exercise: A randomised controlled trial. *Pain* 1998;77:73–79.

76. Majlesi J, Unalan H. High-power pain threshold ultrasound technique in the treatment of active myofascial trigger points: A randomized, double-blind, case-control study. *Arch Phys Med Rehabil* 2004;85:833–836.

77. Esenyel M, Aldemir T, Gursoy E, Esenyel CZ, Demir S, Durmusoglu G. Myofascial pain syndrome: Efficacy of different therapies. *J Back Musculoskel Rehabil* 2007;20:43–47.

78. Smania N, Corato E, Fiaschi A, Pietropoli P, Aglioti SM, Tinazzi M. Repetitive magnetic stimulation: A novel approach for myofascial pain syndrome. *J Neurol* 2005;252:307–314.

79. Hanten WP, Olson SL, Butts NL, Nowicki AL. Effectiveness of a home program of ischemic pressure followed by sustained stretch for treatment of myofascial trigger points. *Phys Ther* 2000;80:997–1003.

80. Fernández-de-las-Peñas C, Alonso-Blanco C, Fernández-Carnero J, Miangolarra-Page JC. The immediate effect of ischemic compression technique and transverse friction on tenderness of active and latent myofascial trigger points: A pilot study. *J Bodywork Movement Ther* 2006;10:3–9.

81. Gemmell H, Miller P, Nordstrom H. Immediate effect of ischaemic compression and trigger point pressure release on neck pain and upper trapezius trigger points: A randomised controlled trial. *Clin Chiropr* 2007;11:30–36.

82. Redmond A, Keenan AM. Understanding statistics: putting *P*-values into perspective. *Australasian Journal of Podiatric Medicine* 2000;34:125–131.

83. Guyatt GH, Osoba D, Wu AW, Wyrwich KW, Norman GR. Methods to explain the clinical significance of health status measures. *Mayo Clinic Proceedings* 2002;77:371–383.

84. Kroeling P, Gross A, Goldsmith CH, Cervical Overview Group. Electrotherapy for neck disorders. *The Cochrane Database of Systematic Reviews*. 2005, Issue 2.

85. Robertson VJ, Baker KG. A review of therapeutic ultrasound: Effectiveness studies. *Phys Ther* 2001;81:1339–1350.

86. Fernández-de-las-Peñas C, Campo MS, Fernández-Carnero J, Miangolarra-Page JC. Manual therapies in myofascial trigger point treatment: A systematic review. *J Bodywork Movement Ther* 2005;9:27–34.

87. Gerwin RD. A review of myofascial pain and fibromyalgia: Factors that promote their persistence. *Acupunct Med* 2005;23:121–134.

88. Simons DG. Understanding effective treatments of myofascial trigger points. *J Bodywork Movement Ther* 2002;6:81–88.

89. Fine PG, Milano R, Hare BD. The effects of myofascial trigger point injections are naloxone reversible. *Pain* 1988;32:15–20.

90. Niddam DM, Chan RC, Lee HS, Yeh TC, Hsieh JC. Central modulation of pain evoked from myofascial trigger point. *Clin J Pain* 2007;23:440–448.

91. McClaflin RR. Myofascial pain syndrome: Primary care strategies for early intervention. *Postgrad Med* 1994;96:56–73.

92. Graff-Radford SB, Reeves JL, Jaeger B: Management of head and neck pain: The effectiveness of altering perpetuating factors in myofascial pain. *Headache* 1986;27:186–190.

93. Hopwood MB, Abram SE. Factors associated with failure of trigger point injections. *Clin J Pain* 1994;10:227–234.
94. Graven-Nielsen T, Arendt-Nielsen L. Peripheral and central sensitization in musculoskeletal pain disorders: An experimental approach. *Curr Rheumatol Rep* 2002;4:313–321.
95. Graff-Radford SB. Myofascial pain: Diagnosis and management. *Curr Pain Headache Rep* 2004;8;463–467.
96. Bajaj P, Graven-Nielsen T, Arendt-Nielsen L. Trigger points in patients with lower limb osteoarthritis. *J Musculoskel Pain* 2001;9:17–33.
97. Shah JP, Phillips TM, Danoff JV, Gerber LH. An in vivo microanalytical technique for measuring the local biochemical milieu of human skeletal muscle. *J Appl Physiol* 2005;99: 1977–1984.
98. Simons DG. Review of Microanalytical in vivo study of biochemical milieu of myofascial trigger points. *J Bodywork Movement Ther* 2006;10:10–11.
99. Millan MJ. The induction of pain: An integrative review. *Progress in Neurobiology* 1999;57:1–164.
100. Campbell JN, Meyer RA. Mechanisms of neuropathic pain. *Neuron* 2006;52:77–92.
101. Quintner JL, Cohen ML. Referred pain of peripheral nerve origin: An alternative to the 'myofascial pain construct.' *Clin J Pain*.1994;10:243–251.
102. Butler D. *The Sensitive Nervous System.* Adelaide, Australia: NOI publications; 2000:65.
103. Moher D, Fortin P, Jadad AR, et al. Completeness of reporting of trials published in languages other than English: Implications for conduct and reporting of systematic reviews. *Lancet* 1996;347:363–366.
104. Rosenthal R. The file drawer problem and tolerance for null results. *Psychological Bulletin* 1979;86:638–641.
105. Alderson P, Green S, Higgins JPT, eds. *Cochrane Reviewers' Handbook 4.2.2* [updated December 2003]. Available at: http://www.cochrane.org/resources/handbook/hbook.htm. Accessed July 9, 2004.
106. Jadad AR, Moore RA, Carroll D, Jenkinson C, Reynolds DJ, Gavaghan DJ. Assessing the quality of reports of randomized clinical trials: Is blinding necessary? *Controlled Clinical Trials* 1996;17:1–12.
107. Berlin JA. Does blinding of readers affect the results of meta-analyses? *Lancet* 1997;350: 185–186.
108. Moher D, Jadad AR, Nichol G, Penman M, Tugwell P, Walsh S. Assessing the quality of randomized controlled trials: an annotated bibliography of scales and checklists. *Controlled Clinical Trials* 1995;16:62–73.
109. Hawk C, Long CR, Reiter R, Davis CS, Cambron JA, Evans R. Issues in planning a placebo-controlled trial of manual methods: results of a pilot study. *J Alternative Complementary Med* 2002;8:21–32.

Chapter 8

# Trigger Point Dry Needling

*Jan Dommerholt, PT, MPS, DPT, DAAPM*

*Orlando Mayoral del Moral, PT*

*Christian Gröbli, PT*

## Introduction

Trigger point dry needling (TrP-DN), also referred to as intramuscular stimulation (IMS), is an invasive procedure in which an acupuncture needle is inserted into the skin and muscle. As the name implies, TrP-DN is directed at myofascial trigger points (MTrPs), which are defined as "hyperirritable spots in skeletal muscle that are associated with a hypersensitive palpable nodule in a taut band."[1] Physical therapists around the world practice TrP-DN as part of their clinical practice and use the technique in combination with other physical therapy interventions. TrP-DN falls within the scope of physical therapy practice in many countries, including Canada, Chile, Ireland, The Netherlands, South Africa, Spain, and the United Kingdom. In 2002, two Dutch medical courts ruled that TrP-DN is within the scope of physical therapy practice in The Netherlands even though the Royal Dutch Physical Therapy Association had expressed the opinion that TrP-DN should not be part of physical therapy practice.[2-4] Of the approximately 9,000 physical therapists in South Africa, over 75% are estimated to employ the technique at least once daily (Stavrou, personal communication, 2006). Physical therapy continuing education programs in TrP-DN in Ireland, Switzerland, and Spain are popular among physical therapists. In Spain, several universities offer academic and specialist certification programs featuring TrP-DN as an integral component of invasive physical therapy.[5]

In the United States and Australia, TrP-DN is not commonly included in physical therapy entry-level educational curricula or postgraduate continuing education programs. Relatively few physical therapists in the United States have received training and employ the technique. The only known U.S. physical therapy academic program that includes course work in TrP-DN is the entry-level doctorate of physical therapy curriculum

Courtesy of John M. Medeiros, PT, PhD, managing editor of the *Journal of Manual and Manipulative Therapy*.

at Georgia State University. Other universities are exploring adding dry needling to their curricula. Physical therapy state boards of Alabama, Colorado, Georgia, Kentucky, Maryland, New Hampshire, New Mexico, Ohio, Oregon, South Carolina, Texas, and Virginia have determined in recent years that TrP-DN does fall within the scope of physical therapy in those states. Several other state boards are currently reviewing whether dry needling should fall within the scope of physical therapy practice, and the Director of Regulations of the State of Colorado has issued a specific "Director's Policy on Intramuscular Stimulation" (**Table 8-1**).[6]

In contrast, the Tennessee Board of Occupational and Physical Therapy concluded in 2002 that TrP-DN is not an acceptable physical therapy technique. The decision of the Tennessee board was "based on the need for education and training," or, in other words, the realization that TrP-DN is not commonly included in the physical therapy curricula of U.S. academic programs.[5,7] Some state laws have defined the practice of physical therapy as noninvasive, which would implicitly put TrP-DN outside the scope of physical therapy in those states. For example, the Hawaii Physical Therapy Practice Act specifies that physical therapists not be allowed to penetrate the skin.[8] The definition of the practice of physical therapy according to a 2009 Florida statute states that, among other things, the practice of physical therapy "means the performance of acupuncture only upon compliance with the criteria set forth by the Board of Medicine, when no penetration of the skin occurs."[9] Whether TrP-DN would be considered as falling under this peculiar definition has not been contested, and the Florida statutes do not provide any guidelines as to how to perform acupuncture without penetration of the skin.[9] In 2008, the Chiropractic Board of Maryland approved dry needling as part of the chiropractic scope of practice.

The introduction of TrP-DN to American physical therapists shares many similarities with the introduction of manual therapy. When New Zealand physical therapist Stanley Paris expressed his interest in manual therapy during the 1960s, he experienced considerable resistance, not only from academia, but also from employers, the American Physical Therapy Association (APTA), and even from Dr. Janet Travell.[10] Paris reported that in 1966 Dr. Travell blocked his membership in the North American Academy of Manipulative Medicine, an organization she had founded with Dr. John Mennell, on the grounds that "manipulation is a diagnostic and therapeutic tool to be reserved for physicians only."[10] Similarly, the 2002 rejection of TrP-DN by the Tennessee Board of Occupational and Physical Therapy was in part based on the testimony of an academic expert witness.[7] In 2006, the APTA omitted an educational activity about physical therapy and dry needling from the tentative agenda of its annual conference, while the Royal Dutch Physical Therapy Association upheld the opinion that TrP-DN should not fall within the scope of physical therapy practice. In October 2006, the Virginia Board of Physical Therapy heard arguments from physician and acupuncture organizations against physical therapists using TrP-DN. Within the context of autonomous physical therapy practice, TrP-DN does seem to fit the current practice model in spite of the reservations of other disciplines and some physical therapy professional organizations. In 2009, the Executive Committee of

**TABLE 8-1   The Colorado Physical Therapy Licensure Rules and Regulations 4 Ccr 732-1, Includes Rule 11—Requirements for Physical Therapists to Perform Dry Needling**

| | |
|---|---|
| A | Dry needling is a physical intervention that uses a filiform needle to stimulate trigger points, diagnose and treat neuromuscular pain and functional movement deficits, is based upon Western medical concepts, requires an examination and diagnosis, and treats specific anatomic entities selected according to physical signs. Dry needling does not include the stimulation of auricular or distal points. |
| B | Dry needling as defined pursuant to this rule is within the scope of practice of physical therapy. |
| C | A physical therapist must have the knowledge, skill, ability, and documented competency to perform an act that is within the physical therapist's scope of practice. |
| D | To be deemed competent to perform dry needling a physical therapist must meet the following requirements:<br>1. Documented successful completion of a dry needling course of study. The course must meet the following requirements:<br>   a. A minimum of 46 hours of face-to-face IMS/dry needling course study; online study is not considered appropriate training.<br>   b. Two years of practice as a licensed physical therapist prior to using the dry needling technique. |
| E | A provider of a dry needling course of study must meet the educational and clinical prerequisites as defined in this rule, D (1) (a) & (b) and demonstrate a minimum of two years of dry needling practice techniques. The provider is not required to be a physical therapist. |
| F | A physical therapist performing dry needling in his/her practice must have written informed consent for each patient where this technique is used. The patient must sign and receive a copy of the informed consent form. The consent form must, at a minimum, clearly state the following information:<br>1. Risks and benefits of dry needling.<br>2. Physical therapist's level of education and training in dry needling.<br>3. The physical therapist will not stimulate any distal or auricular points during dry needling. |
| H | When dry needling is performed this must be clearly documented in the procedure notes and must indicate how the patient tolerated the technique as well as the outcome after the procedure. |
| I | Dry needling shall not be delegated and must be directly performed by a qualified, licensed physical therapist. |

*(continued)*

**TABLE 8-1   The Colorado Physical Therapy Licensure Rules and Regulations 4 Ccr 732-1, Includes Rule 11—Requirements for Physical Therapists to Perform Dry Needling (cont.)**

| | |
|---|---|
| J | Dry needling must be performed in a manner consistent with generally accepted standards of practice, including clean needle techniques and standards of the Center for Communicable Diseases. |
| K | The physical therapist must be able to supply written documentation, upon request by the Director, which substantiates appropriate training as required by this rule. Failure to provide written documentation is a violation of this rule, and is *prima facie* evidence that the physical therapist is not competent and not permitted to perform dry needling. |
| L | This rule is intended to regulate and clarify the scope of practice for physical therapists. |

*Source:* Williams T. Colorado Physical Therapy Licensure Policies of the Director; Policy 3—Director's Policy on Intramuscular Stimulation. Denver, CO: State of Colorado, Department of Regulatory Agencies, 2005.

the American Academy of Orthopaedic Manual Physical Therapists issued a position statement that dry needling falls within the scope of physical therapy practice.

In order to practice TrP-DN, physical therapists need to be able to demonstrate competence or adequate training in the technique and practice in a jurisdiction where TrP-DN is considered within the scope of physical therapy practice. Many country and state physical therapy statutes address the issue of competence by including language such as the following: "physical therapists shall not perform any procedure or function which they are by virtue of education or training not competent to perform."[5] Obviously, physical therapists employing TrP-DN must have excellent knowledge of anatomy and be very familiar with its indications, contraindications, and precautions. This chapter provides an overview of TrP-DN in the context of contemporary physical therapy practice.

## Dry Needling Techniques

Because dry needling techniques emerged empirically, different schools and conceptual models have been developed, including the radiculopathy model, the MTrP model, and the spinal segmental sensitization model.[1,5,11-13] In addition, other less common needling approaches, such as neural acupuncture and automated or electrical twitch-obtaining intramuscular stimulation, exist.[14-22] In neural acupuncture, acupuncture points are infiltrated with lidocaine for the treatment of myofascial pain.[14,15] A medical specialist, Dr. Jennifer Chu, developed electrical twitch-obtaining intramuscular stimulation; this approach combines aspects of the radiculopathy model with the trigger point model.[16-23]

The radiculopathy model will be reviewed briefly, whereas the MTrP model will be discussed in detail. The spinal segmental sensitization model and neural acupuncture are not included in this chapter due to their exclusive use of injections, which are outside the scope of physical therapy practice in most jurisdictions.[5,12]

Another classification is based on the depth of the needle insertion and distinguishes superficial dry needling (SDN) and deep dry needling (DDN).[24,25] Examples of SDN include Baldry's SDN approach and Fu's subcutaneous needling, which fall within the trigger point (TrP) model.[24,26-29] The needling approach advocated by the radiculopathy model is a form of DDN. The TrP model includes both superficial dry needling (TrP-SDN) and deep dry needling (TrP-DDN) (**Table 8-2**).

## Radiculopathy Model

The radiculopathy model is based on empirical observations by Canadian medical physician Dr. Chan Gunn, who was one of the early pioneers of dry needling. A review of TrP-DN would be incomplete without including a brief summary of Gunn's needling approach, although the radiculopathy model no longer includes TrP-DN.[13] Initially, Gunn incorporated MTrPs in his thinking, but fairly soon he moved away from MTrPs and further developed and defined his DDN approach, referred to as intramuscular stimulation, or IMS.[18-20] Gunn introduced the term "IMS" to distinguish his approach from other needling and injection approaches, but the term frequently is used to describe any dry needling technique.[30] According to Gunn's web site, "hundreds of doctors and physiotherapists from all around the world" have been trained in the technique.[31] The web site also mentions that "some practitioners employ altered versions of IMS not endorsed by Professor Gunn or the medical community."[31]

The Gunn IMS technique is based on the premise that myofascial pain syndrome (MPS) is always the result of peripheral neuropathy or radiculopathy, defined by Gunn as "a condition that causes disordered function in the peripheral nerve."[30] In Gunn's view, shortening of the paraspinal muscles, particularly the multifidi muscles, leads to disc compression, narrowing of the intervertebral foramina, or direct pressure on the nerve root, which subsequently would result in peripheral neuropathy and compression of supersensitive nociceptors and pain.

The radiculopathy model is based on Cannon and Rosenblueth's Law of Denervation, which maintains that the function and integrity of innervated structures is dependent upon the free flow of nerve impulses.[32] When the flow of nerve impulses is restricted, all innervated structures, including skeletal muscle, smooth muscle, spinal neurons, sympathetic

| TABLE 8-2 | Models of Needling | | |
| --- | --- | --- | --- |
| | **Trigger Point Model** | **Radiculopathy Model** | **Spinal Segmental Sensitization Model** |
| Superficial dry needling | Yes | No | No |
| Deep dry needling | Yes | Yes | No |
| Injection therapy | Yes | No | Yes |

ganglia, adrenal glands, sweat cells, and brain cells become atrophic, highly irritable, and supersensitive.[30] Gunn suggested that many common diagnoses, such as Achilles tendonitis, lateral epicondylitis, frozen shoulder, chrondromalacia patellae, headaches, plantar fasciitis, temporomandibular joint dysfunction, myofascial pain syndrome (MPS), and others, might in fact be the result of neuropathy.[30] Chu has adapted Gunn's radiculopathy model in that she has recognized that MTrPs are frequently the result of cervical or lumbar radiculopathy.[16,18,22,23]

Gunn[13] maintained that the most effective treatment points are always located close to the muscle motor points or musculotendinous junctions, which are distributed in a segmental or myotomal fashion in muscles supplied by the primary anterior and posterior rami. Because the primary posterior rami are segmentally linked to the paraspinal muscles, including the multifidi, and the primary anterior rami with the remainder of the myotome, the treatment must always include the paraspinal muscles as well as the more peripheral muscles. Gunn found that the tender points usually coincided with painful palpable muscle bands in shortened and contracted muscles. He suggested that nerve root dysfunction is particularly due to spondylotic changes. According to Gunn, relatively minor injuries would not result in severe pain that continues beyond a "reasonable" period, unless the nerve root was already in a sensitized state prior to the injury.[13]

Gunn's assessment technique is based on the evaluation of specific motor, sensory, and trophic changes. The main objective of the initial examination is to find characteristic signs of neuropathic pain and to determine which segmental levels are involved in a given individual. The examination is rather limited and does not include standard medical and physical therapy evaluation techniques, including common orthopaedic or neurological tests, laboratory tests, electromyographic or nerve conduction tests, or radiologic tests, such as MRI, CT, or even x-rays. Motor changes are assessed through a few functional motor tests and through systematic palpation of the skin and muscle bands along the spine and in those peripheral muscles that belong to the involved myotomes. Gunn emphasized evaluating the paraspinal regions for trophic changes, which may include orange peel skin (*peau d'orange*), dermatomal hair loss, and differences in skin folds and moisture levels (dry versus moist skin).[13]

Gunn et al completed one of the first dry needling outcome studies, which demonstrated that IMS can be an effective treatment option, but there are no studies that substantiate the theoretical basis of the radiculopathy model or of the IMS needling interventions.[5,33]

Although Gunn emphasized the importance of being able to objectively verify the findings of neuropathic pain,[34] there also are no interrater reliability studies and no studies that support the idea that the described findings are indeed indicative of neuropathic pain.[5] For example, there is no scientific evidence that an MTrP is always a manifestation of radiculopathy resulting from trauma to a nerve, even though it is conceivable that one possible cause of the formation of MTrPs is indeed nerve damage or dysfunction.[35] Interestingly, Gunn did not regard his model as a hypothesis but rather considered it a mere "description of clinical findings that can be found by anyone who examines a patient for radiculopathy."[34] However, without scientific validation, the radiculopathy model was never developed beyond the hypothetical stage. Gunn's conclusion that relative minor injuries would not result in chronic pain without prior sensitization of the nerve root is inconsistent with many current neurophysiological studies that confirm that persistent and even relatively brief nociceptive input can result in pain-producing plastic dorsal horn changes.[36-42]

## Trigger Point Model

Clinicians practicing from the perspective of the trigger point model specifically target MTrPs. The clinical manifestation of MTrPs is referred to as MPS and is defined as the "sensory, motor, and autonomic symptoms caused by MTrPs."[1] Myofascial trigger points may consist of multiple contraction knots, which are thought to be due to an excessive release of acetylcholine (ACh) from select motor endplates, and can be divided into active and latent MTrPs.[1,43,44] The release of ACh has been associated with endplate noise, a characteristic electromyographic discharge at MTrP sites, consisting of low-amplitude discharges in the order of 10-50 μV and intermittent high-amplitude discharges (up to 500 μV) in painful MTrPs.[45-47] Active MTrPs can spontaneously trigger local pain in the vicinity of the MTrP, or they can refer pain or paresthesiae to more distant locations. They cause muscle weakness, range of motion restrictions, and several autonomic phenomena. Latent MTrPs do not trigger local or referred pain without being stimulated, but they may alter muscle activation patterns and contribute to limited range of motion.[48] Simons, Travell, and Simons documented the referred pain patterns of MTrPs in 147 muscles,[1] while Dejung et al[49] published slightly different referred pain patterns based on their empirical findings. Several case reports and research studies have examined referred pain patterns from MTrPs.[50-71] Following Kellgren's early studies of muscle referred pain patterns, which contributed to Travell's interest in musculoskeletal pain, many studies have been published on muscle referred pain without specifically mentioning MTrPs. This brings up the question as to whether referred pain patterns are characteristic of each muscle or can be established for specific MTrPs.[72-84] MTrPs are identified manually by using either a flat palpation—for example with palpation of the infraspinatus, the masseter, temporalis, and lower trapezius—or a pincer-type palpation technique, for example with palpation of the sternocleidomastoid, the upper trapezius, and the gastrocnemius.[1]

The interrater reliability of identifying MTrPs has been studied by several researchers and was established in a small number of studies.[85-87] Gerwin et al[86] concluded that training is essential to reliably identify MTrPs, while Sciotti et al[87] confirmed the clinically adequate interrater reliability of locating latent MTrPs in the trapezius muscle. As also discussed in Chapter 5, Bron et al reported that three blinded observers were able to reach acceptable agreement on the presence or absence of TrPs in the shoulder region. The authors concluded that palpation of MTrPs is reliable and might be a useful tool in the diagnosis of myofascial pain in patients with nontraumatic shoulder pain.[85] A recent study of the intrarater reliability of identifying MTrPs in patients with rotator cuff tendonitis reached perfect agreement expressed ($\kappa = 1.0$) for the taut band, spot tenderness, jump sign, and pain

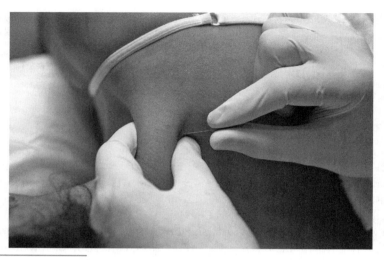

**Figure 8-1**   Trigger point dry needling of the trapezius muscle.

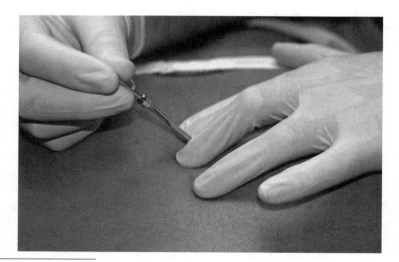

**Figure 8-2**   Trigger point dry needling of the thoracic multifidi muscles using a Japanese needle plunger.

recognition, which the author attributed to methodological rigor.[88] However, considering the small sample size and limited variation in the subjects used in this study, it might have been inappropriate to establish the intrarater reliability using the kappa statistic.[89]

Diagnostically, TrP-DDN can assist in differentiating between pain that originates from a joint, an entrapped nerve, or a muscle. Mechanical stimulation or deformation of a

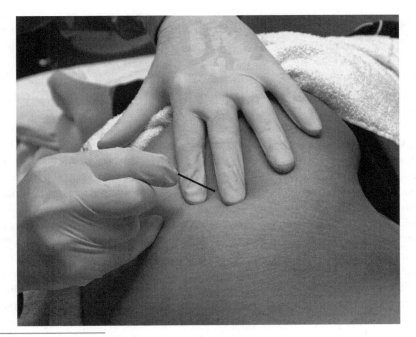

**Figure 8-3**  Trigger point dry needling of the gluteus medius muscle.

sensitized MTrP can reproduce the patient's pain complaint due to MTrPs when the DDN technique is used.[90,91] In most instances, it is relatively easy to trigger the patient's referred pain pattern with TrP-DDN compared to manual techniques. When the pain originates in deeper structures, such as the multifidi, supraspinatus, psoas, or soleus muscles, manual techniques may be inadequate and may not provide sufficient diagnostic information. In addition, myofascial pain may mimic radicular pain syndromes.[55] For example, pain resembling a C8 or L5 radiculopathy may be due to MTrPs in the teres minor muscle or the gluteus minimus muscle, respectively. If needling an MTrP elicits the patient's familiar referred pain down the involved extremity, the cause of at least part of the pain is likely myofascial in nature and not (solely) neurogenic.[55,92] The ability to reproduce the patient's pain has great diagnostic value and can assist in the differential diagnostic process.

One of the unique features of MTrPs is the phenomenon of the so-called local twitch response (LTR), which is an involuntary spinal cord reflex contraction of the muscle fibers in a taut band following palpation or needling of the band or MTrP.[93,94] Local twitch responses can be elicited manually by snapping taut bands that harbor MTrPs. When using invasive procedures like TrP-DDN or injections therapeutically, eliciting LTRs is essential.[95] Not only is the treatment outcome much improved, but LTRs also confirm that the needle was indeed placed into a taut band, which is particularly important when needling MTrPs close to peripheral nerves or viscera, such as the lungs.[25]

## Intramuscular Electrical Stimulation

One of the advantages of TrP-DN is that physical therapists can easily combine the needling procedures with electrical stimulation. Several terms have been used to describe electrical stimulation through acupuncture needles, including percutaneous electrical nerve stimulation (PENS), percutaneous electrical muscle stimulation, percutaneous neuromodulation therapy, and electroacupuncture (EA).[96-99] Mayoral del Moral suggested using the term "intramuscular electrical stimulation" (IES) when applied within the context of physical therapy practice.[25] White et al[99] demonstrated that the best results were achieved when the needles were placed within the dermatomes corresponding to the local pathology. Using the needles as electrodes offers many advantages over more traditional transcutaneous nerve stimulation (TENS). Not only is the resistance of the skin to electrical currents eliminated, but several studies have also demonstrated that PENS provided more pain relief and improved functionality than TENS, for example in patients with sciatica and chronic low back pain.[100,101] Animal experiments have shown that EA can modulate the expression of N-methyl-D-aspartate in primary sensory neurons with involvement of glutamate receptors.[102,103]

Not much is known about the optimal treatment parameters for IES. Although EA units offer many options for amplitude and frequencies, little research has linked these options to the management of pain. Frequencies between 2–4 Hz with high intensity are commonly used in nociceptive pain conditions and may result in the release of endorphins and enkephalins. For neuropathic pain, it is recommended to use currents with a frequency between 80–100 Hz, which are thought to affect release of dynorphin, gamma-aminobutyric acid, and galanin.[104] However, a study examining the effects of high- and low-frequency EA in pain after abdominal surgery found that both frequencies significantly reduced the pain.[105] Another study concluded that high-intensity levels were more effective than low-intensity stimulation.[97] In IES, the negative electrode is usually placed in the MTrP and the positive in the taut band but outside the MTrP. Elorriaga recommended inserting two converging electrodes in the MTrP, while Mayoral del Moral et al suggested inserting the electrodes at both sides of an MTrP inside the taut band.[106,107] Chu developed an electrical stimulation modality that automatically elicits LTRs, which she referred to as "electrical twitch-obtaining intramuscular stimulation," or ETOIMS.[18,21,22] The technique can also be simulated using standard EMG equipment.[23]

## Superficial Dry Needling

In the early 1980s, Baldry was concerned about the risk of causing a pneumothorax when treating a patient with an MTrP in the anterior scalene muscle. Rather than using TrP-DDN, he inserted the needle superficially into the tissue immediately overlying the MTrP. After leaving the needle in for a short time, the exquisite tenderness at the MTrP was abolished and the spontaneous pain was alleviated.[24] Based on this experience,

Baldry expanded the practice of SDN and applied the technique to MTrPs throughout the body with good empirical results, even in the treatment of MTrPs in deeper muscles.[24] He recommended inserting an acupuncture needle into the tissues overlying each MTrP to a depth of 5–10 mm for 30 seconds.[24] Because the needle does not necessarily reach the MTrP, LTRs are not expected. Nevertheless, the patient commonly experiences an immediate decrease in sensitivity following the needling procedure. If there is any residual pain, the needle is reinserted for another 2–3 minutes. When using the TrP-SDN technique, Baldry commented that the amount of needle stimulation depends on an individual's responsiveness. In so-called average responders, Baldry recommended leaving the needle *in situ* for 30–60 seconds. In weak responders, the needle may be left for up to 2–3 minutes. There is some evidence from animal studies that this responsiveness is at least partially genetically determined. Mice deficient in endogenous opioid peptide receptors did not respond well to needle-evoked nerve stimulation.[108] Baldry suggested that weak responders might have excessive amounts of endogenous opioid peptide antagonists.[24] Baldry preferred TrP-SDN over TrP-DDN, but indicated that in cases where MTrPs were secondary to the development of radiculopathy, he would consider using TrP-DDN.[24]

Another SDN technique was developed in 1996 in China.[27,29] Initially, Fu's subcutaneous needling (FSN), also referred to as "floating needling," was developed to treat various pain problems without consideration of MTrPs, such as chronic low back pain, fibromyalgia, osteoarthritis, chronic pelvic pain, postherpetic pain, peripheral neuropathy, and complex regional pain syndrome.[29] In a recent paper, Fu et al[28] applied their needling technique to MTrPs and examined whether the direction of the needle is relevant in that treatment. The needle was either directed across muscle fibers or along muscle fibers toward an MTrP. The authors concluded that FSN had an immediate effect on inactivating MTrPs in the neck, irrespective of the direction of the needle.[28]

The FSN needle consists of three parts: a 31 mm beveled-tip needle with a 1 mm diameter, a soft tube similar to an intravenous catheter, and a cap. The needle is directed toward a painful spot or MTrP at an angle of 20–30° with the skin but does not penetrate muscle tissue. The technique acts solely in the subcutaneous layers. The needle is advanced parallel to the skin surface until the soft tube is also under the skin. At that time, the needle is moved smoothly and rhythmically from side to side for at least 2 minutes, after which the needle is removed from the soft tube, which stays in place. Patients go home with the soft tube still inserted under the skin. The soft tube can move slightly underneath the skin because of patients' movements and is thought to continue to stimulate subcutaneous connective tissues while in place.[27-29] The soft tube is kept under the skin for a few hours for acute injuries and for at least 24 hours for chronic pain problems, after which it is removed.[27,29] According to Fu et al, the technique has no adverse or side effects and usually induces an immediate reduction of pain. The needle technique should not be painful, as subcutaneous layers are poorly innervated.[27-29] Because FSN was only recently introduced to the Western world, the technique has not been used much outside of China, and there are no other clinical outcome studies.

## Effectiveness of Trigger Point Dry Needling

The effectiveness of TrP-DN is, to some extent, dependent upon the ability to accurately palpate MTrPs. Without the required excellent palpation skills, TrP-DN can be a rather random process. In addition to being able to palpate MTrPs before using TrP-DN, it is equally important that clinicians develop the skills to accurately needle the MTrPs identified with palpation. Physical therapists need to learn how to visualize a 3D image of the exact location and depth of the MTrP within the muscle. The level of kinesthetic perception needed to perform TrP-DN safely and accurately is a learned skill. Noë[109] maintained that such perception is constituted in part by sensorimotor knowledge but also depends on having sufficient knowledge of the subject.[109] The ability to perceive the end of the needle and the pathways the needle takes inside the patient's body is a developed skill on the part of the physical therapist, a process Noë referred to as an "enactive" approach to perception.[109] A high degree of kinesthetic perception allows a physical therapist to use the needle as a palpation tool and to appreciate changes in the firmness of those tissues pierced by the needle.[25] For example, a trained clinician will appreciate the difference between needling the skin, the subcutaneous tissue, the anterior lamina of the rectus abdominis muscle, the muscle itself, a taut band in the muscle, the posterior lamina, and the peritoneal cavity, thereby increasing the accuracy of the needling procedure and reducing the risks associated with it.[25]

Considering the invasive nature of TrP-DN, it is very difficult to develop and implement double-blind and randomized placebo-controlled studies.[110-113] When researchers use minimal, sham, superficial, or placebo needling, there is growing evidence that even light touch of the skin can stimulate mechanoreceptors coupled to slow conducting afferents, which causes activity in the insular region and subsequent increased feelings of well-being and decreased feelings of unpleasantness.[114-117] However, several case reports, review articles, and research studies have attested to the effectiveness of TrP-DN. Ingber[118] documented the successful TrP-DN treatment of the subscapularis muscles in three patients diagnosed with chronic shoulder impingement syndrome. One patient required a total of six TrP-DN treatments out of a total of 11 visits. The treatments were combined with a progressive therapeutic stretching program and later with muscle strengthening. The second patient had a 1-year history of shoulder impingement. He required 11 treatments with TrP-DN before returning to playing racquetball. Both patients had failed previous physical therapy treatments, which included ice, electrical stimulation, ultrasound, massage, shoulder limbering, isotonic strengthening, and the use of an upper body ergometer. The third patient was a competitive racquetball player with a 5-month history of sharp anterior shoulder pain, who was unable to play despite medical treatment. After one session of TrP-DN, he was able to compete in a racquetball tournament. Throughout the tournament, he required twice-weekly TrP-DN treatments. Following the tournament, he had just a few follow-up visits. The patient reported a return of full power on serves and forehand strokes.[118]

In 1979, Czech medical physician Karel Lewit published one of the first clinical reports on the subject.[119] Lewit confirmed the findings of Steinbrocker that the effects of needling were primarily due to mechanical stimulation of MTrPs. As early as 1944, Steinbrocker had commented on the effects of needle insertions on musculoskeletal pain without using an injectate.[120] Lewit found that dry needling of MTrPs caused immediate analgesia in nearly 87% of needle sites. In over 31% of cases, the analgesia was permanent, while 20% had several months of pain relief, 22% several weeks, and 11% several days; 14% had no relief at all.[119]

Cummings[121] reported a case of a 28-year-old female with a history of a left axillary vein thrombosis, a subsequent venoplasty, and a trans-axillary resection of the left first rib. The patient developed chronic chest pain with left arm, forearm, and hand pain. The symptoms were initially attributed to traction on the intercostobrachial nerve, rotator cuff atrophy, Raynaud phenomenon, and possible scarring around the C8/T1 nerve root. After 7 months of chronic pain, the patient consulted with a clinician familiar with MTrPs, who identified an MTrP in the left pectoralis major muscle. She was treated with only two gentle and brief needle insertions of 10 seconds each, combined with a home stretching program. After 2 weeks, she had few remaining symptoms. One additional treatment with two TrP-DN insertions resolved the symptoms within 2 hours.[121] In another case report, Cummings described a 33-year-old woman with an 8-year history of knee pain, who was successfully treated with two sessions of EA directed at an MTrP in the ilopsoas muscle.[54]

Weiner and Schmader[64] described the successful use of TrP-DN in the treatment of five persons with postherpetic neuralgia. For example, a 71-year-old female with postherpetic neuralgia for 18 months required only three TrP-DN sessions during which LTRs were elicited. Previous treatments included gabapentin, oxycodone, acetaminophen, chiropractic manipulations, and epidural corticosteroids. Another patient was treated with a combination of cervical percutaneous electrical nerve stimulation and TrP-DN for four sessions, resulting in a dramatic decrease in pain. The authors suggested that prospective studies of the correlation between MTrPs and postherpetic neuralgia are desperately needed.[64] Only one previous report has described the relevance of MTrPs in the symptomatology of postherpetic neuralgia.[52]

A study comparing the effects of therapeutic and placebo dry needling on hip straight leg raising, internal rotation, muscle pain, and muscle tightness in subjects recruited from Australian Rules football clubs found no differences in range of motion and reported pain between the two groups.[122] Unfortunately, the researchers attempted to treat MTrPs in the gluteal muscles of presumably well-trained athletes with a 25 mm needle, which most likely is too short to reach deeper points in conditioned individuals. In other words, both interventions may have been placebos, as direct needling of pertinent MTrPs may not have occurred. At the same time, there are many other muscles that may need to be treated before changes in hip range of motion would be measurable, including the piriformis and other hip rotators, the adductor magnus, and the hamstrings. Hamstring pain is frequently due to MTrPs in the hamstrings or the adductor magnus and not from gluteal MTrPs.[123]

Another Australian study considered the effects of latent MTrPs on muscle activation patterns in the shoulder region.[48] During the first phase of the study, subjects with latent MTrPs were found to have abnormal muscle activation patterns compared to healthy control subjects. The time of onset of muscle activity of the upper and lower trapezius, the serratus anterior, the infraspinatus, and the middle deltoid muscles was determined using surface electromyography. During the second phase, the subjects with latent MTrPs and abnormal muscle activation patterns were randomly assigned to either a treatment group or a placebo group. Subjects in the treatment group were treated with TrP-DN and passive stretching. Subjects in the placebo group received sham ultrasound. After TrP-DN and stretching, the muscle activation patterns of the treated subjects had returned to normal. Subjects in the placebo treatment group did not change after the sham treatment. This study confirmed that latent MTrPs could significantly impair muscle activation patterns.[48] The authors also established that TrP-DN combined with muscle stretches facilitated an immediate return to normal muscle activation patterns, which may be especially relevant when optimal movement efficiency is required in sports participation, musical performance, and other demanding motor tasks, for example.

A 2005 Cochrane review aimed to "assess the effects of acupuncture for the treatment of non-specific low back pain and dry needling for myofascial pain syndrome in the low back region."[124] Cochrane reviews are highly regarded, rigorous reviews of the available evidence of clinical treatments. The reviews become part of the Cochrane Database of Systematic Reviews, which is published quarterly as part of the Cochrane Library. For this 2005 review, the researchers reviewed the CENTRAL, MEDLINE, and EMBASE databases, the Chinese Cochrane Centre database of clinical trials, and Japanese databases from 1996 to February 2003. Only randomized controlled trials were included in this review using the strict guidelines from the Cochrane Collaboration. Although the authors did not find many high-quality studies, they concluded that dry needling might be a useful adjunct to other therapies for chronic low back pain. They did call for more and better quality studies with greater sample sizes.[124]

Recent research by Shah et al[125] at the U.S. National Institutes of Health underscored the importance of eliciting LTRs with TrP-DDN. Those authors sampled and measured the *in vitro* biochemical milieu within normal muscle and at active and latent MTrPs in near real-time at the subnanogram level of concentration; they found significantly increased concentrations of bradykin, calcitonin-gene-related-peptide, substance P, tumor necrosis factor-$\alpha$, interleukin-1$\beta$, serotonin, and norepinephrine in the immediate milieu of active MTrPs only.[125] After the researchers elicited an LTR at the active and latent MTrPs, the concentrations of the chemicals in the immediate vicinity of active MTrPs spontaneously reduced to normal levels. Not only did this study suggest that LTRs might normalize the chemical environment near active MTrPs and reduce the concentration of several nociceptive substances, it also confirmed that the clinical distinction between latent and active MTrPs was associated with a highly significant objective difference in the nociceptive milieu.[125] Another study confirmed the importance of eliciting LTRs with TrP-DDN.[126] In a rabbit study of the effect of LTRs on endplate noise, Chen et al found that eliciting LTRs actually diminished the spontaneous electrical activity associated with MTrPs.[44,126]

Dilorenzo et al[127] conducted a prospective, open-label, randomized study on the effect of DDN on shoulder pain in 101 patients with a cerebrovascular accident. The patients were randomly assigned to a standard rehabilitation-only group or to a standard rehabilitation and DDN group. Subjects in the DDN group received four DDN treatments at

5- to 7-day intervals into MTrPs in the supraspinatus, infraspinatus, upper and lower trapezius, levator scapulae, rhomboids, teres major, subscapularis, latissimus dorsi, triceps, pectoralis, and deltoid muscles. Compared to subjects in the rehabilitation-only group, subjects in the DDN group reported significantly less pain during sleep and during physical therapy treatments, had more restful sleep, and experienced significantly less frequent and less intense pain. They reduced their use of analgesic medications and demonstrated increased compliance with the rehabilitation program. The authors concluded that DDN might provide a new therapeutic approach to managing shoulder pain in patients with hemiparesis.

Several studies have compared SDN to DDN.[128-130] Ceccherelli et al[128] randomly assigned 42 patients with lumbar myofascial pain into two groups. The first group was treated with a shallow needle technique to a depth of 2 mm at five predetermined traditional acupuncture points, while the second group received intramuscular needling at four arbitrarily selected MTrPs. The DDN technique resulted in significantly better analgesia than the SDN technique.[128] Another randomized controlled clinical study compared the efficacy of standard acupuncture, SDN, and DDN in the treatment of elderly patients with chronic low back pain.[129] The standard acupuncture group received treatment at traditional acupuncture points with the needles inserted into the muscle to a depth of 20 mm. The points were stimulated with alternate pushing and pulling of the needle until the subjects felt dull pain, or the "de qi" acupuncture sensation, after which the needle was left in place for 10 minutes. This "de qi" sensation is a desired sensation in traditional acupuncture. The TrP-DN groups received treatment at MTrPs in the quadratus lumborum, iliopsoas, piriformis, and gluteus maximus muscles, among others. In the SDN group, the needles were inserted into the skin over MTrPs to a depth of approximately 3 mm. Once a subject reported dull pain or the "de qi" sensation mentioned above, the needle was kept in place for 10 more minutes. In the DDN group, the needle was advanced an additional 20 mm. Using the same alternate pushing and pulling needle technique, the needle was again kept in place for an additional 10 minutes once an LTR was elicited. The authors concluded that DDN might be more effective in the treatment of low back pain in elderly patients than either standard acupuncture or SDN.[129] While the authors of both studies concluded that DDN might be the most effective treatment option, it is important to realize that the protocols used in these studies for both SDN and DDN do not reflect common clinical practice for either needling technique. For example, needles are rarely kept in place for 10 minutes. Also, Baldry did not recommend inserting the needle to only a 2 mm depth. In the second study, only one LTR was required in the DDN group. In clinical practice, multiple LTRs are elicited per MTrP.[95] The second study had a relatively small sample size of only nine subjects per group, which may make any definitive conclusions somewhat premature. Neither study considered Baldry's notion of differentiating the technique based on the response pattern of the patient.

Edwards and Knowles[131] conducted a randomized prospective study of superficial dry needling combined with active stretching. Subjects received either SDN combined with active stretching exercises, stretching exercises alone, or no treatments. After 3 weeks, there were no statistically significant differences between the three groups. However, after another 3 weeks the SDN group had significantly less pain compared to the no-intervention group and significantly higher pressure threshold measures compared to the active stretching-only group. This study did support the SDN technique, even though not all outcome measures were blinded.[131] Macdonald et al[132] demonstrated the efficacy of SDN in a randomized study of subjects with chronic lumbar MTrPs. The active group received SDN with the needles inserted to a depth of 4 mm over the MTrPs. The control group received sham electrotherapy. The researchers concluded that SDN was significantly better than this placebo.[132] Unfortunately, these studies did not follow Baldry's procedures either. However, the techniques are similar, with some variations in duration and depth of insertion. Lastly, a study comparing superficial versus deep acupuncture found no statistical difference in reduction of idiopathic anterior knee pain between the two methods. Pain measurements decreased significantly for both groups.[133]

## Mechanisms of Trigger Point Dry Needling

In spite of a growing body of literature exploring the etiology and pathophysiology of MTrPs, the exact mechanisms of TrP-DN remain elusive.[5] The finding that LTRs can normalize the chemical environment of active MTrPs and diminish endplate noise associated with MTrPs in rabbits nearly instantaneously, is critical in understanding the effects of TrP-DN, but neither has been explored in depth.[125,126] Simons, Travell, and Simons[1] indicated that the therapeutic effect of TrP-DDN was mechanical disruption of the MTrP contraction knots. Because MTrPs are associated with dysfunctional motor endplates, it is conceivable that TrP-DDN damages or even destroys motor endplates and causes distal axon denervations when the needle hits an MTrP. There is some evidence that this could trigger specific changes in the endplate cholinesterase and ACh receptors as part of the normal muscle regeneration process.[134,135] Needles used in TrP-DDN have a diameter of approximately 160–300 μm, which would cause very small focal lesions without any significant risk of scar tissue formation. In comparison, the diameter of human muscle fibers ranges from 10–100 μm. Muscle regeneration involves satellite cells, which repair or replace damaged myofibers.[136] Satellite cells may migrate from other areas in the muscle and are activated following actual muscle damage but also after light pressure as used in manual trigger point therapy.[134,137] Muscle regeneration following TrP-DN is expected to be complete in approximately 7–10 days.[138] It is not known whether repeated needling during the regeneration phase in the same area of a muscle can exhaust the regenerative capacity of muscle tissue, giving rise to an increase in connective tissue and impairing the reinnervation process.[138] An accurately placed needle may also provide a localized stretch to the contractured cytoskeletal structures, which would allow the involved sarcomeres to resume their resting length by reducing the degree of overlap between actin and myosin filaments.[5] To provide ultra-localized stretch to the contractured structures, it may be beneficial to rotate the needle.[139] In addition, the mechanical pressure exerted via the needle may electrically polarize muscle and connective tissues. A physical characteristic of collagen fibers is their intrinsic piezoelectricity, a property that allows tissues to transform mechanical stress into electrical activity necessary for tissue remodeling.[140]

TrP-SDN involves a very light stimulus aimed at minimizing pain responses.[24] Based on their studies on rats and mice, Swedish researchers have suggested that the reduction of pain after TrP-SDN may partially be due to the central release of oxytocin.[141,142] Baldry suggested that with TrP-SDN, the acupuncture needle stimulates Aδ sensory nerve afferents, an assumption based primarily on the work of Bowsher, who maintained that sticking a needle into the skin is always a noxious stimulus.[143]According to Baldry, Aδ nerve fibers are stimulated for as long as 72 hours after needle insertion. Prolonged stimulation of the sensory afferent Aδ nerve fibers may activate enkephalinergic, serotonergic, and noradrenergic inhibitory systems, which would imply that TrP-SDN could cause opioid-mediated pain suppression.[144] However, other than in so-called "strong responders," TrP-SDN is usually painless even when applied over painful MTrPs. It is therefore questionable that the effects of TrP-SDN can be explained through their alleged stimulation of Aδ fibers. As Millan has summarized in his comprehensive review,[145] Aδ fibers are divided into two types: Type I Aδ fibers are high-threshold, rapidly conducting mechanoreceptors and are activated only by mechanical stimuli in the noxious range, whereas Type II Aδ fibers are more responsive to thermal stimuli. Superficial trigger point dry needling as advocated by Baldry does not seem to be able to stimulate either type of Aδ fiber, unless the patient experiences the needling as a noxious event. As an alternative to invasive procedures, several quartz stimulators have been developed. When pressed against the skin, they cause a small painful spark, similar to an electric barbecue igniter. While these devices are likely to cause Aδ fiber activation, and at least theoretically could be used as an alternative to TrP-SDN, the U.S. Food and Drug Administration has not approved their use.[146]

Skin and muscle needle stimulation of Aδ and C afferent fibers in anesthetized rats was capable of producing an increase in cortical cerebral blood flow, which was thought to be due to a reflex response of the afferent pathway, including group II and IV afferent nerves, and the efferent intrinsic nerve pathway, including cholinergic vasodilators.[147] Superficial needling of certain acupuncture points in patients with chronic pain showed similar changes in cerebral blood flow.[148] Takeshige et al[149] determined that direct needling into the gastrocnemius muscle and into the ipsilateral L5 paraspinal muscles of a guinea pig resulted in significant recovery of the circulation, after ischemia was introduced to the muscle using tetanic muscle stimulation. They also confirmed that needling of acupuncture and nonacupuncture points involved the descending pain inhibitory system, although the actual afferent pathways were distinctly different. Acupuncture analgesia involved the medial hypothalamic arcuate nucleus of the descending pain inhibitory system, whereas nonacupuncture analgesia involved the anterior part of the hypothalamic arcuate nucleus. In both kinds of needle stimulation, the posterior hypothalamic arcuate nucleus was involved.[149-151] Several other acupuncture studies reported specific changes in various parts of the brain with needling of acupuncture points in comparison with control points.[152,153] Although traditional acupuncturists have maintained that acupuncture points have unique clinical effects, the findings of these studies are not specific necessarily to acupuncture but may be more related to the patients' expectations.[154] It is likely that any needling, including TrP-DN, causes similar changes, although there is no research to date that provides definitive evidence for the role of the descending pain inhibitory system when needling MTrPs.[155]

Recent studies by Langevin et al[139,156-161] are of particular interest even though they did not consider TrP-DN in their work. A common finding when using acupuncture needles is the phenomenon of the "needle grasp," which has been attributed to muscle fibers contracting around the needle and holding the needle tightly in place.[162] During needle grasp, a clinician experiences an increased pulling at the needle and an increased resistance to further movement of the inserted needle. The studies by Langevin et al provided evidence that needle grasp is not necessarily due to muscle contractions, but that subcutaneous tissues play a crucial role, especially when the needle is manipulated. Rotation of the needle did not only increase the force required to remove the needle from connective tissues, but it also created measurable changes in connective tissue architecture, due to winding of connective tissue and creation of a tight mechanical coupling between needle and tissue.[159] Even small amounts of needle rotation caused pulling of collagen fibers toward the needle and initiated specific changes in fibroblasts further away from the needle. The fibroblasts responded by changing shape from a rounded appearance to a more spindle-like shape, which the researchers described as "large and sheet-like."[139,156,157,159] The transduction of the mechanical signal into fibroblasts can lead to a wide variety of cellular and extracellular events, including mechanoreceptor and nociceptor stimulation, changes in the actin cytoskeleton, cell contraction, variations in gene expression and extracellular matrix composition, and eventually to neuromodulation.[156,163,164] Although the significance of these studies is not yet clear for TrP-DDN, it is likely that loose connective tissue plays an important role in TrP-SDN. Fu et al[28] attributed the effects of their subcutaneous needle approach to the manipulation of the needle, and referred to this groundbreaking research done by Langevin et al. To increase the effectiveness of TrP-SDN, it may prove beneficial to rotate the needle rather than leave it in place without manipulation, especially in weak responders. Needle rotation may stimulate Aδ fibers and activate enkephalinergic, serotonergic, and noradrenergic inhibitory systems.[24,143] With TrP-DDN, rotation of a needle placed within an MTrP can facilitate the eliciting of typical referred pain patterns. More research is needed to determine the various aspects of the mechanisms of TrP-DN.

## Trigger Point Dry Needling versus Injection Therapy

The term "dry needling" is used to differentiate this technique from MTrP injections. Myofascial trigger point injections are performed with a variety of injectables, such as procaine, lidocaine, and other local anesthetics, isotonic saline solutions, nonsteroidal anti-inflammatories, corticosteroids, bee venom, botulinum toxin, and serotonin antagonists.[165-173] There is no evidence that MTrP injections with steroids are superior to lidocaine injections.[174] In fact, intramuscular steroid injections may lead to muscle breakdown and degeneration.[175,176] Travell preferred to use procaine.[173,177] Because procaine is difficult to obtain, it is now recommended to use a 0.25% lidocaine solution.[169] Recent studies in Germany demonstrated that injections with tropisetron, which is a serotonin receptor antagonist, were superior to injections with local anesthetics.[171,178] However, injectable serotonin receptor antagonists are not available in the United States. Myofascial trigger point injections are generally limited to medical practice only, although in some jurisdictions, such as South Africa and the State of Maryland, physical therapists are legally allowed to perform MTrP injections. Similarly, physical therapists in the United Kingdom are allowed to perform joint and soft-tissue injections.[179]

When comparing MTrP injection therapy with TrP-DN, many authors have suggested that "dry needling of the MTrP provides as much pain relief as injection of lidocaine but causes more post-injection soreness."[180] Usually, these authors reference a study by Hong[95] comparing lidocaine injections with TrP-DN; however, Hong compared lidocaine injections with TrP-DN using a syringe and not an acupuncture needle. Recently, Kamanli et al[181] updated the 1994 Hong study and compared the effects of lidocaine injections, botulinum toxin injections, and TrP-DN. In this study, the researchers also used a syringe and not an acupuncture needle, and they did not consider LTRs. In clinical practice, TrP-DN is typically performed with an acupuncture needle. There are no scientific studies that compare TrP-DN with acupuncture needles to MTrP injections with syringes. Based on published research studies, the assumption that TrP-DN would cause more post-needling soreness when compared to lidocaine injections cannot be substantiated when acupuncture needles are used.

Prior to the development of TrP-DN, MTrPs were treated primarily with injections, which explains why many clinical outcome studies are based on injection therapy.[67,165,166,169,174,176,182-188] Several recent studies have confirmed that TrP-DN is equally effective as injection therapy, which may justify extrapolating the effects of injection therapy to TrP-DN.[25,95,176,181,189,190] Cummings and White[190] concluded, "the nature of the injected substance makes no difference to the outcome, and wet needling is not therapeutically superior to dry needling." A possible exception may be the use of botulinum toxin for those MTrPs that have not responded well to other interventions.[166,191-196] A recent consensus paper specifically recommended that botulinum toxin should only be used after trials of physical therapy and TrP-DN do not provide satisfactory relief.[193] Botulinum toxin does not only prevent the release of ACh from cholinergic nerve endings, but there is also growing evidence that it inhibits the release of other selected neuropeptide transmitters from primary sensory neurons.[192,197,198]

Frequently, patients with chronic pain conditions report having received previous MTrP injections. However, many also report that they never experienced LTRs, which raises the question as to how well trained and skilled physicians are in identifying and injecting MTrPs. A recent study revealed that MTrP injections were the second most common procedure used by Canadian anesthesiologists after epidural steroid injections. The study did not mention whether these anesthesiologists had received any training in the identification and treatment of MTrPs with injections.[199]

## Trigger Point Dry Needling versus Acupuncture

Although some patients erroneously refer to TrP-DN as a form of acupuncture, TrP-DN did not originate as part of the practice of traditional Chinese acupuncture. When Gunn started exploring the use of acupuncture needles in the treatment of persons with chronic pain problems, he used the term "acupuncture" in his earlier papers. However, his thinking was grounded in neurology and segmental relationships, and he did not consider the more esoteric and metaphysical nature of traditional acupuncture.[200-202] As reviewed previously, Gunn advocated needling motor points instead of traditional acupuncture points.[33,203,204] Baldry has not advocated using the traditional system of Chinese acupuncture with energy pathways or meridians either, and he has described them as "not of any practical importance."[24]

A few researchers have attempted to link the two needling approaches.[205-211] In an older study, Melzack et al[206,211] concluded that there was a 71% overlap between MTrPs and acupuncture points based on their anatomic location. This study had a profound impact, particularly on the development of the theoretical foundations of acupuncture. Many researchers and clinicians quoted this study by Melzack et al as evidence that acupuncture had an established physiologic basis and that acupuncture practice could be based on reported correlations with MTrPs.[205] More recently, Dorsher[207] compared the anatomic and clinical relationships between 255 MTrPs described by Travell and Simons and 386 acupuncture points described by the Shanghai College of Traditional Medicine and other acupuncture publications. He concluded that there is significant overlap between MTrPs and acupuncture points and argued that "the strong correspondence between trigger point therapy and acupuncture should facilitate the increased integration of acupuncture into contemporary clinical pain management." Although these studies appear to provide evidence that TrP-DN could be considered a form of acupuncture, both studies assume that there are distinct anatomic locations of MTrPs and that acupuncture points have point specificity.

It is questionable whether MTrPs have distinct anatomic locations and whether these can be reliably used in comparisons with other points.[212] In part, the *Trigger Point Manuals* are to blame for suggesting that MTrPs have distinct locations.[1,213] Simons, Travell, and Simons[1] described specific MTrPs in numbered sequences based on their "approximate order of appearance" and may have contributed to the widely accepted impression that indeed MTrPs do have distinct anatomic locations. There is no scientific research that validates the notion that MTrPs have distinctive anatomic locations, other than their close proximity to motor endplate zones. Based on empirical evidence, the numbering sequences are inconsistent with clinical practice and do not reflect patients' presentations. However, Dorsher's observation[207] that MTrP referred pain patterns have striking similarities with described courses of acupuncture meridians may be of interest. But the same dilemma arises: Are referred pain patterns MTrP-specific or should they be described for muscles in general or perhaps for certain parts of muscles? Recent studies of experimentally induced referred pain have suggested that referred pain patterns might be characteristic of muscles rather than of individual MTrPs, as Simons, Travell, and Simons suggested.[1,77,82,83,214]

Birch[205] reassessed the Melzack et al 1977 paper and concluded that the study was based on several "poorly conceived aspects" and "questionable" assumptions. According to Birch, Melzack et al mistakenly assumed that all acupuncture points must exhibit pressure pain and that local pain indications of acupuncture points are sufficient to establish a correlation. He determined that only approximately 18–19% of acupuncture points examined in the 1977 study could possibly correlate with MTrPs, but he did suggest that there may be a relevant correlation between the so-called "Ah Shi" points and MTrPs. In traditional acupuncture, the Ah Shi points belong to one of three major classes of acupuncture points. There are 361 primary acupuncture points referred to as "channel" points. There are hundreds of secondary class acupuncture points, known as "extra" or "nonchannel" points. The third class of acupuncture points is referred to as "Ah Shi" points. By definition, Ah Shi points must have pressure pain. They are used primarily for pain and spasm conditions. Melzack et al did not consider the Ah Shi points in their study but focused exclusively on the channel points and extra points. Hong,[209] as well as Audette and Binder,[210] agreed that acupuncturists might well be treating MTrPs whenever they are treating Ah Shi points.

Whether TrP-DN could be considered a form of acupuncture depends partially on how acupuncture is defined. For example, the New Mexico Acupuncture and Oriental Medicine Practice Act defined acupuncture in a rather generic and broad fashion as "the use of needles inserted into and removed from the human body and the use of other devices, modalities, and procedures at specific locations on the body for the prevention, cure, or correction of any disease, illness, injury, pain, or other condition by controlling and regulating the flow and balance of energy and functioning of the person to restore and maintain health."[215] According to this definition of acupuncture, nearly all physical therapy and medical interventions could be considered a form of acupuncture, including TrP-DN, but also any other modality or procedure. Physicians and nurses could be accused of practicing acupuncture as they "insert and remove needles." From a physical therapy perspective, TrP-DN has no similarities with traditional acupuncture other than the tool. The objective of TrP-DN is not to control and regulate the flow and balance of energy and is not based on Eastern esoteric and metaphysical concepts. Trigger point dry needling and other physical therapy procedures are based on scientific neurophysiological and biomechanical principles that have no similarities with the hypothesized control and regulation of the flow and balance of energy.[5,24] In fact, there is growing evidence against the notion that acupuncture points have unique and reproducible clinical effects.[155] Three recent well-designed randomized controlled clinical trials with 302, 270, and 1,007 patients, respectively, demonstrated that acupuncture and sham acupuncture treatments were more effective than no treatment at all, but there was no statistically significant difference between acupuncture and sham acupuncture.[216-218] As Campbell pointed out, acupuncture does not appear to have unique effects on the central nervous system, or on pain and pain modulation, which implies that the discussion of whether TrP-DN is a form of acupuncture becomes irrelevant.[155]

## Conclusion

Trigger point dry needling is a relatively new treatment modality used by physical therapists worldwide. The introduction of trigger point dry needling to American physical therapists has many similarities with the introduction of manual therapy during the 1960s. During the past few decades, much progress has been made toward the understanding of the nature of MTrPs, and thereby of the various treatment options. Trigger point dry needling has been recognized by prestigious organizations such as the Cochrane Collaboration and is recommended as an option for the treatment of persons with chronic low back pain. Several clinical outcome studies have demonstrated the effectiveness of trigger point dry needling. However, questions remain regarding the mechanisms of needling procedures. Physical therapists are encouraged to explore using trigger point dry needling techniques in their practices.

## References

1. Simons DG, Travell JG, Simons LS. *Travell & Simons' Myofascial Pain and Dysfunction: The Trigger Point Manual*. Vol 1. 2nd ed. Baltimore, MD: Lippincott Williams & Wilkins; 1999.
2. Uitspraken van het RTG Amsterdam [Dutch; Decisions regional medical disciplinary committee]. Available at: http://www.tuchtcollege-gezondheidszorg.nl/regionaal_files/amsterdam/uitspraken/00222F.ASD.htm. Accessed November 21, 2006.
3. Uitspraken van het CTG inzake fysiotherapeuten 2001.141 [Dutch; Decisions regional medical disciplinary committee with regard to physical therapists 2001.141]. Available at: http://www.tuchtcollege-gezondheidszorg.nl/,2002. Accessed November 21, 2006.
4. Dommerholt J, Bron C, Franssen J. Myofasciale triggerpoints: Een aanvulling [Dutch; Myofascial trigger points: Additional remarks]. *Fysiopraxis* 2005;Nov:36–41.
5. Dommerholt J. Dry needling in orthopedic physical therapy practice. *Orthop Phys Ther Pract* 2004;16(3):15–20.
6. Williams T. *Colorado Physical Therapy Licensure Policies of the Director. Policy 3: Director's Policy on Intramuscular Stimulation*. Denver, CO: State of Colorado, Department of Regulatory Agencies; 2005.
7. Tennessee Board of Occupational and Physical Therapy. Committee of Physical Therapy Minutes. 2002.
8. Hawaii Revised Statutes. Chapter 461J; Physical Therapy Practice Act. Article §461J-2.5 Prohibited practices, 2006.
9. The 2006 Florida Statutes. Title XXXII: Regulation of Professions and Occupations. Chapter 486: Physical Therapy Practice. Article 486.021, 11, 2006.
10. Paris SV. In the best interest of the patient. *Phys Ther* 2006;86:1541–1553.
11. Fischer AA. New approaches in treatment of myofascial pain. In: Fischer AA, ed. *Myofascial Pain: Update in Diagnosis and Treatment*. Philadelphia, PA: W.B. Saunders; 1997;153–170.
12. Fischer AA. Treatment of myofascial pain. *J Musculoskel Pain* 1999;7(1–2):131–142.
13. Gunn CC. *The Gunn Approach to the Treatment of Chronic Pain*. 2nd ed. New York, NY: Churchill Livingstone; 1997.
14. Frobb MK. Neural acupuncture: A rationale for the use of lidocaine infiltration at acupuncture points in the treatment of myofascial pain syndromes. *Med Acupunct* 2003;15(1):18–22.
15. Frobb MK. Neural acupuncture and the treatment of myofascial pain syndromes. *Acupunct Canada* 2005;Spring:1–3.

16. Chu J. Dry needling (intramuscular stimulation) in myofascial pain related to lumbosacral radiculopathy. *Eur J Phys Med Rehabil* 1995;5(4):106–121.

17. Chu J. The role of the monopolar electromyographic pin in myofascial pain therapy: Automated twitch-obtaining intramuscular stimulation (ATOIMS) and electrical twitch-obtaining intramuscular stimulation (ETOIMS). *Electromyogr Clin Neurophysiol* 1999;39:503–511.

18. Chu J. Twitch-obtaining intramuscular stimulation (TOIMS): Long-term observations in the management of chronic partial cervical radiculopathy. *Electromyogr Clin Neurophysiol* 2000;40:503–510.

19. Chu J. Early observations in radiculopathic pain control using electrodiagnostically derived new treatment techniques: Automated twitch-obtaining intramuscular stimulation (ATOIMS) and electrical twitch-obtaining intramuscular stimulation (ETOIMS). *Electromyogr Clin Neurophysiol* 2000;40:195–204.

20. Chu J, Schwartz I. The muscle twitch in myofascial pain relief: Effects of acupuncture and other needling methods. *Electromyogr Clin Neurophysiol* 2002;42:307–311.

21. Chu J, Takehara I, Li TC, Schwartz I. Electrical twitch-obtaining intramuscular stimulation (ETOIMS) for myofascial pain syndrome in a football player. *Br J Sports Med* 2004;38(5): E25.

22. Chu J, Yuen KF, Wang BH, Chan RC, Schwartz I, Neuhauser D. Electrical twitch-obtaining intramuscular stimulation in lower back pain: A pilot study. *Am J Phys Med Rehabil* 2004;83: 104–111.

23. Chu J. Does EMG (dry needling) reduce myofascial pain symptoms due to cervical nerve root irritation? *Electromyogr Clin Neurophysiol* 1997;37:259–272.

24. Baldry PE. *Acupuncture, Trigger Points and Musculoskel Pain*. Edinburgh, UK: Churchill Livingstone; 2005.

25. Mayoral del Moral O. Fisioterapia invasiva del síndrome de dolor miofascial [Spanish; Invasive physical therapy for myofascial pain syndrome]. *Fisioterapia* 2005;27(2):69–75.

26. Baldry P. Superficial versus deep dry needling. *Acupunct Med* 2002;20(2–3):78–81.

27. Fu ZH, Chen XY, Lu LJ, Lin J, Xu JG. Immediate effect of Fu's subcutaneous needling for low back pain. *Chin Med J (Engl)* 2006;119(11):953–956.

28. Fu Z-H, Wang J-H, Sun J-H, Chen X-Y, Xu J-G. Fu's subcutaneous needling: Possible clinical evidence of the subcutaneous connective tissue in acupuncture. *J Altern Complement Med* 2007;13:47–51.

29. Fu Z-H, Xu J-G. A brief introduction to Fu's subcutaneous needling. *Pain Clinical Updates* 2005;17(3):343–348.

30. Gunn CC. Radiculopathic pain: Diagnosis, treatment of segmental irritation or sensitization. *J Musculoskel Pain* 1997;5(4):119–134.

31. Gunn CC. Available at: *http://www.istop.org/infopages/practitioners.htm*. 2006. Accessed November 21, 2006.

32. Cannon WB, Rosenblueth A. *The Supersensitivity of Denervated Structures: A Law of Denervation*. New York, NY: MacMillan; 1949.

33. Gunn CC, Milbrandt WE, Little AS, Mason KE. Dry needling of muscle motor points for chronic low-back pain: A randomized clinical trial with long-term follow-up. *Spine* 1980;5: 279–291.

34. Gunn CC. Reply to Chang-Zern Hong. *J Musculoskel Pain* 2000;8(3):137–142.

35. Hong C-Z. Comment on Gunn's "radiculopathy model of myofascial trigger points." *J Musculoskel Pain* 2000;8(3):133–135.

36. Arendt-Nielsen L, Graven-Nielsen T. Deep tissue hyperalgesia. *J Musculoskel Pain* 2002;10(1–2): 97–119.

37. Curatolo M, Arendt-Nielsen L, Petersen-Felix S. Evidence, mechanisms, and clinical implications of central hypersensitivity in chronic pain after whiplash injury. *Clin J Pain* 2004;20: 469–476.

38. Graven-Nielsen T, Arendt-Nielsen L. Peripheral and central sensitization in musculoskeletal pain disorders: An experimental approach. *Curr Rheumatol Rep* 2002;4:313–321.

39. Mense S. The pathogenesis of muscle pain. *Curr Pain Headache Rep* 2003;7:419–425.

40. Ji RR, Woolf CJ. Neuronal plasticity and signal transduction in nociceptive neurons: Implications for the initiation and maintenance of pathological pain. *Neurobiol Dis* 2001;8:1–10.

41. Woolf CJ. The pathophysiology of peripheral neuropathic pain: Abnormal peripheral input and abnormal central processing. *Acta Neurochir* 1993;58(suppl):125–130.

42. Woolf CJ, Mannion RJ. Neuropathic pain: Aetiology, symptoms, mechanisms, and management. *Lancet* 1999;353(9168):1959–1964.

43. Simons DG. Do endplate noise and spikes arise from normal motor endplates? *Am J Phys Med Rehabil* 2001;80:134–140.

44. Simons DG, Hong C-Z, Simons LS. Endplate potentials are common to midfiber myofascial trigger points. *Am J Phys Med Rehabil* 2002;81:212–222.

45. Hubbard DR, Berkoff GM. Myofascial trigger points show spontaneous needle EMG activity. *Spine* 1993;18:1803–1807.

46. Simons DG. Review of enigmatic MTrPs as a common cause of enigmatic musculoskeletal pain and dysfunction. *J Electromyogr Kinesiol* 2004;14:95–107.

47. Weeks VD, Travell J. How to give painless injections. In: *AMA Scientific Exhibits*. New York, NY: Grune & Stratton, 1957:318–322.

48. Lucas KR, Polus BI, Rich PS. Latent myofascial trigger points: Their effect on muscle activation and movement efficiency. *J Bodywork Movement Ther* 2004;8:160–166.

49. Dejung B, Gröbli C, Colla F, Weissmann R. *Triggerpunkttherapie*. [German: Trigger Point Therapy]. Bern, Switzerland: Hans Huber; 2003.

50. Archibald HC. Referred pain in headache. *Calif Med* 1955;82(3):186–187.

51. Bajaj P, Bajaj P, Graven-Nielsen T, Arendt-Nielsen L. Trigger points in patients with lower limb osteoarthritis. *J Musculoskel Pain* 2001;9(3):17–33.

52. Chen SM, Chen JT, Kuan TS, Hong CZ. Myofascial trigger points in intercostal muscles secondary to herpes zoster infection of the intercostal nerve. *Arch Phys Med Rehabil* 1998;79: 336–338.

53. Çimen A, Çelik M, Erdine S. Myofascial pain syndrome in the differential diagnosis of chronic abdominal pain. *Agri* 2004;16(3):45–47.

54. Cummings M. Referred knee pain treated with electroacupuncture to iliopsoas. *Acupunct Med* 2003;21(1–2):32–35.

55. Facco E, Ceccherelli F. Myofascial pain mimicking radicular syndromes. *Acta Neurochir* 2005;92(suppl):147–150.

56. Fernández-de-las-Peñas C, Alonso-Blanco C, Cuadrado ML, Pareja JA. Myofascial trigger points in the suboccipital muscles in episodic tension-type headache. *Man Ther* 2006;11:225–230.

57. Fernández-de-las-Peñas C, Alonso-Blanco C, Cuadrado ML, Gerwin RD, Pareja JA. Trigger points in the suboccipital muscles and forward head posture in tension-type headache. *Headache* 2006;46:454–460.

58. Fernández-de-las-Peñas CF, Cuadrado ML, Gerwin RD, Pareja JA. Referred pain from the trochlear region in tension-type headache: A myofascial trigger point from the superior oblique muscle. *Headache* 2005;45:731–737.

59. Fernández-de-Las-Peñas C, Alonso-Blanco C, Cuadrado ML, Gerwin RD, Pareja JA. Myofascial trigger points and their relationship to headache clinical parameters in chronic tension-type headache. *Headache* 2006;46:1264–1272.

60. Fernández-de-Las-Peñas C, Ge HY, Arendt-Nielsen L, Cuadrado ML, Pareja JA. Referred pain from trapezius muscle trigger points shares similar characteristics with chronic tension-type headache. *Eur J Pain* 2007;11:475–482.

61. Fricton JR, Kroening R, Haley D, Siegert R. Myofascial pain syndrome of the head and neck: A review of clinical characteristics of 164 patients. *Oral Surg Oral Med Oral Pathol* 1985;60:615–623.

62. Kern KU, Martin C, Scheicher S, Muller H. Auslosung von Phantomschmerzen und -sensationen durch muskulare Stumpftriggerpunkte nach Beinamputationen [German; Referred pain from amputation stump trigger points into the phantom limb]. *Schmerz* 2006;20: 300–306.

63. Travell J. Referred pain from skeletal muscle: The pectoralis major syndrome of breast pain and soreness and the sternomastoid syndrome of headache and dizziness. *NY State J Med* 1955;55:331–340.

64. Weiner DK, Schmader KE. Post-herpetic pain: More than sensory neuralgia? *Pain Med* 2006;7:243–249.

65. Mascia P, Brown BR, Friedman S. Toothache of nonodontogenic origin: A case report. *J Endod* 2003;29:608–610.

66. Reeh ES, elDeeb ME. Referred pain of muscular origin resembling endodontic involvement: Case report. *Oral Surg Oral Med Oral Pathol* 1991;71:223–227.

67. Hong CZ, Kuan TS, Chen JT, Chen SM. Referred pain elicited by palpation and by needling of myofascial trigger points: A comparison. *Arch Phys Med Rehabil* 1997;78:957–960.

68. Hong C-Z, Chen Y-N, Twehous D, Hong DH. Pressure threshold for referred pain by compression on the trigger point and adjacent areas. *J Musculoskel Pain* 1996;4(3):61–79.

69. Vecchiet L, Vecchiet J, Giamberardino MA. Referred muscle pain: Clinical and pathophysiologic aspects. *Curr Rev Pain* 1999;3:489–498.

70. Travell J. Temporomandibular joint pain referred from muscles of the head and neck. *J Prosthet Dent* 1960;10:745–763.

71. Travell JG, Rinzler SH. The myofascial genesis of pain. *Postgrad Med* 1952;11:452–434.

72. Kellgren JH. Observations on referred pain arising from muscle. *Clin Sci* 1938;3:175–190.

73. Kellgren JH. A preliminary account of referred pains arising from muscle. *BMJ* 1938;1:325–327.

74. Kellgren JH. Deep pain sensibility. *Lancet* 1949;1:943–949.

75. Arendt-Nielsen L, Graven-Nielsen T, Svensson P, Jensen TS. Temporal summation in muscles and referred pain areas: An experimental human study. *Muscle Nerve* 1997;20:1311–1313.

76. Arendt-Nielsen L, Laursen RJ, Drewes AM. Referred pain as an indicator for neural plasticity. *Prog Brain Res* 2000;129:343–356.

77. Cornwall J, Harris AJ, Mercer SR. The lumbar multifidus muscle and patterns of pain. *Man Ther* 2006;11:40–45.

78. Gibson W, Arendt-Nielsen L, Graven-Nielsen T. Delayed onset muscle soreness at tendon-bone junction and muscle tissue is associated with facilitated referred pain. *Exp Brain Res* 2006;174:351–360.

79. Gibson W, Arendt-Nielsen L, Graven-Nielsen T. Referred pain and hyperalgesia in human tendon and muscle belly tissue. *Pain* 2006;120:113–123.

80. Graven-Nielsen T, Arendt-Nielsen L. Induction and assessment of muscle pain, referred pain, and muscular hyperalgesia. *Curr Pain Headache Rep* 2003;7:443–451.

81. Graven-Nielsen T, Arendt-Nielsen L, Svensson P, Jensen TS. Quantification of local and referred muscle pain in humans after sequential i.m. injections of hypertonic saline. *Pain* 1997;69:111–117.

82. Hwang M, Kang YK, Kim DH. Referred pain pattern of the pronator quadratus muscle. *Pain* 2005;116:238–242.

83. Hwang M, Kang YK, Shin JY, Kim DH. Referred pain pattern of the abductor pollicis longus muscle. *Am J Phys Med Rehabil* 2005;84:593–597.

84. Witting N, Svensson P, Gottrup H, Arendt-Nielsen L, Jensen TS. Intramuscular and intradermal injection of capsaicin: A comparison of local and referred pain. *Pain* 2000;84:407–412.

85. Bron C, Wensing M, Franssen JLM, Oostendorp RAB. Interobserver reliability of palpation of myofascial trigger points in shoulder muscles. *J Manual Manipulative Ther* 2007;15:203–215.

86. Gerwin RD, Shannon S, Hong CZ, Hubbard D, Gevirtz R. Interrater reliability in myofascial trigger point examination. *Pain* 1997;69:65–73.

87. Sciotti VM, Mittak VL, DiMarco L, Ford LM, Plezbert J, Santipadri E, Wigglesworth J, Ball K. Clinical precision of myofascial trigger point location in the trapezius muscle. *Pain* 2001;93:259–266.

88. Al-Shenqiti AM, Oldham JA. Test-retest reliability of myofascial trigger point detection in patients with rotator cuff tendonitis. *Clin Rehabil* 2005;19:482–487.

89. Simons DG, Dommerholt J. Myofascial pain syndromes: Trigger points. *J Musculoskel Pain* 2005;13(4):39–48.

90. Dommerholt J. Muscle pain syndromes. In: RI Cantu, AJ Grodin, eds. *Myofascial Manipulation*. Gaithersburg, MD: Aspen; 2001:93–140.

91. Fryer G, Hodgson L. The effect of manual pressure release on myofascial trigger points in the upper trapezius muscle. *J Bodywork Movement Ther* 2005;9:248–255.

92. Escobar PL, Ballesteros J. Teres minor: Source of symptoms resembling ulnar neuropathy or C8 radiculopathy. *Am J Phys Med Rehabil* 1988;67:120–122.

93. Hong C-Z. Persistence of local twitch response with loss of conduction to and from the spinal cord. *Arch Phys Med Rehabil* 1994;75:12–16.

94. Hong C-Z, Torigoe Y. Electrophysiological characteristics of localized twitch responses in responsive taut bands of rabbit skeletal muscle. *J Musculoskel Pain* 1994;2:17–43.

95. Hong C-Z. Lidocaine injection versus dry needling to myofascial trigger point: The importance of the local twitch response. *Am J Phys Med Rehabil* 1994;73:256–263.

96. Ahmed HE, White PF, Craig WF, Hamza MA, Ghoname ES, Gajraj NM. Use of percutaneous electrical nerve stimulation (PENS) in the short-term management of headache. *Headache* 2000;40:311–315.

97. Barlas P, Ting SL, Chesterton LS, Jones PW, Sim J. Effects of intensity of electroacupuncture upon experimental pain in healthy human volunteers: A randomized, double-blind, placebo-controlled study. *Pain* 2006;122:81–89.

98. Mayoral O, Torres R. Tratamiento conservador y fisioterápico invasivo de los puntos gatillo miofasciales [Spanish: Conservative treatment and invasive physical therapy of myofascial trigger points]. In: *Patología de Partes Blandas en el Hombro* [Spanish; *Soft-Tissue Pathology in Man*]. Madrid, Spain: Fundación MAPFRE Medicina; 2003.

99. White PF, Craig WF, Vakharia AS, Ghoname E, Ahmed HE, Hamza MA. Percutaneous neuromodulation therapy: Does the location of electrical stimulation affect the acute analgesic response? *Anesth Analg* 2000;91:949–954.

100. Ghoname EA, Craig WF, White PF, Ahmed HE, Hamza MA, Henderson BN, Gajraj NM, Huber PJ, Gatchel RJ. Percutaneous electrical nerve stimulation for low back pain: A randomized crossover study. *JAMA* 1999;281:818–823.

101. Ghoname EA, White PF, Ahmed HE, Hamza MA, Craig WF, Noe CE. Percutaneous electrical nerve stimulation: An alternative to TENS in the management of sciatica. *Pain* 1999;83: 193–199.

102. Wang L, Zhang Y, Dai J, Yang J, Gang S. Electroacupuncture (EA) modulates the expression of NMDA receptors in primary sensory neurons in relation to hyperalgesia in rats. *Brain Res* 2006;1120:46–53.

103. Choi BT, Lee JH, Wan Y, Han JS: Involvement of ionotropic glutamate receptors in low-frequency electroacupuncture analgesia in rats. *Neurosci Lett* 2005;377(3):185–188.

104. Lundeberg T, Stener-Victorin E. Is there a physiological basis for the use of acupuncture in pain? *Int Congress Series* 2002;1238:3–10.

105. Lin JG, Lo MW, Wen YR, Hsieh CL, Tsai SK, Sun WZ. The effect of high- and low-frequency electroacupuncture in pain after lower abdominal surgery. *Pain* 2002;99:509–514.

106. Elorriaga A. The 2-needle technique. *Med Acupunct* 2000;12(1):17–19.

107. Mayoral del Moral O, De Felipe JA, Martínez JM. Changes in tenderness and tissue compliance in myofascial trigger points with a new technique of electroacupuncture: Three preliminary case reports. *J Musculoskel Pain* 2004;12(suppl):33.

108. Peets JM, Pomeranz B. CXBK mice deficient in opiate receptors show poor electroacupuncture analgesia. *Nature* 1978;273(5664):675–676.

109. Noë A. *Action in Perception*. Cambridge, MA: MIT Press; 2004.

110. Dincer F, Linde K. Sham interventions in randomized clinical trials of acupuncture: A review. *Complement Ther Med* 2003;11(4):235–242.

111. Streitberger K, Kleinhenz J. Introducing a placebo needle into acupuncture research. *Lancet* 1998;352(9125):364–365.

112. White P, Lewith G, Hopwood V, Prescott P. The placebo needle: Is it a valid and convincing placebo for use in acupuncture trials? A randomised, single-blind, cross-over pilot trial. *Pain* 2003;106:401–409.

113. Goddard G, Shen Y, Steele B, Springer N. A controlled trial of placebo versus real acupuncture. *J Pain* 2005;6:237–242.

114. Cole J, Bushnell MC, McGlone F, Elam M, Lamarre Y, Vallbo A, Olausson H. Unmyelinated tactile afferents underpin detection of low-force monofilaments. *Muscle Nerve* 2006;34:105–107.

115. Lund I, Lundeberg T. Are minimal, superficial or sham acupuncture procedures acceptable as inert placebo controls? *Acupunct Med* 2006;24(1):13–15.

116. Olausson H, Lamarre Y, Backlund H, Morin C, Wallin BG, Starck G, Ekholm S, Strigo I, Worsley K, Vallbo AB, Bushnell MC. Unmyelinated tactile afferents signal touch and project to insular cortex. *Nat Neurosci* 2002;5:900–904.

117. Mohr C, Binkofski F, Erdmann C, Buchel C, Helmchen C. The anterior cingulate cortex contains distinct areas dissociating external from self-administered painful stimulation: A parametric fMRI study. *Pain* 2005;114:347–357.

118. Ingber RS. Iliopsoas myofascial dysfunction: A treatable cause of "failed" low back syndrome. *Arch Phys Med Rehabil* 1989;70:382–386.

119. Lewit K. The needle effect in the relief of myofascial pain. *Pain* 1979;6:83–90.

120. Steinbrocker O. Therapeutic injections in painful musculoskeletal disorders. *JAMA* 1944;125:397–401.

121. Cummings M. Myofascial pain from pectoralis major following trans-axillary surgery. *Acupunct Med* 2003;21(3):105–107.

122. Huguenin L, Brukner PD, McCrory P, Smith P, Wajswelner H, Bennell K. Effect of dry needling of gluteal muscles on straight leg raise: A randomised, placebo-controlled, double-blind trial. *Br J Sports Med* 2005;39:84–90.

123. Gerwin RD. A standing complaint: Inability to sit. An unusual presentation of medial hamstring myofascial pain syndrome. *J Musculoskel Pain* 2001;9(4):81–93.

124. Furlan A, Tulder M, Cherkin D, Tsukayama H, Lao L, Koes B, Berman B. Acupuncture and dry-needling for low back pain: An updated systematic review within the framework of the Cochrane Collaboration. *Spine* 2005;30:944–963.

125. Shah JP, Phillips TM, Danoff JV, Gerber LH. An *in vivo* microanalytical technique for measuring the local biochemical milieu of human skeletal muscle. *J Appl Physiol* 2005;99: 1980–1987.

126. Chen JT, Chung KC, Hou CR, Kuan TS, Chen SM, Hong C-Z. Inhibitory effect of dry needling on the spontaneous electrical activity recorded from myofascial trigger spots of rabbit skeletal muscle. *Am J Phys Med Rehabil* 2001;80:729–735.

127. Dilorenzo L, Traballesi M, Morelli D, Pompa A, Brunelli S, Buzzi MG, Formisano R. Hemiparetic shoulder pain syndrome treated with deep dry needling during early rehabilitation: A prospective, open-label, randomized investigation. *J Musculoskel Pain* 2004;12(2):25–34.

128. Ceccherelli F, Rigoni MT, Gagliardi G, Ruzzante L. Comparison between superficial and deep acupuncture in the treatment of lumbar myofascial pain: A double-blind randomized controlled study. *Clin J Pain* 2002;18:149–153.

129. Itoh K, Katsumi Y, Kitakoji H.Trigger point acupuncture treatment of chronic low back pain in elderly patients: A blinded RCT. *Acupunct Med* 2004;2(4):170–177.

130. Karakurum B, Karaalin O, Coskun O, Dora B, Ucler S, Inan L. The "dry-needle technique": Intramuscular stimulation in tension-type headache. *Cephalalgia* 2001;21:813–817.

131. Edwards J, Knowles N. Superficial dry needling and active stretching in the treatment of myofascial pain: A randomised controlled trial. *Acupunct Med* 2003;21(3 SU):80–86.

132. Macdonald AJ, Macrae KD, Master BR, Rubin AP. Superficial acupuncture in the relief of chronic low back pain. *Ann R Coll Surg Engl* 1983;65:44–46.

133. Naslund J, Naslund UB, Odenbring S, Lundeberg T. Sensory stimulation (acupuncture) for the treatment of idiopathic anterior knee pain. *J Rehabil Med* 2002;34:231–238.

134. Sadeh M, Stern LZ, Czyzewski K. Changes in end-plate cholinesterase and axons during muscle degeneration and regeneration. *J Anat* 1985;140(Pt 1):165–176.

135. Gaspersic R, Koritnik B, Erzen I, Sketelj J. Muscle activity-resistant acetylcholine receptor accumulation is induced in places of former motor endplates in ectopically innervated regenerating rat muscles. *Int J Dev Neurosci* 2001;19:339–346.

136. Schultz E, Jaryszak DL, Valliere CR. Response of satellite cells to focal skeletal muscle injury. *Muscle Nerve* 1985;8:217–222.

137. Teravainen H. Satellite cells of striated muscle after compression injury so slight as not to cause degeneration of the muscle fibres. *Z Zellforsch Mikrosk Anat* 1970;103:320–327.

138. Reznik M. Current concepts of skeletal muscle regeneration. In: CM Pearson, FK Mostofy, eds. *The Striated Muscle.* Baltimore, MD: Williams & Wilkins; 1973:185–225.

139. Langevin HM, Churchill DL, Cipolla MJ. Mechanical signaling through connective tissue: A mechanism for the therapeutic effect of acupuncture. *FASEB J* 2001;15:2275–2282.

140. Liboff AR. Bioelectromagnetic fields and acupuncture. *J Altern Complement Med* 1997;3(suppl 1): S77–S87.

141. Lundeberg T, Uvnas-Moberg K, Agren G, Bruzelius G. Antinociceptive effects of oxytocin in rats and mice. *Neurosci Lett* 1994;170:153–157.

142. Uvnas-Moberg K, Bruzelius G, Alster P, Lundeberg T. The antinociceptive effect of non-noxious sensory stimulation is mediated partly through oxytocinergic mechanisms. *Acta Physiol Scand* 1993;149:199–204.

143. Bowsher D. Mechanisms of acupuncture. In: J Filshie, A White, eds. *Western Acupuncture: A Western Scientific Approach.* Edinburgh, UK: Churchill Livingstone; 1998.

144. Baldry PE. *Myofascial Pain and Fibromyalgia Syndromes*. Edinburgh, UK: Churchill Livingstone; 2001.
145. Millan MJ. The induction of pain: An integrative review. *Prog Neurobiol* 1999;57:1–164.
146. FDA Topics and Answers. Available at: http://www.fda.gov/bbs/topics/ANSWERS/ ANS00817. html.1997. Accessed November 15, 2005.
147. Uchida S, Kagitani F, Suzuki A, Aikawa Y. Effect of acupuncture-like stimulation on cortical cerebral blood flow in anesthetized rats. *Jpn J Physiol* 2000;50:495–507.
148. Alavi A, LaRiccia PJ, Sadek AH, Newberg AB, Lee L, Reich H, Lattanand C, Mozley PD. Neuroimaging of acupuncture in patients with chronic pain. *J Altern Complement Med* 1997;3(suppl 1):S47–S53.
149. Takeshige C, Kobori M, Hishida F, Luo CP, Usami S. Analgesia inhibitory system involvement in nonacupuncture point-stimulation-produced analgesia. *Brain Res Bull* 1992;28:379–391.
150. Takeshige C, Sato T, Mera T, Hisamitsu T, Fang J. Descending pain inhibitory system involved in acupuncture analgesia. *Brain Res Bull* 1992;29:617–634.
151. Takeshige C, Tsuchiya M, Zhao W, Guo S. Analgesia produced by pituitary ACTH and dopaminergic transmission in the arcuate. *Brain Res Bull* 1991;26:779–788.
152. Hui KK, Liu J, Makris N, Gollub RL, Chen AJ, Moore CI, Kennedy DN, Rosen BR, Kwong KK. Acupuncture modulates the limbic system and subcortical gray structures of the human brain: Evidence from fMRI studies in normal subjects. *Hum Brain Mapp* 2000;9:13–25.
153. Wu MT, Hsieh JC, Xiong J, Yang CF, Pan HB, Chen YC, Tsai G, Rosen BR, Kwong KK. Central nervous pathway for acupuncture stimulation: Localization of processing with functional MR imaging of the brain—Preliminary experience. *Radiol* 1999;212:133–141.
154. Wager TD, Rilling JK, Smith EE, Sokolik A, Casey KL, Davidson RJ, Kosslyn SM, Rose RM, Cohen JD. Placebo-induced changes in FMRI in the anticipation and experience of pain. *Science* 2004;303(5661):1162–1167.
155. Campbell A. Point specificity of acupuncture in the light of recent clinical and imaging studies. *Acupunct Med* 2006;24(3):118–122.
156. Langevin HM, Bouffard NA, Badger GJ, Churchill DL, Howe AK. Subcutaneous tissue fibroblast cytoskeletal remodeling induced by acupuncture: Evidence for a mechanotransduction-based mechanism. *J Cell Physiol* 2006;207:767–774.
157. Langevin HM, Bouffard NA, Badger GJ, Iatridis JC, Howe AK. Dynamic fibroblast cytoskeletal response to subcutaneous tissue stretch *ex vivo* and *in vivo*. *Am J Physiol Cell Physiol* 2005; 288:C747–C756.
158. Langevin HM, Churchill DL, Fox JR, Badger GJ, Garra BS, Krag MH. Biomechanical response to acupuncture needling in humans. *J Appl Physiol* 2001;91:2471–2478.
159. Langevin HM, Churchill DL, Wu J, Badger GJ, Yandow JA, Fox JR, Krag MH. Evidence of connective tissue involvement in acupuncture. *Faseb J* 2002;16:872–874.
160. Langevin HM, Konofagou EE, Badger GJ, Churchill DL, Fox JR, Ophir J, Garra BS. Tissue displacements during acupuncture using ultrasound elastography techniques. *Ultrasound Med Biol* 2004;30:1173–1183.
161. Langevin HM, Storch KN, Cipolla MJ, White SL, Buttolph TR, Taatjes DJ. Fibroblast spreading induced by connective tissue stretch involves intracellular redistribution of alpha- and beta-actin. *Histochem Cell Biol* 2006;125:487–495.
162. Gunn CC, Milbrandt WE. The neurological mechanism of needle-grasp in acupuncture. *Am J Acupuncture* 1977;5(2):115–120.
163. Chiquet M, Renedo AS, Huber F, Fluck M. How do fibroblasts translate mechanical signals into changes in extracellular matrix production? *Matrix Biol* 2003;22:73–80.

164. Langevin HM. Connective tissue: A body-wide signaling network? *Med Hypotheses* 2006;66: 1074–1077.

165. Byrn C, Borenstein P, Linder LE. Treatment of neck and shoulder pain in whiplash syndrome patients with intracutaneous sterile water injections. *Acta Anaesthesiol Scand* 1991;35: 52–53.

166. Cheshire WP, Abashian SW, Mann JD. Botulinum toxin in the treatment of myofascial pain syndrome. *Pain* 1994;59:65–69.

167. Frost A. Diclofenac versus lidocaine as injection therapy in myofascial pain. *Scand J Rheumatol* 1986;15:153–156.

168. Hameroff SR, Crago BR, Blitt CD, Womble J, Kanel J. Comparison of bupivacaine, etidocaine, and saline for trigger-point therapy. *Anesth Analg* 1981;60:752–755.

169. Iwama H, Akama Y. The superiority of water-diluted 0.25% to near 1% lidocaine for trigger-point injections in myofascial pain syndrome: A prospective, randomized, double-blinded trial. *Anesth Analg* 2000;91:408–409.

170. Iwama H, Ohmori S, Kaneko T, Watanabe K. Water-diluted local anesthetic for trigger-point injection in chronic myofascial pain syndrome: Evaluation of types of local anesthetic and concentrations in water. *Reg Anesth Pain Med* 2001;26:333–336.

171. Müller W, Stratz T. Local treatment of tendinopathies and myofascial pain syndromes with the 5-HT3 receptor antagonist tropisetron. *Scand J Rheumatol Suppl* 2004;119:44–48.

172. Rodriguez-Acosta A, Pena L, Finol HJ, and Pulido-Mendez M. Cellular and subcellular changes in muscle, neuromuscular junctions and nerves caused by bee (Apis mellifera) venom. *J Submicrosc Cytol Pathol* 2004;36:91–96.

173. Travell J. Basis for the multiple uses of local block of somatic trigger areas (procaine infiltration and ethyl chloride spray). *Miss Valley Med* 1949;71:13–22.

174. Frost FA, Jessen B, Siggaard-Andersen J. A control, double-blind comparison of mepivacaine injection versus saline injection for myofascial pain. *Lancet* 1980;1:499–501.

175. Fischer AA. New developments in diagnosis of myofascial pain and fibromyalgia. In: Fischer AA, ed. *Myofascial Pain: Update in Diagnosis and Treatment*. Philadelphia, PA: W.B. Saunders, 1997:1–21.

176. Garvey TA, Marks MR, Wiesel SW. A prospective, randomized, double-blind evaluation of trigger-point injection therapy for low-back pain. *Spine* 1989;14:962–964.

177. Travell J, Bobb AL. Mechanism of relief of pain in sprains by local injection techniques. *Fed Proc* 1947;6:378.

178. Ettlin T. Trigger point injection treatment with the 5-HT3 receptor antagonist tropisetron in patients with late whiplash-associated disorder: First results of a multiple case study. *Scand J Rheumatol Suppl* 2004;119:49–50.

179. Saunders S, Longworth S. *Injection Techniques in Orthopaedics and Sports Medicine: A Practical Manual for Doctors and Physiotherapists*. 3rd ed. Edinburgh, UK: Churchill Livingstone; 2006.

180. Borg-Stein J. Treatment of fibromyalgia, myofascial pain, and related disorders. *Phys Med Rehabil Clin N Am* 2006;17(2):491–510, viii.

181. Kamanli A, Kaya A, Ardicoglu O, Ozgocmen S, Zengin FO, Bayik Y. Comparison of lidocaine injection, botulinum toxin injection, and dry needling to trigger points in myofascial pain syndrome. *Rheumatol Int* 2005;25:604–611.

182. Fischer AA. Local injections in pain management: Trigger point needling with infiltration and somatic blocks. In: GH Kraft, SM Weinstein, eds. *Injection Techniques: Principles and Practice*. Philadelphia, PA: W.B. Saunders; 1995.

183. McMillan AS, Blasberg B. Pain-pressure threshold in painful jaw muscles following trigger point injection. *J Orofacial Pain* 1994;8:384–390.

184. Tschopp KP, Gysin C. Local injection therapy in 107 patients with myofascial pain syndrome of the head and neck. *ORL* 1996;58:306–310.

185. Ling FW, Slocumb JC. Use of trigger point injections in chronic pelvic pain. *Obstet Gynecol Clin North Am* 1993;20:809–815.

186. Padamsee M, Mehta N, White GE. Trigger point injection: A neglected modality in the treatment of TMJ dysfunction. *J Pedod* 1987;12:72–92.

187. Tsen LC, Camann WR. Trigger point injections for myofascial pain during epidural analgesia for labor. *Reg Anesth* 1997;22:466–468.

188. Ney JP, Difazio M, Sichani A, Monacci W, Foster L, Jabbari B. Treatment of chronic low back pain with successive injections of botulinum toxin over 6 months: A prospective trial of 60 patients. *Clin J Pain* 2006;22:363–369.

189. Jaeger B, Skootsky SA. Double-blind, controlled study of different myofascial trigger point injection techniques. *Pain* 1987;4(suppl):S292.

190. Cummings TM, White AR. Needling therapies in the management of myofascial trigger point pain: A systematic review. *Arch Phys Med Rehabil* 2001;82:986–992.

191. Wheeler AH, Goolkasian P, Gretz SS. A randomized, double-blind, prospective pilot study of botulinum toxin injection for refractory, unilateral, cervicothoracic, paraspinal, myofascial pain syndrome. *Spine* 1998;23:1662–1666.

192. Mense S. Neurobiological basis for the use of botulinum toxin in pain therapy. *J Neurol* 2004;251(suppl 1):I1–I7.

193. Reilich P, Fheodoroff K, Kern U, Mense S, Seddigh S, Wissel J, Pongratz D. Consensus statement: Botulinum toxin in myofascial pain. *J Neurol* 2004;251(suppl 1):I36–I38.

194. Lang AM. Botulinum toxin therapy for myofascial pain disorders. *Curr Pain Headache Rep* 2002;6:355–360.

195. Kern U, Martin C, Scheicher S, Müller H. Langzeitbehandlung von Phantom- und Stumpfschmerzen mit Botulinumtoxin Typ A über 12 Monate: Eine erste klinische Beobachtung. [German; Prolonged treatment of phantom and stump pain with Botulinum Toxin A over a period of 12 months: A preliminary clinical observation.] *Nervenarzt* 2004;75: 336–340.

196. Göbel H, Heinze A, Reichel G, Hefter H, Benecke R. Efficacy and safety of a single botulinum type A toxin complex treatment (Dysport) for the relief of upper back myofascial pain syndrome: Results from a randomized double-blind placebo-controlled multicentre study. *Pain* 2006;125:82–88.

197. Aoki KR. Review of a proposed mechanism for the antinociceptive action of botulinum toxin type A. *Neurotoxicology* 2005;26:785–793.

198. Aoki KR. Pharmacology and immunology of botulinum neurotoxins. *Int Ophthalmol Clin* 2005;45(3):25–37.

199. Peng PW, Castano ED. Survey of chronic pain practice by anesthesiologists in Canada. *Can J Anaesth* 2005;52(4):383–389.

200. Gunn CC. Transcutaneous neural stimulation, needle acupuncture and "the Ch'I" phenomenon. *Am J Acupuncture* 1976;4:317–322.

201. Gunn CC. Type IV acupuncture points. *Am J Acupuncture* 1977;5(1):45–46.

202. Gunn CC, Ditchburn FG, King MH, Renwick GJ. Acupuncture loci: A proposal for their classification according to their relationship to known neural structures. *Am J Chin Med* 1976;4:183–195.

203. Gunn CC, Milbrandt WE. Tenderness at motor points: An aid in the diagnosis of pain in the shoulder referred from the cervical spine. *J Am Osteopath Assoc* 1977;77(3):196–212.

204. Gunn CC. Motor points and motor lines. *Am J Acupuncture* 1978;6:55–58.

205. Birch S. Trigger point: Acupuncture point correlations revisited. *J Altern Complement Med* 2003;9:91–103.
206. Melzack R. Myofascial trigger points: Relation to acupuncture and mechanisms of pain. *Arch Phys Med Rehabil* 1981;62:114–117.
207. Dorsher P. Trigger points and acupuncture points: Anatomic and clinical correlations. *Med Acupunct* 2006;17(3):21–25.
208. Kao MJ, Hsieh YL, Kuo FJ, Hong C-Z. Electrophysiological assessment of acupuncture points. *Am J Phys Med Rehabil* 2006;85:443–448.
209. Hong C-Z: Myofascial trigger points: Pathophysiology and correlation with acupuncture points. *Acupunct Med* 2000;18(1):41–47.
210. Audette JF, Binder RA. Acupuncture in the management of myofascial pain and headache. *Curr Pain Headache Rep* 2003;7(5 suppl):395–401.
211. Melzack R, Stillwell DM, Fox EJ. Trigger points and acupuncture points for pain: Correlations and implications. *Pain* 1977;3:3–23.
212. Simons DG, Dommerholt J. Myofascial pain syndromes: Trigger points. *J Musculoskel Pain* 2006 (in press).
213. Travell JG, Simons DG. *Myofascial Pain and Dysfunction: The Trigger Point Manual.* Vol 2. Baltimore, MD: Williams & Wilkins; 1992.
214. Ge HY, Madeleine P, Wang K, Arendt-Nielsen L. Hypoalgesia to pressure pain in referred pain areas triggered by spatial summation of experimental muscle pain from unilateral or bilateral trapezius muscles. *Eur J Pain* 2003;7:531–537.
215. New Mexico Statutes Annotated 1978. Chapter 61: Professional and Occupational Licenses. Article 14A: Acupuncture and Oriental Medicine Practice. 3: Definitions, 1978.
216. Linde K, Streng A, Jurgens S, Hoppe A, Brinkhaus B, Witt C, Wagenpfeil S, Pfaffenrath V, Hammes MG, Weidenhammer W, Willich SN, Melchart D. Acupuncture for patients with migraine: A randomized controlled trial. *JAMA* 2005;293:2118–2125.
217. Melchart D, Streng A, Hoppe A, Brinkhaus B, Witt C, Wagenpfeil S, Pfaffenrath V, Hammes M, Hummelsberger J, Irnich D, Weidenhammer W, Willich SN, Linde K. Acupuncture in patients with tension-type headache: Randomised controlled trial. *BMJ* 2005;331(7513):376–382.
218. Scharf HP, Mansmann U, Streitberger K, Witte S, Kramer J, Maier C, Trampisch HJ, Victor N. Acupuncture and knee osteoarthritis: A three-armed randomized trial. *Ann Intern Med* 2006;145:12–20.

Chapter 9

# Physical Therapy Diagnosis and Management of a Patient with Chronic Daily Headache: A Case Report

*Tamer S. Issa, PT, BSc, DPT, OCS*

*Peter A. Huijbregts, PT, MSc, MHSc, DPT, OCS, FAAOMPT, FCAMT*

## Introduction

Headaches are one of the most common reasons people seek medical attention. They constitute the leading cause for neurology visits, accounting for one-third of outpatient visits.[1] No data are available on the prevalence of headache as a cause for orthopaedic physical therapy visits; however, Boissonnault[2] reported headache as a comorbidity in 22% of patients presenting for outpatient physical and occupational therapy services. Most relevant to the physical therapist are those headaches that to some extent have (or may have) a neuromusculoskeletal etiology, because those are the headache types that could logically be expected to benefit from physical therapy (PT) diagnosis and management. The International Headache Society (IHS) has long aimed to improve upon the understanding, diagnosis, and management of headache disorders. The IHS published the first internationally accepted and clinically useful headache classification system in 1988 with the first edition of the *International Classification of Headache Disorders* (ICHD); a second edition (ICHD-II) was published in 2004.[3] The ICHD-II has classified hundreds of different types of headaches into two categories: primary headaches and secondary headaches. Primary headaches are the most common headache type and have no other underlying cause. They include migraine headache (MH), tension-type headache (TTH), cluster headache and additional trigeminal autonomic cephalalgias, and other primary headaches. Secondary headaches are classified according to their causes and are classified into 10 separate categories. Of the primary headaches, mounting evidence in the scientific literature indicates that TTH and—to

Courtesy of John M. Medeiros, PT, PhD, Managing Editor of the *Journal of Manual and Manipulative Therapy*.

a lesser extent MH—may have an underlying neuromusculoskeletal contribution. Secondary headaches with a neuromusculoskeletal etiology include cervicogenic headache (CGH), occipital neuralgia (ON), and headache associated with temporomandibular disorder (TMD).

TTH is the most common yet least studied of the primary headaches.[4,5] It was once thought to be primarily psychogenic, but now there is evidence of a neurobiological component. Recent studies aimed at understanding the etiology and mechanism of TTH have looked at the role of muscle contraction, the significance of pericranial muscle tenderness, and the combined influence of these peripheral inputs with central etiologic features.[6,7] Pericranial muscle tenderness is the most well-documented abnormality found in TTH.[6-8] It has been proposed that in patients with chronic TTH, prolonged nociceptive stimuli from pericranial myofascial tissue contribute to supraspinal facilitation leading to central sensitization, which in turn results in an increased general pain sensitivity.[6,7,9] Central sensitization arises from the amplification of receptiveness of central pain-signaling neurons to input from low-threshold mechanoreceptors and is clinically characterized by the presence of hyperalgesia and/or allodynia.[10,11] **Table 9-1** lists the ICHD-II diagnostic criteria for some of the TTH forms.

It has been hypothesized that part of the continued peripheral nociceptive input leading to central sensitization in patients with TTH originates in myofascial trigger points (MTrPs). Referred pain originating in these MTrPs may also contribute to the clinical presentation of patients with TTH.[12-15] An MTrP is defined as a hypersensitive nodule within a taut band in skeletal muscle, which is painful on compression and which may cause characteristic referred pain, tenderness, or autonomic phenomena.[12-14,16-18] Myofascial trigger points can be found in a specific muscle or group of muscles and can limit the flexibility of the affected muscles.[12] Active MTrPs cause clinical symptoms of pain and restricted motion, whereas latent trigger points may not contribute to pain but still influence muscle fatigue and mobility.[12-14,16-19] Several muscles of the head and neck have referral pain patterns into the head that can cause or contribute to pain distribution patterns commonly associated not only with TTH but also with MH and secondary headaches such as CGH, occipital neuralgia, and TMD. Other trigger–point-related symptoms include tinnitus, eye symptoms, and torticollis.[12-21]

MH is a common disabling headache with a strong genetic basis. This headache type can be divided into two categories: migraine with or without aura (Table 9-1). The pathophysiology of MH is believed to be a neurovascular disorder of the trigeminovascular system in which a dysfunctional vasodilation in the brainstem mechanically irritates sensory fibers of the trigeminal nerve, resulting in the release of inflammatory substances and the activation of meningeal nociceptors. Release of substance P and calcitonin gene-related peptide further contributes to vasodilation and neurogenic inflammation, leading to an increased activation of neurons in the trigeminal ganglion and subsequent transmission of pain signals to the brain. During the progression of an MH episode, the spinal and supraspinal nervous centers become sensitized, resulting in increased pain and sensitivity to stimuli.[22]

**TABLE 9-1 Competing Primary Headaches⁴ (Migraine, Tension-Type, New Daily Persistent)**

| Type | Diagnostic Criteria |
|---|---|
| Migraine without aura (1.1) | A. At least five attacks fulfilling criteria B–D |
| | B. Headache attacks lasting 4–72 hours (untreated or unsuccessfully treated) |
| | C. Headache has at least two of the following characteristics: |
| |   1. Unilateral location |
| |   2. Pulsating quality |
| |   3. Moderate or severe pain intensity |
| |   4. Aggravation by or causing avoidance of routine physical activity (e.g., walking or climbing stairs) |
| | D. During headache at least one of the following: |
| |   1. Nausea and/or vomiting |
| |   2. Photophobia and phonophobia |
| | E. Not attributed to another disorder |
| Typical aura with migraine (1.2.1) | A. At least two attacks fulfilling criteria B–D |
| | B. Aura consisting of at least one of the following, but no motor weakness: |
| |   1. Fully reversible visual symptoms including positive features (e.g., flickering lights, spots or lines) and/or negative features (i.e., loss of vision) |
| |   2. Fully reversible sensory symptoms including positive features (i.e., pins and needles) and/or negative features (i.e., numbness) |
| |   3. Fully reversible dysphasic speech disturbance |
| | C. At least two of the following: |
| |   1. Homonymous visual symptoms and/or unilateral sensory symptoms |
| |   2. At least one aura symptom develops gradually over ≥5 minutes and/or different aura symptoms occur in succession over ≥5 minutes |
| |   3. Each symptom lasts ≥5 and ≤60 minutes |
| | D. Headache fulfilling criteria B–D for 1.1 *Migraine without aura* begins during the aura or follows aura within 60 minutes. |
| | E. Not attributed to another disorder |

*(continued)*

TABLE 9-1 Competing Primary Headaches[4] (Migraine, Tension-Type, New Daily Persistent) (cont.)

| Type | Diagnostic Criteria |
|---|---|
| Chronic migraine (1.5.1) | A. Headache fulfilling criteria C and D for 1.1 *Migraine without aura* on ≥15 days/month for >3 months |
| | B. Not attributed to another disorder |
| Probable migraine without aura (1.6.1) | A. Attacks fulfilling all but one of criteria A–D for 1.1 *Migraine without aura* |
| | B. Not attributed to another disorder |
| Infrequent episodic tension-type headache (2.1) | A. At least 10 episodes occurring on <1 day per month on average (<12 days per year) and fulfilling criteria B–D |
| | B. Headache lasting from 30 minutes to 7 days |
| | C. Headache has at least two of the following characteristics: |
| |    1. Bilateral location |
| |    2. Pressing/tightening (nonpulsating) quality |
| |    3. Mild or moderate intensity |
| |    4. Not aggravated by routine physical activity such as walking or climbing stairs |
| | D. Both of the following: |
| |    1. No nausea or vomiting (anorexia may occur) |
| |    2. No more than one of photophobia or phonophobia |
| | E. Not attributed to another disorder |
| Frequent episodic tension-type headache (2.2) | A. At least 10 episodes of occurring on ≥1 but <15 days per month for at least 3 months and fulfilling criteria B–D |
| | B. Headache lasting from 30 minutes to 7 days |
| | C. Headache has at least two of the following characteristics: |
| |    1. Bilateral location |
| |    2. Pressing/tightening (nonpulsating) quality |
| |    3. Mild to moderate intensity |
| |    4. Not aggravated by routine physical activity such as walking or climbing stairs |
| | D. Both of the following: |
| |    1. No nausea and/or vomiting (anorexia may occur) |
| |    2. No more than one of photophobia and phonophobia |
| | E. Not attributed to another disorder |

*(continued)*

## TABLE 9-1   Competing Primary Headaches[4] (Migraine, Tension-Type, New Daily Persistent) (cont.)

| Type | Diagnostic Criteria |
|---|---|
| Chronic tension-type headache (2.3) | A. Headache occurring on ≥15 days per month on average for >3 months and fulfilling criteria B–D |
| | B. Headache lasts hours or may be continuous |
| | C. Headache has at least two of the following characteristics: |
| |   1. Bilateral location |
| |   2. Pressing/tightening (nonpulsating) quality |
| |   3. Mild to moderate intensity |
| |   4. Not aggravated by routine physical activity such as walking or climbing stairs |
| | D. Both of the following: |
| |   1. No more than one of photophobia, phonophobia, or mild nausea |
| |   2. Neither moderate or severe nausea nor vomiting |
| | E. Not attributed to another disorder |
| Chronic tension-type headache associated with pericranial tenderness (2.3.1) | A. Headache fulfilling criteria A–E for 2.3 *Chronic tension-type headache* |
| | B. Increased pericranial tenderness on manual palpation |
| Chronic tension-type headache not associated with pericranial tenderness (2.3.2) | A. Headache fulfilling criteria A–E for 2.3 *Chronic tension-type headache* |
| | B. No increased pericranial tenderness |
| Cluster headache (3.1) | A. At least five attacks fulfilling criteria B–D |
| | B. Severe or very severe unilateral orbital, supraorbital, and/or temporal pain lasting 15–180 minutes if untreated |
| | C. Headache is accompanied by at least one of the following: |
| |   1. Ipsilateral conjunctival injection and/or lacrimation |
| |   2. Ipsilateral nasal congestion and/or rhinorrhoea |
| |   3. Ipsilateral eyelid edema |
| |   4. Ipsilateral forehead and facial sweating |
| |   5. Ipsilateral miosis and/or ptosis |
| |   6. A sense of restlessness or agitation |

*(continued)*

TABLE 9-1    Competing Primary Headaches[4] (Migraine, Tension-Type, New Daily Persistent) (cont.)

| Type | Diagnostic Criteria |
|---|---|
| | D. Attacks have a frequency from one every other day to eight per day |
| | E. Not attributed to another disorder |
| New daily persistent headache (4.8) | A. Headache >3 months fulfilling criteria B–D |
| | B. Headache is daily and unremitting from onset or from <3 days from onset |
| | C. At least two of the following pain characteristics: |
| |     1. Bilateral location |
| |     2. Pressing/tightening (nonpulsating) quality |
| |     3. Mild or moderate intensity |
| |     4. Not aggravated by routine physical activity such as walking or climbing stairs |
| | D. Both of the following: |
| |     1. No more than one of photophobia, phonophobia, or mild nausea |
| |     2. Neither moderate or severe nausea nor vomiting |
| | E. Not attributed to another disorder |

The proposed etiology of CGH is based on the convergence of afferent sensory input into the cervicotrigeminal nucleus from structures that are innervated by the first three spinal nerves or the trigeminal nerve. A subsequent "misinterpretation" of nociceptive signals originating in the cervical somatosensory structures as coming from the structures in the head innervated by the trigeminal nerve is thought to be responsible for this type of headache.[23-27] Musculoskeletal structures in the neck that are innervated by the first three spinal nerves that may refer pain into the head include the atlanto-occipital joints, joints and ligaments of the atlanto-axial joint, the C2–C4 zygapophyseal joints, the C2–C3 intervertebral disk, and muscles innervated by C1–C3.[23-29] **Table 9-2** lists the diagnostic criteria for CGH.

Temporomandibular disorder describes a variety of conditions affecting the temporomandibular joint (TMJ) and the muscles of mastication.[30] Symptoms include jaw and facial pain, limited TMJ mobility, joint sounds, tinnitus, and—most relevant to this case report—headaches.[15,16,30,31] A classification of TMD into two subtypes provides a better understanding of the disorder and possible treatment options.[30] Arthralgia encompasses impairments related to the joint biomechanics, internal derangements, degenerative

## TABLE 9-2 Competing Secondary Headaches[4] (Related to Whiplash, Head/Neck Trauma, Cervical Spine, Temporomandibular Joint)

| Type | Diagnostic Criteria |
|---|---|
| Chronic headache attributed to whiplash injury (5.4) | A. Headache, not typical characteristics known, fulfilling criteria C and D |
| | B. History of whiplash (sudden and significant acceleration/deceleration movement of the neck) associated at the time with neck pain |
| | C. Headache develops within 7 days after whiplash injury |
| | D. Headache persists for >3 months after whiplash injury |
| Chronic headache attributed to other head and/or neck trauma (5.6.2) | A. Headache, no typical characteristics known, fulfilling criteria C and D |
| | B. Evidence of head and/or neck trauma of a type not described above |
| | C. Headache develops in close temporal relation to, and/or other evidence exists to establish a causal relationship with, the head and/or neck trauma |
| | D. Headache persist for >3 months after the head and/or neck trauma |
| Cervicogenic headache (11.2.1) | A. Pain, referred from a source in the neck and perceived in one or more regions of the head and/or face, fulfilling criteria C and D |
| | B. Clinical, laboratory and/or imaging evidence of a disorder or lesion within the cervical spine or soft tissues of the neck known to be, or generally accepted as, a valid cause of headache |
| | C. Evidence that the pain can be attributed to the neck disorder or lesion based on at least one of the following: |
| |   1. Demonstration of clinical signs that implicate a source of pain in the neck |
| |   2. Abolition of headache following diagnostic blockade of a cervical structure or its nerve supply using placebo or other adequate controls |
| | D. Pain resolves within 3 months after successful treatment of the causative disorder or lesion |

*(continued)*

TABLE 9-2 Competing Secondary Headaches[4] (Related to Whiplash, Head/Neck Trauma, Cervical Spine, Temporomandibular Joint) (Cont.)

| Type | Diagnostic Criteria |
|---|---|
| Headache or facial pain attributed to temporo-mandibular joint (TMJ) disorder (11.7) | A. Recurrent pain in one or more regions of the head and/or face fulfilling criteria C and D<br><br>B. X-ray, MRI and/or bone scintigraphy demonstrate TMJ disorder<br><br>C. Evidence that pain can be attributed to the TMJ disorder, based on at least one of the following:<br><br>  1. Pain is precipitated by jaw movements and/or chewing of hard or tough food<br><br>  2. Reduced range of or irregular jaw movements<br><br>  3. Noise from one or both TMJs during jaw movements<br><br>  4. Tenderness of the joint capsule(s) of one or both TMJs<br><br>D. Headache resolves within 3 months, and does not recur, after successful treatment of the TMJ disorder |

Note: TMJ: Temporomandibular joint.

changes, developmental defects, and other pathologies related to the TMJ.[30] Myalgia is related to impairments and pain in the musculature surrounding the TMJ.[30] Table 9-2 lists the diagnostic criteria for TMD-related headache.

Data on the epidemiology of headache further underscore the need for knowledge related to headache. We noted that headaches are one of the most common reasons for people to seek medical attention. Headaches are more prevalent in women than in men but prevalence tends to decrease with age.[1,32,33] Up to one adult in 20 has a headache every day or nearly every day.[1] Most of the population studies and research have focused on MH: European and American studies have shown a 1 year prevalence of MH in 6–8% of males and 15–18% of females.[1] One in four American households has a migraine sufferer, totaling approximately 29.5 million people.[32] TTH is even more prevalent: It affects two-thirds of males and over 80% of females in developed countries.[1] Episodic TTH is the most common headache type reported in over 70% of some populations; chronic TTH is found in 1–3%.[1] Approximately 78% of adults will suffer from a TTH at least once in their lives.[32] The prevalence of CGH has been reported to be 0.4–2.5% in the general population and as high as 15–20% in those with chronic headaches.[23] The prevalence of TMD in the Western population ranges from 10–40%.[15] TMD can be episodic, but it is often a chronic condition affecting women more than men,[15] and can be associated with headaches. Medication-overuse headache is a chronic headache form that affects up to 5% of the population.[1] Chronic daily headache is perhaps the most disabling of the headache groups. It signifies those who experience a headache daily or nearly daily (15 days or more per month), and affects up to one in 20 adults worldwide.[1]

Headache also has a significant socioeconomic impact. Persons with chronic headaches report disabling complaints that interfere with daily activities. Work capacity and social activity is reduced in 60% of TTH patients and in almost all MH patients.[33] A 2001 report by the World Health Organization (WHO) stated that MH contributed to 1.4% of all years lived with disability (YLDs), ranking it as the 19th highest cause of disability in both sexes of all ages.[33] Among women, it contributed to 2.0% of YLDs, which ranked it 12th among causes of disability.[33] The financial impact of headaches on the sufferer and society is of considerable concern. Health-care costs are 70% higher in families with migraine sufferers in the United States.[34] Outpatient health-care costs in the United States were 80% higher for "migraine families" than for "nonmigraine families."[34] Pharmacy costs accounted for 20% of total health-care costs in migraine families, compared to 15% in nonmigraine families.[34] The prevalence of MH is highest between the ages of 25 to 55 years, corresponding to an individual's most productive years.[34] In the United Kingdom, some 25 million working days or school days are lost every year because of MH.[1] It has been reported that 8.3% of patients with episodic TTH lost an average of 8.9 work days and that 11.8% of patients with chronic TTH lost an average of 27.4 work days.[35]

Headache can be difficult to evaluate, and an individual may present with multiple forms of the condition. As indicated above and in Tables 9-1 and 9-2, TTH, MH, CGH, and TMD share many similar signs and symptoms. Muscle tenderness to palpation is a common finding among them, making it difficult to differentiate between them. To further complicate matters with regard to differential diagnosis, some authors believe that MH and TTH are in fact headaches on the same continuum, whereas others believe they are separate entities.[3,6] There is also overlap between various headaches and TMJ pain, because the head and face share a common innervation and vascular supply, leading to similar pain patterns in cases of dysfunction or disease.[30] There is a close relationship between the increase of bruxism (grinding or clenching of teeth) and parafunction (excessive or unnecessary function related to the jaw) found in TMD and an increase in TTH frequency.[30] One review looked at the CGH diagnostic criteria and concluded that there was insufficient specificity to separate CGH from MH patients.[36] Another study looked at the association between MH and TMD and concluded that they were two clearly differentiated diagnostic entities.[30] Various authors agree that there are neuromuscu-loskeletal abnormalities that play a role in the pathogenesis and presentation of TTH,[6-8,12-16,20,24-26,37,38] MH,[26,37,38] CGH,[16,24-26,28-30,37,38] TMD-related headaches,[15,16,30,31,38] and occipital neuralgia headaches,[21] further exacerbating the difficulty faced by the clinician with regard to differential diagnosis.[16,21]

Despite the high prevalence of headache disorders and their socioeconomic and personal impact, headache disorders continue to be underestimated in scale, poorly diagnosed, and undertreated by the medical community.[1,33] The patient described in this case report presented with a medical diagnosis of MH and chronic TTH with an onset of a new type of chronic daily headache potentially related to a history of motor vehicle accident (MVA) and/or possibly caused by TMD. The etiology of various headaches is often difficult to determine with potential combined influences of neurologic, musculoskeletal, neurovascular, psychological, and nutritional factors and chemical imbalances in the brain. Some headaches are indicative of an underlying disease process; some of these are life-threatening and others benign. Thus, a thorough medical evaluation is necessary with any new onset or ongoing headache. Likewise, a thorough PT examination should aim to rule out serious pathology by way of a systems review approach, to determine the type of headache, and to define the neuromusculoskeletal factors that may be contributing to the headache. An accurate differential diagnosis is imperative in determining whether a headache is neuromusculoskeletal in origin, which is treatable, or whether it is another type of headache that requires medical consultation and (co)management. The purposes of this chapter describing a patient with chronic daily headache are to:

1. Describe the PT differential diagnosis and decision-making process

2. Provide a treatment rationale and description of subsequent PT management using a combination of myofascial trigger point dry needling, orthopaedic manual physical therapy (OMPT), exercise therapy, and patient education

## Case Description

### History

The patient described in this chapter was a married 48-year-old-female with four teenage children, two dogs, one cat, and a horse, which made for a busy home life. She was referred to PT within a multidisciplinary pain management practice with a medical diagnosis of common MH, chronic TTH, and TMD. The patient worked as a full-time general counsel attorney and had been at her current job for 6 months. Work environment was sedentary with physical demands related to sitting deskwork with some time spent using the computer and telephone. She had not lost any work time because of her headaches. The patient was a nonsmoker and drank two glasses of wine per week and one cup of caffeinated coffee per day. The wine and coffee were not reported as triggers for her headaches. Recreational activities included yoga once a week, aerobic and resistance training three times a week, and reading. Prior to the initial evaluation, the patient was asked to complete a pain drawing (**Figure 9-1**) and two outcome assessment tools: the *Henry Ford Hospital Headache Disability Inventory* [HDI] (**Figure 9-2**) and the *Neck Disability Index* [NDI] (**Figure 9-3**). The HDI and NDI were chosen as outcome measures to assess the response to treatment on the patient's headache and neck-related self-perceived disability.

The HDI is a 25-item questionnaire that aims to measure the self-perceived disabling effects of headache on daily life. The questionnaire contains two subgroups of questions, thereby creating emotional and functional subscale scores and a total score. Two additional items on the questionnaire ask the patient to rate the severity of his/her headache as (1) mild, (2) moderate, or (3) severe and the frequency as (1) less than or equal to one per month, (2) more

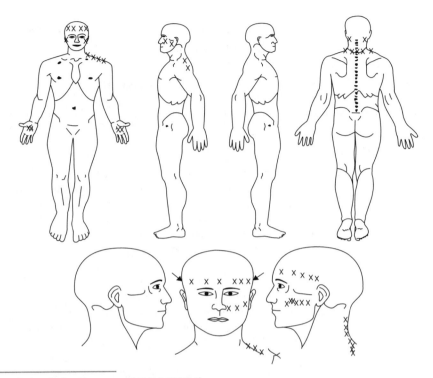

**Figure 9-1** Pain diagram (10/18/2004).

than one but less than four per month, or (3) four or more times per month. The results of the HDI for this patient (Figure 9-2) indicated severe headache intensity, headache frequency greater than one per week, and a total score of 56/100 (emotional 26/52, functional 30/48). The HDI has good internal consistency reliability; correlations between the emotional and functional subscale scores and the total score were both excellent ($r = 0.89$).[39] It also has good short-term (1-week) ($r = 0.93$–$0.95$)[40] and generally good long-term (2-month) test-retest reliability ($r = 0.83$)[39] for the total scores. The HDI also exhibits good internal construct validity ($P <0.001$).[39] A minimal detectable change ($MDC_{95}$) score at 1-week retest is 16 points; this value for the $MDC_{95}$ indicates that a clinician can be 95% confident that a true change has occurred with a change in the HDI score $\geq 16$ points.[40] Similarly, a 29-point score improvement constitutes the $MDC_{95}$ over a 2-month time period.[39] The HDI test is simple to administer and takes little time to complete. This self-reporting outcome measure is useful in periodically and reliably assessing the effects of treatment intervention in patients with disabling headaches.[39,40]

The NDI is a 10-item questionnaire that aims to measure the self-perceived disabling effects of neck pain on daily life. It is a modification of the *Oswestry Low Back Pain Index*, which has been used as a self-reporting outcome measure for low-back pain disability.

Name:                    Record #:                  Date: <u>10/18/04</u>

### Headache Disability Index

**INSTRUCTIONS:** Please CIRCLE the correct response.

1. I have headache: (1) 1 per month (2) more then 1 but less than 4 per month (3) more than one per week
2. My headache is: (1) mild        (2) moderate                (3) severe

**Please read carefully:** The purpose of the scale is to identify difficulties that you may be experiencing because of your headache. Please check off "Yes," "SOMETIMES," or "NO" to each item. Answer each question as it pertains to your headache only.

| YES | SOMETIMES | NO | | |
|---|---|---|---|---|
| | ✓ | | E1. | Because of my headaches I feel handicapped. |
| | ✓ | | F2. | Because of my headaches I feel restricted in performing my routine daily activities. |
| | ✓ | | E3. | No one understands the effect my headaches have on my life. |
| ✓ | | | F4. | I restrict my recreational activities (e.g., sports, hobbies, etc.) because of my headaches. |
| ✓ | | | E5. | My headaches make me angry. |
| ✓ | | | E6. | Sometimes I feel that I am going to lose contrct because of my headaches. |
| ✓ | | | F7. | Because of my headaches I am less likely to socialize. |
| | ✓ | | E8. | My spouse (significant other), or family and friends have no idea what I am going through because of my headaches. |
| | ✓ | | E9. | My headaches are so bad that I feel that am going to go insane. |
| | ✓ | | E10. | My outlook on the world is affected by my headaches. |
| | | ✓ | E11. | I am afraid to go outside when I feel that a headache is starting. |
| | ✓ | | E12. | I feel desperate because of my headaches. |
| ✓ | | | F13. | I am concerned that I am paying penalties at work at home because of my headaches. |
| | ✓ | | E14. | My headaches place stress on my relationships with family or friends. |
| | ✓ | | F15. | I avoid being around people when I have a headache. |
| ✓ | | | F16. | I believe my headaches are making it difficult for me to achieve my goals in life. |
| | | ✓ | F17. | I am unable to think clearly because of my headaches. |
| ✓ | | | F18. | I get tense (e.g. muscle tension) because of my headaches. |
| | | ✓ | F19. | I do not enjoy social gatherings because of my headaches. |
| ✓ | | | F20. | I feel irritable because of my headaches. |
| | | ✓ | F21. | I avoid traveling because of my headaches. |
| | | ✓ | E22. | My headaches make me feel confused. |
| ✓ | | | E23. | My headaches make me feel frustrated. |
| | ✓ | | F24. | I find it difficult to read because of my headaches. |
| | | ✓ | F25. | I find it difficult to focus my attention away from my headaches and on other things. |
| 36 | 20 | 0 | = | 56/100 |

**Figure 9-2** Initial headache disability index.[39]

Name:                   Record #:               Date: <u>10/18/04</u>

## Neck Disability Index

This questionnaire is designed to help us better understand how your neck pain affects your ability to manage everyday-life activities. Please mark in each section the **one box** that applies to you. Although you may consider that two of the statements in any one section relate to you, please mark the box that most closely describes your present-day situation.

### Section 1: Pain Intensity

0☐ I have no pain at the moment.
1☑ The pain is very mild at the moment.
2☐ The pain is moderate at the moment.
3☐ The pain is fairly severe at the moment.
4☐ The pain is very severe at the moment.
5☐ The pain is the worst imaginable at the moment.

### Section 2: Personal Care

0☐ I can look after myself normally without causing extra pain.
1☑ I can look after myself normally but it causes extra pain.
2☐ It is painful to look after myself, and I am slow and careful.
3☐ I need some help but can manage most of my personal care.
4☐ I need help every day in most aspects of self-care.
5☐ I do not get dressed, wash with difficulty and stay in bed.

### Section 3: Lifting

0☐ I can lift heavy weights without causing extra pain.
1☐ I can lift heavy weights, but it gives me extra pain.
2☑ Pain prevents me from lifting heavy weights off the floor, but I can manage if they are conveniently placed, i.e. on a table.
3☐ Pain prevents me from lifting heavy weights but I can manage light to medium weights if they are conveniently positioned.
4☐ I can only lift very light weights.
5☐ I can not lift or carry anything at all.

### Section 4: Work

0☐ I can do as much work as I want.
1☑ I can only do my usual work, but no more.
2☐ I can do most of my usual work, but no more.
3☐ I can't do my usual work.
4☐ I can hardly do any work at all.
5☐ I can't do any work at all.

### Section 5: Headaches

0☐ I have no headaches at all.
1☐ I have slight headaches that come infrequently.
2☐ I have moderate headaches that come infrequently.
3☐ I have moderate headaches that come frequently.
4☐ I have severe headaches that come frequently.
5☑ I have headaches almost all the time.

### Section 6: Concentration

0☐ I concentrate fully without difficulty.
1☑ I can concentrate fully with slight difficulty.
2☐ I have a fair degree of difficulty concentrating.
3☐ I have a lot of difficulty concentrating.
4☐ I have a great deal of difficulty concentrating.
5☐ I can't concentrate at all.

### Section 7: Sleeping

0☑ I have no trouble sleeping.
1☐ My sleep is slightly disturbed for less that 1 hour.
2☐ My sleep is mildly disturbed for up to 1–2 hours.
3☐ My sleep is moderately distributed for up to 2–3 hours.
4☐ My sleep is greatly disturbed for up to 3–5 hours.
5☐ My sleep is completely disturbed for up to 5–7 hours.

### Section 8: Driving

0☐ I can drive my car without neck pain.
1☐ I can drive as long as I want with slight neck pain.
2☐ I can drive as long as I want with moderate neck pain.
3☑ I can't drive as long as I want because of moderate neck pain.
4☐ I can hardly drive at all because of severe neck pain.
5☐ I can't drive my car at all because of neck pain.

### Section 9: Reading

0☐ I can read as much as I want with no neck pain.
1☐ I can read as much as I want with slight neck pain.
2☐ I can read as much as I want with moderate neck pain.
3☑ I can't read as much as I want because of moderate neck pain.
4☐ I can't read as much as I want because of severe neck pain.
5☐ I can't read at all.

### Section 10: Recreation

0☐ I have no neck pain during all recreational activities.
1☐ I have some neck pain with all recreation activities.
2☑ I have some neck pain with a few recreational activities.
3☐ I have neck pain with most recreational activities.
4☐ I can hardly do recreational activities due to neck pain.
5☐ I can't do any recreational activities due to neck pain.

38/100

**Figure 9-3** Initial neck disability index.

Interpretation is possible through scoring intervals as follows: 0–4 = no disability, 5–14 = mild, 15–24 = moderate, 25–34 = severe, and above 34 = complete disability.[41] To arrive at a percentage disability, the total score can be multiplied by two. The NDI questionnaire results for this patient (Figure 9-3) indicated a 38% score (i.e., moderate disability). The NDI has moderate test-retest reliability (ICC = 0.68).[42] Construct validity of the NDI as an outcome measure for neck pain has been demonstrated by comparing it to other tests or measures. Cleland et al[42] showed that a 7-point (14%) change in the NDI constituted a minimally clinically important difference (MCID) for the NDI in patients with cervical radiculopathy.

On the pain drawing (Figure 9-1), the patient indicated headache, facial pain, and neck pain. The headaches were located in the bilateral frontal head region, the facial pain was in the left cheek and jaw region, and the neck pain was in the bilateral suboccipital region, lower neck, and left back of neck. The headache was described as severe, daily, and bandlike across the front of the head with tenderness of the head and occasional ringing in the left ear. The neck pain was described as tenderness. The patient denied complaints of dizziness, loss of consciousness, loss of balance, sensation disturbances, weakness, nausea and vomiting, or visual disturbances. These symptoms were asked about in order to screen for central nervous system dysfunction—including cord compression, cranial nerve dysfunction due to undiagnosed central processes, vertebral or carotid artery compromise, postconcussive syndrome, and other intracranial pathology—that might be causing the current complaints of headache.[43] The diagnostic accuracy of these symptoms for implicating the mentioned pathologies has not been validated.

The patient reported that symptoms were improved by local application of heat, stretching, sometimes doing nothing, and sumatriptan if it was a migraine-type headache. The patient identified this migraine-type headache as the headache that caused pain behind her left eye; this identification was confirmed by the positive response to medication specific for an MH (i.e., sumatriptan). However, the patient noted that the use of sumatriptan did not always relieve the present headache, which would seem to indicate the presence of more than one type of headache. Symptoms were aggravated by bright light, certain smells, hunger, hot weather, exercise, and change in barometric pressure. No diurnal pattern of symptoms was noted. Sleep was undisturbed in a habitual left and/or right sidelying position with use of a cervical pillow.

A review of the available physician medical records and radiological reports indicated a history of MH since age 17. The onset time and cause of her neck pain was unknown. Onset of the newly described headache was 3 years before, and a neurologist who specialized in headache management supervised its diagnosis and management. Follow-up with the physician had occurred approximately 1 year prior because of the onset of left tinnitus. The patient was then referred to a dentist due to suspicion of TMD. The dentist prescribed a night splint, which the patient wore on and off. She continued to see her dentist regularly until her mother died in February of 2004. Headaches had become more intense in March of 2004 and continued to become progressively worse over the next 6 months.

The patient was unable to relate possible reasons contributing to the onset or worsening of the complaints.

Her neurologist then referred the patient to a pain management outpatient practice in August 2004, where a physician who was a neurologist and pain management specialist saw her. This physician reported increased and abnormal tone of the left arm and pronounced slowness of finger tapping of the left hand. He was concerned with the facts of increasing severity of headaches, worsening of symptoms lying down compared to being upright, and motor dysfunction with the left arm when raised. The physician ordered a magnetic resonance imaging (MRI) study; findings showed no focal signal abnormality or mass lesions in the brain. MRI and magnetic resonance angiography (MRA) studies of the brain done approximately 2 years earlier were again evaluated and found normal. The patient had a follow-up visit with the same physician 1 month later with continued complaints of headache more than 50% of the time. At the time of the initial physical therapy evaluation, the headache was daily during some weeks but at other times the patient could go several days without a headache. At times she took the sumatriptan (Imitrex) daily or even twice daily but the effect varied from none to satisfactory headache relief. The TMJ remained uncomfortable, but the dentist told the patient that improvement as a result of wearing the splint would take time. The neurologist had recommended botulinum toxin injections for selected neck, shoulder, and facial muscles in combination with PT, but the patient elected against these injections.

The medical history for this patient included MH, asthma, depression, and a fractured pelvis and nose as a result of an MVA 5 years before. Her surgical history included tubal ligation, laser surgery for cervix dysplagia, and tonsillectomy. Current medications included citalopram 20 mg once a day (QD) (antidepressant), sumatriptan 50 mg as needed (PRN), tizanidine hydrochloride PRN (short-acting muscle relaxant), fluticasone QD (asthma treatment), and drospirenone/ethinyl estradiol (birth control). A screening examination using a systems approach revealed that the patient was receiving psychological counseling once a week. The patient's family history included the father alive at 69 with high blood pressure and diabetes and the mother deceased at age 69 from an overdose. The patient provided no further details on her mother's death. There was no indication in the family history of headaches, including MH. First-degree relatives of persons who never had MH are at no increased risk of MH without aura (relative risk = 1.11 [95% confidence interval (CI) 0.83–1.39]) or with aura (relative risk = 0.65 [95% CI: 0.36–0.94]).[44]

## Physical Examination

The patient stood 5′7″ at 155 lbs with a mesomorphic body type. Postural observation of this patient from the side using a 3-point grading system (increased, normal, decreased) revealed decreased lumbar lordosis, increased thoracic kyphosis, and increased craniocervical extension resulting in a forward head posture (FHP). Observation from the back revealed symmetrical iliac crest and shoulder heights; the head was side-bent to the right.

Fedorak et al[45] noted fair intra- ($\kappa = 0.50$) and poor interrater reliability ($\kappa = 0.16$) for visual assessment of cervical and lumbar lordosis using a similar 3-point rating system.

Craniocervical, cervical, and upper thoracic spine active range of motion (AROM) testing in a sitting position assessed quality of motion, range, and pain provocation; limitations were estimated visually with the following findings:

- Craniocervical flexion limited by 50%; extension not limited.
- C1–C2 rotation right limited by 50%.
- Cervical flexion limited by 25% with tightness reported in the upper back; extension hypermobility with an apex of the curve observed at C5–C6.
- Cervical side-bending right (SBR) limited by 75% with tightness in the contralateral neck; SBL limited by 25% with restriction noted ipsilateral.
- Cervical rotation right (RR) limited by 25% with contralateral tightness; RL limited by 75% with no symptoms.
- Upper-thoracic (T1–T4) and mid-thoracic (T4–T8) extension limited without pain; all other directions were within normal limits.

Bilateral shoulder functional AROM assessed also by way of visual estimation was within normal limits. Interrater reliability for visual estimation of cervical ROM is poor overall compared to goniometric techniques.[46] Interrater agreement for visual estimation of shoulder AROM tests is poor to good (ICC = 0.15–0.88) but decreases when pain and disability are present. However, with the exception of horizontal adduction, it is suitable for distinguishing between the affected and normal side, indicating that its use here as a screening tool was appropriate.[47]

A neuroconductive examination yielded bilateral normal (5/5) results for C2–T1 myotomal muscle strength tests. Reflex testing yielded a 2+ bilateral for the brachioradialis, biceps, and triceps deep tendon reflexes. Sensation testing for bilateral C1–C5 distribution was normal for light touch and pinprick. Spine compression through the head in sitting was negative for pain reproduction. Spine distraction in sitting was negative for pain reproduction or pain relief. Extension quadrant AROM to the right revealed slight limitation with complaints of left anterior neck tightness but to the left produced no limitations or symptoms. Jepsen et al[48] noted fair to good ($\kappa = 0.25$–$0.72$) interrater reliability for upper-limb manual muscle testing; Bertilson et al[49] reported poor to moderate ($\kappa = 0.20$–$0.57$) reliability for myotomal (C2–C8) strength tests and poor interrater reliability ($\kappa = -0.09$) for reflex testing. Sensitivity to pain with use of a pinwheel has shown moderate to substantial ($\kappa = 0.46$–$0.79$) interrater reliability.[49] Using a 3-point rating scale, Jepsen et al[50] reported median interrater (values of 0.69 for sensitivity to light touch and 0.48 for sensitivity to pin prick. Neck compression and traction tests for reproduction or traction tests for relief have shown moderate ($\kappa = 0.44$, $\kappa = 0.41$, and $\kappa = 0.63$, respectively) interrater reliability.[49]

Palpation for condition of the cervical spine in sitting revealed no aberrant findings for skin temperature, skin moisture, paravertebral muscle tone, or swelling. Palpation for soft-tissue condition of the spine, neck, and head was also performed in supine and prone positions. This revealed myofascial hypertonicity characterized by palpable taut bands and active MTrPs using clinical diagnostic criteria (**Table 9-3**)[12] in bilateral upper trapezius (UT) (left worse than the right), sternocleidomastoid (SCM), splenius capitis (SpCap), suboccipital (SO), and left masseter and temporalis muscles. Trigger point palpation of the UT produced referred pain into the upper neck, and palpation of the SCM caused referred pain into the forehead. Reliability studies looking at the various clinical aspects of MTrPs have been varied, and clinically relevant agreement in identifying the presence or absence of trigger points has proven to be difficult to achieve.[51] Gerwin et al[52] found good interrater reliability among four expert clinicians for the identification of tenderness, presence of a taut band, referred pain, local twitch response, reproduction of the patient's pain, and when a global assessment was made regarding the presence of a trigger point. Lew et al[53] showed poor interrater reliability for locating latent MTrPs in the UT; in contrast, Sciotti et al[54] found acceptable (G-coef ≥0.8) interrater reliability for the same procedure. Schöps et al[55] reported κ values of 0.46–0.63 and 0.31–0.37 for the interrater agreement on pain on palpation for the SCM and UT, respectively. Interrater agreement on muscle tone for these muscles yielded κ values of 0.22–0.37 and 0.20–0.30, respectively. Lending validity to the diagnosis of MTrPs, the primary author later confirmed above manual identification of MTrPs with the elicitation of local twitch responses (LTR) during treatment; Hong et al[56] concluded that an LTR was more frequently elicited by needling than by palpation. They also noted that there was a significant ($P$ <0.01) correlation between the incidence of referred pain and the pain intensity of an active trigger point and the occurrence of an LTR.

---

**TABLE 9-3  Temporomandibular Disorders Diagnostic Criteria for Myofascial Pain[82]**

**Essential Criteria**

1. Palpable taut band (if muscle accessible)
2. Exquisite spot tenderness of a nodule within the taut band
3. Pressure of tender nodule elicits patient's current pain complaint (identifies an active trigger point)
4. Painful limitation to full range of motion stretch

**Confirmatory Findings**

1. Visual or tactile identification of a local twitch response
2. Referred pain or altered sensation with pressure of tender nodule
3. EMG demonstration of spontaneous electrical activity in the tender nodule of a taut band
4. Imaging of a local twitch response induced by needle penetration of tender nodule

Palpation for position in sitting revealed a decreased functional space between the occiput and spinous process of C2. Without reference to research, Rocabado[57] noted that this functional space is adequate if a minimum of two fingers can be placed between the base of the occiput and the C2 spinous process. Palpation for position of the C1 in sitting revealed that the right transverse process of the C1 was anterior and superior compared to the left and was tender to palpation compared to the left. Positional palpation of C1 has moderate interrater reliability ($\kappa = 0.63$).[58] Palpation for position in supine revealed no aberrant findings for palpation of the articular pillars of the cervical spine, bony landmarks of the scapula, or for the first and second ribs. Lewis et al[59] noted surface palpation as a valid tool for determining scapular position.

Palpation for passive mobility of the cervical spine was performed in supine and of the thoracic spine in prone. Passive intervertebral motion (PIVM) was tested using the Paris grading system[60] (**Table 9-4**). This yielded the following findings:

- C0–C1: Pain-free grade 1 restriction for flexion and SBL
- C1–C2: Painful grade 1 restriction for RR
- T1–T4: Pain-free grade 1 restriction for extension
- T4–T8: Pain-free grade 2 restriction for extension

Palpation for mobility is used by manual medicine clinicians to identify mobility dysfunctions that may contribute to spinal disorders.[61-66] Palpation for mobility in the cervical and thoracic spine has demonstrated both intra- and interrater agreement varying from no better than chance to perfect.[65] Most relevant to this case report, however, Jull et al[61] reported near excellent to perfect interrater agreement ($\kappa = 0.78$–$1.00$) for identifying a C0-C3 joint restriction considered relevant to CGH. Jull et al[67] also examined construct validity of cervical palpation for mobility tests and found 100% sensitivity and

TABLE 9-4    Grading System for Passive Intervertebral Mobility (PIVM) Tests[60]

| Grade | Description |
| --- | --- |
| 0 | Ankylosis or no detectable movement |
| 1 | Considerable limitation in movement |
| 2 | Slight limitation in movement |
| 3 | Normal (for the individual) |
| 4 | Slight increase in motion |
| 5 | Considerable increase in motion |
| 6 | Unstable |

specificity when comparing palpation tests with single facet blocks. Zito et al[68] reported 80% sensitivity for a finding of painful upper cervical joint dysfunction with manual examination in the differential diagnosis of patients with CGH from those with MH and controls. Aprill et al[69] found a 60% positive predictive value for occipital headaches originating in the C1–C2 joint with a combination of findings including pain in the (sub)occipital region, tenderness on palpation of the lateral C1–C2 joint, and restricted C1–C2 rotation.

All tests above were performed during the initial visit. A TMJ evaluation on the 14th visit revealed decreased AROM of mouth opening (MO) to 30 mm measured with a ruler. During mouth opening, the primary author noted lateral anterior translation of the left condyle. There was also maximal limitation with right lateral excursion (LE), moderate limitation with left LE, and moderate limitation for protrusion (Pro). The latter three movements were evaluated using visual estimation on a 4-point scale (none, minimal, moderate, and maximal). Bilateral TMJ traction and compression tests were negative. Tenderness was evident with palpation of the left TMJ. At this time—and different from the first visit—myofascial hypertonicity and MTrPs were noted in bilateral masseter and temporalis muscles. Walker et al[70] noted near-perfect interrater agreement for measuring mouth opening with a ruler (ICC = 0.99). Manfredini et al[71] noted moderate agreement ($\kappa$ = 0.48–0.53) for palpation for pain of the TMJ. Lobbezoo-Scholte et al[72] reported moderate interrater agreement ($\kappa$ = 0.40) for pain on compression and near-absent agreement for restriction ($\kappa$ = 0.08) and endfeel ($\kappa$ = 0.07) with traction and translation tests. Pain on palpation of the lateral and posterior aspects of the TMJ carried a positive likelihood ratio of 1.16–1.38 for the presence of TMJ synovitis;[73,74] absence of joint crepitus carried a negative likelihood ratio of 0.70 with regard to TMJ osteoarthritis.[73]

## Evaluation and Diagnosis

The evaluation and diagnosis of this patient with a complex presentation involved answering two questions:

- Was this patient appropriate for PT management or was a referral for medical diagnosis and (co)management warranted?

- If appropriate for PT management, which were the relevant neuromusculoskeletal impairments and resultant limitations in activity and restrictions in participation amenable to interventions within the PT scope of practice?

Determining whether this patient was appropriate for PT management required the therapist to both exclude with a sufficient degree of diagnostic confidence potential serious pathology responsible for the current presentation and to ascertain that the provided medical headache diagnoses fit with the signs and symptoms noted during the history and physical examination.

In the authors' clinical opinion, serious pathology was ruled out sufficiently by the comprehensive examination of the referring neurologist and the findings from the history and examination noted above. However, it should be noted that data on the diagnostic accuracy of history items and physical examination as discussed above is either absent or insufficient to confidently exclude central nervous system pathology potentially capable of producing similar signs and symptoms. Therefore, this decision was based mainly on clinician experience and interpretation of the tests based on a pathophysiologic rather than research-based rationale.

This patient came with medical diagnoses of chronic TTH, MH, and TMD. As discussed above, these as well as many other headache types within the ICHD-II could potentially present with the same signs and symptoms as collected during the history and physical examination. Although it is not the role of the physical therapist to make a medical diagnosis, it is his or her responsibility to ascertain that the provided medical diagnosis fits with the history and physical examination findings. Discrepancies between the diagnosis provided and the signs and symptoms observed should lead to medical referral. Only when the signs and symptoms observed fit with the diagnosis provided will a PT examination and diagnosis indicate whether the patient might benefit from PT intervention. A clinical decision-making process was performed to confirm or cast doubt on the provided medical diagnosis. In this case, key differential diagnostic data were derived from the headache's onset, nature, severity, chronicity, characteristics, associated symptoms, and physical examination findings.

Of the primary headache groups noted in the ICDH-II, only MH and TTH required further diagnostic consideration (Table 9-1).[4] With the given patient presentation, the diagnostic criteria for *migraine without aura* (1.1) were not met entirely met. The patient had at least five attacks (criterion A), the headaches lasted 4–72 hours (criterion B), and the headaches were of severe intensity (criterion 4C). However, she did not fulfill a second characteristic out of the four in criterion C: She did describe a unilateral location (behind the left eye), but this was not part of her primary headache. The patient described aggravation by exercise, but not aggravation by or avoidance of routine physical activity (e.g., walking or climbing stairs). She also did not describe a pulsating quality to her headaches. With regard to criterion D, the patient described aggravation by bright light (photophobia), but she did not mention phonophobia, nausea, or vomiting (see Table 9-1). *Typical aura with migraine* (1.2.1) was not a consideration mainly because her symptoms were not accompanied by any aura. She did not meet the frequency and chronic nature of *chronic migraine* (1.5.1), as outlined in criterion A. However, with a report of symptomatic relief of her unilateral headache with a Triptan-class medication, a diagnosis of MH without aura was considered likely despite the patient not meeting all diagnostic criteria.

*Episodic* (2.1) and *frequent episodic TTH* (2.2) could be eliminated because the frequency per month of her headaches exceeded criteria for both, leaving *chronic TTH* (2.3) and *new daily-persistent headache* (4.8). Their criteria are very similar, and the patient's headache fulfilled criteria for both types; however, new daily-persistent headache (4.8) is daily and unremitting since or very close to a time of onset that is clearly recalled and unambiguous.[4] This was not evident with the onset of daily headache for this patient, being described as insidious and vague. Chronic TTH (2.3) exists in two forms: *associated* (2.3.1) and *not associated with pericranial tenderness* (2.3.2), described as local tenderness to manual palpation by the second and third finger on muscles of the head and neck (i.e., frontalis, temporalis, masseter, pterygoid, SCM, splenius, and trapezius muscles).[4] Palpation of the neck and head musculature in this patient revealed tenderness, characterized by palpable taut bands and active MTrPs, making a diagnosis of chronic TTH associated with pericranial tenderness (2.3.1) very plausible.

A medical history of suspected TMD and an MVA 5 years prior, during which the patient sustained a fractured nose, and neuromusculoskeletal impairments found during the examination warranted further inquiry of the secondary headache groups. Whether to classify a secondary headache depends on a few factors. If a headache is a new headache that presents with another disorder known to be capable of causing it, then it is described as a secondary headache.[4] If a primary headache already exists, factors that support adding a secondary headache diagnosis include a close temporal relation to a causative disorder, a discernible worsening of the primary headache, good evidence that the causative disorder can exacerbate the primary headache, and improvement or resolution of the headache after relief of the presumed causative disorder.[4] In respect to the improvement or resolution of the headache, in many cases there is insufficient follow-up time or a diagnosis needs to be made prior to the end of expected time for remission. In these cases, it is recommended to describe the headache as a headache probably attributed to [the disorder]; a definitive diagnosis can only be made once the time-sensitive outcome criterion D is fulfilled.[4]

Of the secondary headache groups, *headache attributed to head and/or neck trauma* and *headache or facial pain attributed to a disorder of cranium, neck, eyes, ears, nose, sinuses, teeth, mouth, or other facial or cranial structures* required further investigation for this patient (Table 9-2).[4] The presentation did not fulfill *chronic headache attributed to whiplash injury* (5.4), because the patient did not describe a discernable whiplash injury after her MVA and the headache did not develop within 7 days after a possible or suspected whiplash injury. A fractured nose might constitute possible head trauma, but there was no evidence that the headache developed in close temporal relation to the trauma, thereby making *chronic headache attributed to other head and/or neck trauma* (5.6.2) unlikely. Although the primary author suspected headache due to TMD and this suspicion was to some degree substantiated later based on the examination findings for the TMJ noted above, this case did not meet the established criteria for *headache or facial pain attributed to temporomandibular joint disorder* (11.7); evidence of TMD established by way of x-ray, MRI, and/or bone scintigraphy was not available (criterion B). Also the time-dependent outcome criterion D could not be met. *Cervicogenic headache* (11.2.1) was a possible secondary headache diagnosis because the examination findings met criteria A, B, and C1. Again, the time-sensitive outcome criterion D could not be confirmed. Clinical findings that supported the diagnosis of CGH included FHP, suboccipital tenderness, and upper cervical positional abnormalities and limited mobility.

In summary, after the initial evaluation, the relevant signs and symptoms associated with the patient's headaches seemed to be consistent with and fulfill ICDH-II diagnostic criteria[4] for:

- Chronic TTH associated with pericranial tenderness
- Probable MH without aura
- Probable cervicogenic headache

The ICHD-II is an update of the original 1988 classification and includes expanded definitions and clarifications.[3,4] Few studies have examined the reliability and validity of this new edition. Relevant to this patient is the fact that there is considerable symptom overlap between the diagnostic criteria for TTH and CGH,[23] yet some evidence shows that they are distinct disorders.[75,76] It should be noted that the absence of data on diagnostic accuracy of the ICHD-II does and should affect the level of diagnostic confidence with regard to the established headache diagnoses.

After excluding serious underlying undiagnosed pathology and establishing the seeming appropriateness of the headache diagnoses provided by the referring physician, the next step in the diagnostic process was to ascertain whether neuromusculoskeletal impairments caused or contributed to the patient's headaches and neck pain. The patient presented with several physical examination findings of the musculoskeletal system of the head and neck that have been shown to contribute to various headache types. Myofascial trigger points have been noted to cause referred pain to the head, neck, and face, contributing to TTH, MH, and CGH.[12-21] Cervical spine joint dysfunction has been noted to contribute to CGH due to referred pain from the facet joints and influence of neural and vascular structures of the head and neck.[23-29,77-79] FHP with posterior rotation of the cranium may lead to adverse affects on the structure and function of the cervical spine and TMJ, increasing the incidence of neck, interscapular, and headache pain.[18,31,37,78,80,81]

In light of this complex patient presentation, the primary author decided to assess for a suspected TMD at a later date due to a lack of time and a lower assigned priority. TMD constitutes a variety of conditions involving the TMJ, muscles of mastication, and other associated structures. The diagnosis of TMD is varied, and agreement has not been met on the pathophysiologic mechanisms involved.[15] At some point during the course of treatment, the patient mentioned the onset of jaw pain. It was at that time that a TMJ evaluation was performed. The American Academy of Orofacial Pain (AAOFP)'s diagnostic criteria for TMD classify two major subgroups:[82]

1. Temporomandibular joint articular disorders, including congenital and developmental disorders, disc derangement disorders, dislocation, inflammatory conditions, arthritides, ankylosis, and fracture

2. Masticatory muscle disorders divided into myofascial pain, myositis, myospasm, myofibrotic contracture, local myalgia (unclassified), myofibrotic contracture, and neoplasia

The TMJ evaluation indicated diagnoses of myofascial pain and left condylar hypermobility based on the history and on active and passive movement and palpation findings. The patient reported being under high stress and complained of jaw pain, stiffness, and pain with chewing. Limitations were present during mouth opening with anterior-lateral translation of the left condyle, bilateral lateral excursion (right worse than left), and protrusion. Palpation revealed myofascial hypertonicity and pain in the muscles of mastication and over the left TMJ. No joint sounds were noted. Therefore, the patient clearly met the diagnostic inclusion criteria for TMJ myofascial pain (**Table 9-5**).[82] However, the myofascial pain diagnosis did not explain the anterior-lateral translation of the left condyle, the discrepancy between left and right lateral excursion, and the pain with palpation of the left TMJ. Further investigation of the TMJ articular disorders did not show any plausible diagnosis for which all inclusion criteria were met. With the absence of joint sounds and without radiographic imaging, disc displacement disorders, inflammatory and osteoarthritic disorders could not be excluded nor included.[82] The diagnosis of left condylar hypermobility is not a classified disorder named by the AAOFP, but it has been used to describe an articular condition that is likely to precede disc derangement disorders of the TMJ.[57] It is characterized by excessive condylar rotation (anterior translation) with mouth opening and could explain the lateral excursion restrictions as well as the TMJ palpable pain.[57]

It should be noted that data on diagnostic accuracy for most tests used in the examination are limited to reliability data; frequently, interrater reliability is insufficient for clinical

---

**TABLE 9-5    Recommended Criteria for Identifying Latent and Active Trigger Points[12]**

1.  Regional dull, aching pain; pain aggravated by mandibular function when the muscles of mastication are involved

2.  Hyperirritable sites (trigger points) frequently palpated within a taut band of muscle tissue or fascia; provocation of these trigger points altering the pain complaint and often revealing a pattern of pain referral

3.  Greater than 50% reduction of pain with vapocoolant spray or local anesthetic injection of the trigger point followed by stretch

**The following may accompany the above:**

1.  Sensation of muscle stiffness

2.  Sensation of acute malocclusion not verified clinically

3.  Ear symptoms, tinnitus, vertigo, toothache, tension-type headache

4.  With masticatory muscle involvement, decreased mouth opening; passive stretching of the elevator muscles increasing mouth opening by more than 4 mm (soft endfeel)

5.  Hyperalgesia in the region of the referred pain

decision making, thereby encouraging us to question our test results. The patient met all three criteria (pain suboccipital region, pain on palpation right C1, and restricted C1–C2 rotation) for CGH originating in C1–C2,[69] and the painful C1–C2 restriction also indicated CGH rather than MH as the cause of at least some of the headache complaints.[68] However, it should be again noted that a positive predictive value of 60% and a positive finding in light of data only on sensitivity might be considered insufficient for confident diagnostic decision making. The AAOFP TMD-classification system has not been studied for reliability or validity. The assumption made here that the patient presented with a muscular and not as much an articular TMD was neither supported nor contradicted by the likelihood ratios noted above for pain on TMJ palpation and the absence of joint crepitus; values close to 1.0 as discussed above do little to affect post-test probability either way. However, in the authors' opinion, for this patient the psychometric data on MTrP palpation and especially on palpation for mobility permitted a physical therapy diagnosis with regard to MTrPs and segmental mobility dysfunction that had sufficient diagnostic confidence to identify impairments potentially amenable to PT intervention.

The International Classification of Functioning, Disability, and Health (ICF) disablement model[83] was used to describe the patient's diagnosis, current functioning, and level of disability (**Figure 9-4**), because the full personal impact of headache disorders can be illustrated well using the ICF classification.[33] ICF terms and definitions are described in **Table 9-6**. Stucki[84] suggested that the ICF is moving toward becoming the generally accepted framework and classification system in medicine, specifically rehabilitation medicine.[84] **Table 9-7** summarizes the involved health conditions, impairments, activity limitations, and participation restrictions in accordance with the ICF.

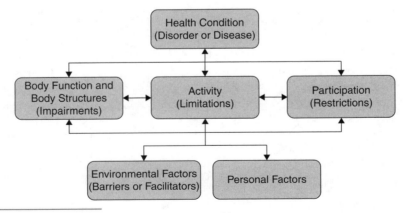

**Figure 9-4** ICF—biopsychosocial framework.[84]

*Source:* Adapted from Stucki G. International Classification of Functioning, Disability, and Health (ICF): A promising framework and classification for rehabilitation medicine. *Am J Phys Med Rehabil* 2005;84:733–740.

## TABLE 9-6   ICF Definition of Terms[83]

**Health condition:** Diseases, disorders, injuries.

**Body functions:** The physiological functions of body systems, including psychological functions. *Impairments* are problems in body function as a significant deviation or loss.

**Body structures:** Anatomic parts of the body, such as organs, limbs, and their components. *Impairments* are problems in structure as a significant deviation or loss.

**Activity:** The execution of a task or action by an individual. Activities may be *limited* in nature, duration, or quality.

**Participation:** The involvement in a life situation. Participation may be *restricted* in nature, duration, or quality.

**Environmental factors:** The make up of the physical, social, and attitudinal environment in which people live and conduct their lives; includes *barriers* or *facilitators*.

**Personal factors:** Factors that impact on functioning (e.g., lifestyle, habits, social background, education, life events, race/ethnicity, sexual orientation, and assets of the individual).

Another diagnostic framework used increasingly within PT in the United States is the preferred practice patterns contained in the *Guide to Physical Therapist Practice.*[85] For this patient, diagnosis using this model with regard to the cervical and thoracic spine included:

1. Pattern B: Impaired posture
2. Pattern D: Impaired joint mobility, motor function, muscle performance, and range of motion associated with connective tissue dysfunction

The PT diagnosis with regard to the TMD, again following the second edition of the *Guide to Physical Therapist Practice,*[85] was pattern D (impaired joint mobility, motor function, muscle performance, and range of motion associated with connective tissue dysfunction). Although promoted for use in PT diagnosis, prognosis, and treatment planning, this diagnostic framework has not been studied for reliability and validity.

## Prognosis

The patient described in this case report presented with a number of poor prognostic indicators. It was not clear if this patient had suffered a whiplash injury during the MVA 5 years before or if her chronic neck pain should be attributed to previous neck injury or chronic TTH. Patients with chronic neck pain and chronic pain and disability related to "late whiplash syndrome" often present with central sensitization. Central sensitization has also been implicated in the etiology of chronic TTH, as discussed above. Signs of central sensitization include hyperalgesia, allodynia, and widespread and stimulus-independent pain.[86]

## TABLE 9-7 Physical Therapy Diagnosis in Accordance with the ICF Format

| | | |
|---|---|---|
| Health condition | Headaches | Chronic tension-type headache associated with pericranial tenderness |
| | | Cervicogenic headache |
| | | Probable migraine headache |
| | Neck pain | Impaired joint mobility, motor function, muscle performance, and range of motion associated with connective tissue dysfunction |
| | | Impaired posture |
| Body function and structure (Impairments) | Active MTrPs contributing to myofascial hypertonicity and tenderness | Bilateral: upper trapezius, sternocleidomastoid, splenius capitis, and suboccipitals |
| | | Left: Masseter and temporalis |
| | Spinal mobility restrictions | Left C0/C1 for FB and SBL |
| | | Left C1/C2 for RR |
| | | U/T and M/T for BB and axial extension |
| | Decreased muscle flexibility | Bilateral: Upper trapezius, sternocleidomastoid, cervical/thoracic paraspinals and suboccipitals |
| | Postural dysfunction | Forward head posture with craniocervical extension |
| | Stress/Tension | Related to busy home and work life, and possible grieving over death of her mother earlier in the year |
| | Craniomandibular disorder | Assessed at a later date |
| Activity (Limitations) | Functional limitations with: | Routine daily activities, personal care, lifting, work activities, concentration, reading, recreational activities, driving |
| | Emotional feelings of being: | Handicapped, isolated, angry, tense, irritable, frustrated, insane, desperate, unable to maintain control |
| Participation (Restrictions) | Restrictions with life situations | Less likely to socialize |
| | | Concerned about consequences on work, home, and relationships with others |
| | | Perceived difficulty achieving life goals |

Central sensitization as might exist in this patient poses an obstacle to therapeutic success due to the negative consequences of maintained pain perception and the increased excitatory state of the central nervous system in response to peripheral inputs.

Emotional stress and depression are relevant psychological impairments that serve as poor prognostic indicators for this patient diagnosed with both TTH and MH. High levels of depression and anxiety are common in patients with chronic TTH.[87,88] Significant functional and well-being impairments have been noted in chronic TTH patients, including adversely affected sleep, energy levels, emotional well-being, and performance in daily responsibilities. In contrast, work and social functioning are generally only severely impaired in a small minority.[88] Leistad et al[89] showed the deleterious effect of cognitive stress on electromyography (EMG) muscle activity and reported on pain noted in patients with MH and TTH and in healthy controls. Although EMG peak activity revealed no between-group differences, the TTH patients recorded higher pain responses in the temporalis and frontalis muscles, a higher increase of pain during the cognitive test, and delayed pain recovery in all muscle regions when compared to controls. They also had delayed EMG recovery in the trapezius compared with controls and MH patients. The MH patients developed more pain in the splenius and temporalis than did the controls; pain responses were higher in the neck and trapezius compared to patients with TTH with delayed pain recovery in the trapezius and temporalis muscles.[89] In this patient, the history revealed both multiple emotional stressors and a history of depression. First, her mother died earlier in the year from a medication overdose: Headache symptoms became worse a month after her death. The patient had a 30-year history of MH as a physical stressor. Also, the patient had a history of depression and was seeing a therapist and used antidepressive medication. She noted work and home-related stress to her physicians and physical therapist, yet she maintained a successful career as an attorney and managed a household of four teenage children and three pets. The responses to her perceived emotional and functional disability on the HDI and NDI questionnaires were revealing with regard to perceived stress levels (Table 9-7). The patient reported feeling handicapped, isolated, angry, tense, irritable, frustrated, insane, desperate, and unable to maintain control. From a functional standpoint, she reported limitations with routine daily activities, personal care, lifting, work activities, concentration, reading, recreational activities, and driving. All of these findings were significant in that they most likely contributed to pain through a stress-related increase of muscular tension and pain perception.

The prolonged nature of complaints and the worsening of the condition over time despite the medical management by various health-care providers seemed to also indicate an unfavorable prognosis. The patient had increased her headache medication intake to daily use and sometimes twice daily. One had to surmise that to expect this patient's chronic pain condition to improve with time on its current course and without specific therapeutic intervention would be unrealistic.

However, this patient did present with a number of musculoskeletal impairments that might indicate the potential for successful treatment of the chronic headache and neck pain by way of an OMPT approach. Manual therapy techniques to address spine dysfunction and soft-tissue/myofascial restrictions, combined with exercise therapy to address postural imbalances and poor cervical muscle activation/endurance, have been noted to be effective treatment approaches both individually and collectively in the treatment of headaches.[38, 77–79, 90–93] Studies have shown that trigger point dry needling relieved symptoms related to myofascial pain[51] and that it improved headache indices, tenderness, and neck mobility in TTH patients.[93] In some studies, spinal manipulation has been shown to be efficacious in the treatment of chronic TTH, MH, and CGH.[92] In this patient, the noted moderate to high headache intensity and chronic nature of headaches were not predictors of a negative outcome in the treatment of CGH using therapeutic exercise and manipulative therapy.[94]

Another positive prognostic indicator—although not known at the time of the evaluation—were the significant within-session improvements of pain and neck mobility observed early in the intervention period. Tuttle[95] reported that positive within-session changes in cervical mobility and pain could predict between-session changes for PT treatment of the cervical spine: Odds ratios (OR) for within-session changes to predict between-session changes using an *improved/not improved* categorization for cervical mobility ranged from 2.5 (95% CI: 0.6–4.3) to 21.3 (95% CI: 10.1–96.1); for pain intensity, the OR was 4.5 (95% CI: 1.2–14.4). The positive likelihood ratio for cervical mobility improvements ranged from 2.1 (95% CI: 0.7–6.2) to 5.0 (95% CI: 2.6–9.9); for pain intensity improvements, it was 2.5 (95% CI: 1.3–4.6).

## Intervention

Following the initial evaluation, the patient was initially seen twice a week for approximately 6 weeks for a total of 11 visits, after which period she was out of town for almost 3 weeks. After this absence from therapy, she was seen 9 times over the next 3 months and finally 1 month later, for a total of 21 visits. As noted above, specific assessment and treatment of the TMD began on the 14th visit. The patient was reassessed at each visit, and treatment on that visit was dependent on subjective reporting and objective reassessments.

The treatment progression was based on the therapist's clinical experience. After the initial evaluation, the findings, recommended treatment plan, and expected outcome were outlined to the patient using charts and other skeletal aids. In the authors' opinion, educating a patient on her problem and how it will be treated may be extremely important for optimal success and patient compliance with exercise and self-management concepts. This also established patient responsibility with regard to self-management.

The initial therapy focus was to decrease pain by addressing the most pertinent myofascial and spinal dysfunctions, to initiate a home exercise program (HEP) for relaxation and flexibility, and to establish whether continuation of the plan of care was indeed warranted indicated by patient progress. The progression of therapy emphasized monitoring self-perceived disability ratings, addressing remaining myofascial dysfunctions established upon each new re-evaluation, monitoring and maintaining spinal mobility, progressing the HEP for mobility and coordination of movement, and further assessing and treating the TMD. It was the primary author's belief that treating the myofascial and upper cervical spine restrictions first would improve the probability of successfully addressing any possible TMD that might be present or that might be contributing to the patient's headaches.

Once a plateau of improvement was reached as indicated by a decrease of headache frequency to one or less per month of mild intensity, the last one to two visits were intended to finalize the patient's HEP, aiming at preventing the onset or exacerbation of the patient's complaints. The following paragraphs will explain in more detail the therapeutic interventions used during follow-up visits (**Table 9-8**).

*Dry Needling*

Trigger point dry needling (TrPDN) is a technique used for "releasing" MTrPs; this release is hypothesized to occur as a result of the elicitation of LTRs with subsequent inactivation of the MTrP. The TrPDN treatment utilizes fine solid acupuncture needles, but the technique is in all other aspects different from traditional acupuncture (**Table 9-9**).[96] Other terminology used in the literature describing similar techniques includes intramuscular stimulation (IMS), twitch-obtaining intramuscular stimulation, and deep dry needling. Other variations of dry needling include superficial dry needling, which involves placing an acupuncture needle in the skin overlying a MTrP, and electrical twitch-obtaining intramuscular stimulation, which applies electricity through a monopolar EMG needle electrode at motor endplate zones. Sometimes the term IMS is used to refer to a specific system of diagnosis and treatment for myofascial pain of hypothesized radiculopathic origin, as developed by Gunn.[96]

Travell first described the use of MTrP injections in the treatment of myofascial pain in a 1942 paper.[97] Her work subsequently led to the development of the TrPDN technique, which is different from trigger point injections in that no substance is injected. In 1979, Lewitt described the "needle effect" as the immediate analgesia that was produced by needling the painful spot. Both Travell and Lewitt, as well as many others, agreed that it is the mechanical stimulus of the needle that likely results in beneficial therapeutic effects and not necessarily the substance being injected.[12,98-100] TrPDN is a technique within the scope of and used by physical therapists in many countries, including Canada, Switzerland, South Africa, Australia, Spain, and the United Kingdom, among others.[101] Physical therapists in the United States are mostly unfamiliar with the technique, but an increasing number are trained and are using TrPDN to treat a variety of acute and chronic neuromusculoskeletal conditions. It is often wrongly assumed that dry needling techniques fall under the exclusive scopes of medical practice, oriental medicine, or acupuncture;[101] several US states, including Colorado, Georgia, Kentucky, Maryland, New Hampshire, New Mexico, South Carolina, and Virginia and more recently also Alabama, Oregon, Texas, and Ohio have declared that dry needling does fall within the scope of PT practice.[101] Several case reports have described dry needling techniques in the treatment of various musculoskeletal conditions by other medical professionals,[102-109] but to date, few case reports in the PT literature exist on the inclusion of the TrPDN technique in PT intervention.

Although there are few reported cases of complications related to dry needling, and despite the differences noted above between dry needling and acupuncture (Table 9-9), precautions

**TABLE 9-8  Physical Therapy Visits and Treatment Interventions**

| Treatment Date | Myofascial OMPT Techniques | Articular OMPT Techniques | Exercise Therapy | Education |
|---|---|---|---|---|
| 10/18/04 (initial eval.)<br>NDI: 38/100<br>HDI: 56/100 | (Trial Treatment)<br>1. TrPDN: Lt UT & SCM<br>2. STM & PIR | | 1. Self-Stretch: UT & SCM for HEP | Eval findings & recommended Tx plan.<br>Postural instruction in sitting. |
| 10/25/04<br>Comments:<br>Significant initial improvement of HA complaints. | 1. TrPDN: Rt UT & SCM<br>2. STM & PIR | 1. Reverse NAGS: T1–T4<br>2. LAD: C0–C2<br>3. Rt lateral glide (Gr. IV): C0/C1<br>4. SNAG: C1/C2 RR 3x | 1. Self-stretch: SOs & SpCap for HEP<br>2. Review of HEP | 1. Education for stress reduction through breathing and relaxation of head, neck, and jaw. |
| 10/28/04<br>Comments:<br>MTrPs reproduced HA pain. | 1. TrPDN: Bil UT & Lt SCM<br>2. STM & PIR | 1. Reverse NAGS: T1–T4<br>2. PA (Prog. Osc.): T4–T8<br>3. Rt lateral glide (Gr. IV): C0/C1<br>4. SNAG: C1/C2 RR 5x | Review of HEP | |

| | | | |
|---|---|---|---|
| 11/01/2004<br>Comments:<br>Onset of mid-back pain. Pain in mid-back with axial extension. Patient brought in her cervical pillow from home. | 1. TrPDN: Lt LT<br>2. STM & PIR: Bil UT, SCM, SpCap, SOs<br>3. SID | Reverse NAGS: T1–4<br>PA (Prog. Osc.): T4–8<br>LAD: C0–2<br>Rt lateral glide (Gr. IV): C0/C1<br>SNAG: C1/C2 RR 5x | 1. Self-stretch: lower trapezius for HEP<br><br>1. Education for proper neck and head positioning during sleep with use of towel roll.<br>2. Education for sub-occipital released self-treatment. |
| 11/04/04 | TrPDN: Rt SCM<br>STM & PIR: Bil UT, SCM, SpCap, SOs<br>SID | 1. PA (Prog. Osc.):<br>T1–T8 | 1. Review of self-Tx for SO release. |
| 11/08/04 | STM & PIR: Bil UT, SCM, SOs<br>SID | 1. PA (Prog. Osc.):<br>T1–T8 | 1. Neck clocks<br>2. AROM AR of the head/axial extension<br>3. Shoulder clocks |
| 11/11/04<br>NDI: 28/100<br>HDI: 42/100<br>Comments:<br>Notes overall improvement. | TrPDN: Bil UT, Lt SCM<br>STM & PIR<br>SID | PA (Prog. Osc.): T1–T8 | 1. Review of exercises issued last visit |

*(continued)*

TABLE 9-8 Physical Therapy Visits and Treatment Interventions

| Treatment Date | Myofascial OMPT Techniques | Articular OMPT Techniques | Exercise Therapy | Education |
|---|---|---|---|---|
| 11/18/04 | TrPDN: Lt UT & LT STM & PIR SID | 1. Traction Mob Gr. V: T4–T8 | | |
| 11/29/04 | TrPDN: Lt UT & LT STM & PIR SID | 1. Traction Mob Gr. V: T4–T8 | | |
| 12/02/04 | TrPDN: Bil temporalis, masseter, SCM STM & PIR (mouth opening) | | | 1. Proper tongue position, resting jaw position, and nasal diaphragmatic breathing.<br>2. Self-STM of temporalis and masseter for HEP. |
| 12/7/04 Comments: Noted excellent improvement. | TrPDN: Bil temporalis, masseter STM & PIR (mouth opening) SID | 1. LAD: C0–C2 | | |

nterruption of physical therapy intervention due to vacation and holiday obligations.

| 1/03/05 | TrPDN: Lt UT | Traction Mob Gr. V: T1-8 |
| | | LAD: C0-2 |
| Comments: | STM: UT, SCM, SOs | |
| Recent exacerbation of pain complaints. | SID | |

| 13/05 | TrPDN: Bil UT | 1. Traction Mob Gr. V: T1-8 |
| NDI: 12/100 | STM & PIR: SCM, SOs, masseter, temporalis | 2. LAD: C0-2 |
| HDI: 24/100 | SID | |

Interruption of physical therapy intervention of headaches and neck pain due to acute onset of left anterior-lateral shoulder pain.

| 2/8/05 | 1. TrPDN: Bil masseter, temporalis | 1. LAD, medial glide, lateral glide Gr. 3: Bil TMJ | 1. AROM: 10 mm MO, 10 mm Rt LE, 10 mm MO in Rt LE | 1. Patient education for TMJ findings and self-care. |
| Interim History: Series of headaches in past week. Most likely due to stress. Jaw pain in past week. Pain with chewing. TMJ examination performed. | 2. STM & PIR (mouth opening) | | | |

| 2/10/05 | 1. TrPDN: Bil masseter, temporalis | 1. LAD, medial glide, lateral glide Gr. 3: Bil TMJ | 1. AROM: 10mm MO, 10 mm Rt LE, 10 mm MO in Rt LE | |
| Comments: Reports much less pain and tightness of her jaw. Decrease in HA intensity and frequency. | 2. STM & PIR (mouth opening) | | | |

(continued)

TABLE 9-8 Physical Therapy Visits and Treatment Interventions

| Treatment Date | Myofascial OMPT Techniques | Articular OMPT Techniques | Exercise Therapy | Education |
|---|---|---|---|---|
| 2/16/05<br>Comments:<br>Reports improvement of jaw pain and mouth opening, but still with some soreness and headaches. | 1. STM: Bil masseter, temporalis, SCM, SOs<br>2. PIR: mouth opening | 1. LAD, medial glide, lateral glide Gr. 3: Bil TMJ | 1. AROM: 10 mm MO, 10 mm Rt LE, 10 mm MO in Rt LE | 1. Proper tongue position, resting jaw position, and nasal diaphragmatic breathing.<br>2. Self STM of masseter and temporalis |
| 2/18/05<br>Comments:<br>Reports some return of jaw pain and headaches. | 1. TrPDN: Bil masseter, temporalis<br>2. STM & PIR (mouth opening) | 1. LAD, medial glide, lateral glide Gr. 3: Bil TMJ | 1. AROM of TMJ for HEP | 1. Review of postural positioning and breathing education. |
| 2/23/05<br>Comments:<br>Reports much improved mouth opening, less jaw pain, and resolution of headaches. Minimal limitation with Lt LE and Pro, and moderate limitation with mouth opening and Rt LE. Good condylar stability with mouth opening. Hypertonicity of Bil masseter and temporalis improved. | 1. TrPDN: Bil UT, SCM<br>2. STM: Bil UT, SCM masseter, temporalis<br>3. SID | 1. FB, SB, Rot Gr. IV Passive Mobs: upper cervical spine | | |

**3/24/05**

1. TrPDN: Bil UT, SCM
2. STM: Bil UT, SCM masseter, temporalis
3. SID

1. FB, SB, Rot Gr. IV
   Passive Mobs: upper cervical spine

Comments:
Continued improvement of mouth opening, jaw pain, and headaches.

**3/31/05**

NDI: 20/100
HDI: 20/100

1. STM: Bil UT
2. SID

1. FB, SB, Rot Gr. IV
   Passive Mobs: upper cervical spine

Comments:
Reports some neck soreness with one HA.

**4/25/05**

1. Traction Mob Gr. V: T4-8

1. Issued neck program
2. Reviewed & performed the relaxation and postural aspects of program

1. Next visit will review, perform, and finalize the flexibility and strength aspects of the neck program.

Comments:
Doing very well. No HA in the past month.

*Note:* OMPT = orthopaedic manual therapy; HA = headache; TMJ = temporomandibular joint; eval = evaluation; Tx = treatment; HEP = home exercise program; NDI = neck disability index; HDI = headache disability inventory; Lt = left; Rt = right; Bil = bilateral; UT = upper trapezius; SCM = sternocleidomastoid; LT = lower trapezius; SpCap = splenius capitus; Sos = suboccipitals; TrPDN = trigger point dry needling; STM = soft-tissue manipulation; PIR = postisometric relaxation; SID = subcranial inhibitive distraction; NAGS = natural apophyseal glides; LAD = long axis distraction; SNAG = sustained natural apophyseal glide; PA (Prog. Osc.) = posterior/anterior progressive oscillations; Gr = grade; Mob = mobilization; AROM = active range of motion; FB = forward bending; SB = side bending; Rot = rotation; MO = mouth opening; LE = lateral excursion; Pro = protrusion.

TABLE 9-9  Differences between Traditional Acupuncture and Dry Needling/Intramuscular Stimulation[96]

| Acupuncture | Dry Needling/Intramuscular Stimulation |
| --- | --- |
| Medical diagnosis not relevant. | Medical diagnosis is pertinent. |
| Medical examination not pertinent. | Medical examination essential. |
| Needle insertions along nonscientific meridians according to Chinese philosophy. | Needled insertions in trigger points/motor points according to examination. |
| Knowledge of anatomy not pertinent. | Knowledge of anatomy essential. |
| No immediate objective changes anticipated. | Immediate subjective and objective effects often expected. |

and complications related to the insertion of acupuncture needles must be considered. Contraindications to dry needling include acute trauma with hematoma, local or generalized circulatory problems (i.e., varicosis, thrombosis, and ulceration), diminished coagulation, and local or generalized skin lesions or infections.[110] Complications related to dry needling may include vasodepressive syncope, hematoma, penetration of visceral organs such as lung, bowel, or kidney, increased spasm and pain of the muscle treated, and muscle edema.[110] Serious complications related to acupuncture are rare but include pneumothorax, cardiac tamponade (compression of the heart caused by blood or fluid accumulation in the space between the myocardium and the pericardium), and spinal cord lesions.[111] Serious injuries to abdominal viscera, perhipheral nerves, and blood vessels are also rare.[111] A prospective survey study of adverse events following acupuncture of 32,000 consultations by 78 acupuncturists reported 2,178 events (i.e., an incidence of 684 per 10,000 consultations).[112] Most included minor events with the following mean incidence per 10,000 (95% CI): bleeding or hematoma in 310 cases (160–590), needling pain in 110 (48–247), aggravation of complaints in 96 (43–178), faintness in 29 (22–37), drowsiness after treatment in 29 (16–49), stuck or bent needle in 13 (0–42), headache in 11 (6–18), and sweating in 10 cases (6–16).[112] Forty-three events were considered significant minor adverse events, a rate of 14 per 10,000 (95% CI: 8–20), and one seizure event was considered serious.[112] Another prospective study of 34,000 consultations by 574 practitioners revealed similar findings:[113] transient minor events, 15% (95% CI: 14.6–15.3), included mild bruising, pain, bleeding, and aggravation of symptoms. Forty-three significant minor events were reported (i.e., a rate of 13 per 10,000; 95% CI: 0.9–1.7).[113] Significant minor events included severe nausea and fainting, severe, unexpected, and prolonged exacerbation of symptoms, prolonged pain and bruising, and psychological and emotional reactions.[113] No serious major adverse events that required a hospital admission or a prolonged hospital stay or that caused permanent disability or death were reported (95% CI: 0–1.1 per 10,000 treatments).[113] The most common side effects of dry needling include soreness, hematoma, and muscle edema.[110] General precautions for dry needling include establishing competence through adequate training and competency testing, clinical experience, and—last but not least—using common sense. Although there is limited evidence to suggest a significant risk of spread of infection through acupuncture, universal precautions are still important.[114] Specific precautions that should be taken include proper patient positioning, use of surgical gloves to protect the clinician against needle stick injuries, knowledge of detailed clinical anatomy, and knowledge of muscle-specific precautions.[110] Training programs for physical therapists wanting to use dry needling/IMS are available in the United States, Canada, Switzerland, Spain, Chile, Norway, Australia, The Netherlands, Belgium, Germany, Great Britain, Ireland, South Africa, and other countries.

For this patient, the initial trial treatment using dry needling was meant to serve two purposes:

- Confirm the clinical diagnosis of active MTrPs through reproducing or relieving the patient's symptoms.
- Assess patient tolerance during and after treatment to this sometimes painful procedure.

For this reason, the initial trial was performed for a minimal period of time (i.e., approximately 5 minutes). The patient was thoroughly educated on the basic premise of TrPDN treatment, how this technique differs from traditional acupuncture, what to expect during and after the treatment, the type of needle used, precautions used, possible side effects, and expected outcomes. Clinician education, training, and clinical experience with TrPDN were made clear to the patient. The patient provided informed consent for the suggested treatment including TrPDN. In this case, the UT and SCM were chosen for the trial treatment, because manual palpation of the MTrPs in these muscles causes referred pain into the neck, head, and face that was similar to the patient's complaints. Treating these muscles first could then serve as a diagnostic indicator for the contribution of MTrPs to the patient's total presentation.

For this patient, individually packaged stainless steel acupuncture needles in plastic insertion tubes were used. The needle sizes (diameter × length) used were 0.30 × 30 mm, 0.30 × 50 mm, and 0.20 × 13 mm. The taut band and MTrP were identified by palpation with the dominant or nondominant hand; the needle in its tube was then fixed against the suspected area by the nondominant hand either by using a pincer grip or flat palpation, depending on the muscle orientation, location, and direction of penetration. With the dominant hand, the needle was gently loosened from the tube and then a flick or tap of the top of the needle was performed to quickly penetrate the layers of the skin. This is done to ensure pain-free penetration of the needle. The needle was then guided toward the taut band until resistance was felt at a particular direction and depth. Gentle, small amplitude withdrawals and penetrations of the needle were performed until a trigger point zone had been found that was clinically identified by the elicitation of an LTR. Within the context of TrPDN, the elicitation of an LTR is considered essential in obtaining a desirable therapeutic effect.[12,96,99,115-118] The needle was focused in this area or other areas by drawing the needle back toward the skin and then redirecting the needle toward suspected areas. Numerous LTRs can generally be reproduced; sometimes >20 LTRs can be elicited from several MTrPs in a focused trigger point zone. The needle was removed once few LTRs were attained (none in three to five passes) or until palpable and/or visible release of the taut band had been determined. The needle could be placed back in the tube to be used immediately on the same patient or discarded in a sharps container while pressure was being applied to the treated area with the nondominant hand for approximately 10–30 seconds. Generally, if the needle had been used twice or if it had been bent or dulled during the procedure, it was discarded. During the procedure, the patient was closely monitored for tolerance and for reproduction of local or referred pain sensations. If the patient had not tolerated the treatment due to numerous or strong LTRs, the treatment would have been paused for several seconds until the patient indicated the ability to continue. As clearly communicated to the patient, the treatment would be stopped at any time upon her request or if it was clear that she was not tolerating the treatment.

Immediately after TrPDN, manual myofascial therapy was performed to relieve soreness, to increase circulation, to decrease myofascial hypertonicity, and to improve flexibility. The application of a cold pack or moist heat was used at the end of the session dependent on the outcome of that session. A cold pack was used if treatment was intensive and edema was visible or palpable. Moist heat was used if no visible or palpable edema was present. At the end of the TrPDN session, the patient was educated as to the following post-treatment care. The patient should expect soreness in the treated area typically for 1–2 days (occasionally more than 2 days). This soreness should be clearly identified as due to treatment and should always resolve. Soreness might make it difficult to judge previous complaints, but the effects would be easy to judge once soreness had subsided. Post-treatment soreness could be decreased with moist heat, gentle massage of the treated area, self-stretch, and over-the-counter pain medication, as necessary.

For the UT muscle, TrPDN was performed with patient in sidelying and/or supine (for the anterior fibers) and the therapist was standing to the side or at the head of the patient (**Figures 9-5** and **9-6**). The pincer grip was used in sidelying, and the taut band and contraction knot was grasped with the nondominant hand while the dominant hand performed the needling procedure in the inferior-lateral, anterior-superior, or anterior-lateral direction. The therapist took care only to needle the muscle fibers accessible between the thumb and index finger. Using flat palpation, the UT taut band and contraction knot were fixed in between the index and middle finger against the superior portion of the scapula. Using the pincer grip in supine, the muscle was needled in the posterior direction towards the index finger. For this technique, the 0.30 × 30 mm and 0.30 × 50 mm needle are used depending on patient physical make-up, location, and direction of treated area. Precautions included that the needle should never be directed in the anterior-medial or inferior direction to avoid puncturing the apex of the lung.

For the SCM muscle, TrPDN was performed in supine or sidelying with the neck and head adequately supported and with the therapist standing to the side or at the head of

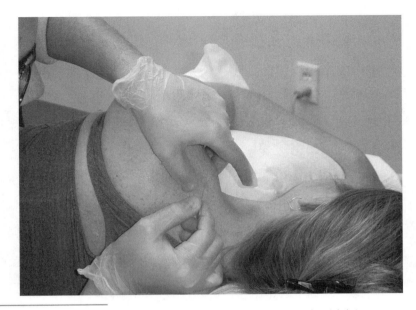

**Figure 9-5** Trigger point dry needling upper trapezius muscle sidelying.

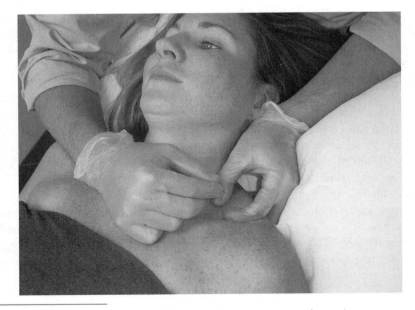

**Figure 9-6** Trigger point dry needling upper trapezius muscle supine.

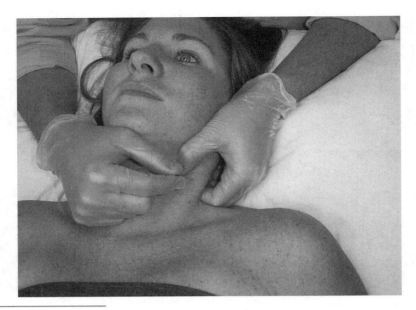

**Figure 9-7**　Trigger point dry needling sternocleidomastoid muscle.

the patient (**Figure 9-7**). In supine, the pincer grip was used to grasp both heads of the muscle while the needle was directed from the medial side to the posterior-lateral and/or anterior to posterior direction between the thumb and index finger. For this muscle, the 0.30 × 30 mm needle was used. Precautions for dry needling of the SCM included that the carotid artery should be identified medial to the SCM and that the direction of the needle should not be in the medial direction to avoid puncturing said artery.

For the lower trapezius (LT) muscle, TrPDN was performed in sidelying or prone with the therapist standing to the treated side (**Figure 9-8**). The diagonally oriented taut band was fixed between the index and middle finger with the contraction knot firmly over a rib. The index finger and middle finger were subsequently located in the intercostal space. The needle was directed anteriorly against the rib or laterally at a shallow angle tangential to the chest wall. For this muscle the 0.30 × 30 mm needle was again used. Precautions for needling this muscle included avoiding penetration of the lung by needling over a rib or tangentially to the chest wall.

For the masseter muscle, TrPDN was performed in sidelying or supine with the neck and head supported by a pillow and with the therapist standing to the side or at the head of patient (**Figure 9-9**). The taut bands and sensitive knots in the superficial and deep masseter muscle were identified by pincer grip or flat palpation. The treated area was fixed between the index and middle fingers and the needle was directed between the fingers. For this technique, the 0.20 × 13 mm needle was used, as precautions included avoiding needle stick injury to the facial nerve.

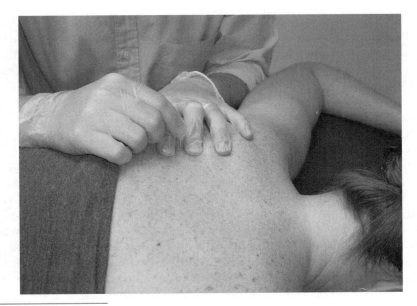

**Figure 9-8** Trigger point dry needling lower trapezius muscle.

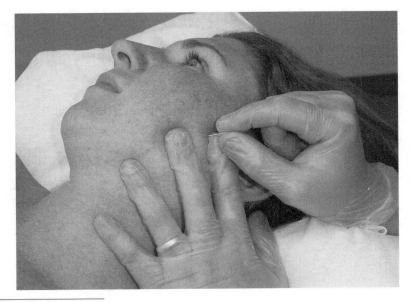

**Figure 9-9** Trigger point dry needling masseter muscle.

For the temporalis muscle, TrPDN was performed in sidelying or supine with the neck and head supported by a pillow and with the therapist again standing to the side or at the head of the patient (**Figure 9-10**). The temporal artery was first palpated and then the taut bands and sensitive knot were identified and fixed against the temporal bone between the index and middle finger. The needle was then directed towards the contraction knot. The 0.20 × 13 mm needle was used, as the precaution for this technique was avoidance of the superficial temporal artery.

*Orthopaedic Manual Physical Therapy*
Well integrated into physical therapy, OMPT includes manipulation techniques with purported effects on either soft tissue or joints. Soft-tissue manipulation uses manual techniques aimed at relaxing muscles, increasing circulation, breaking up adhesions or scar tissue, and easing pain in the soft tissues. Soft tissue manipulation techniques include manual trigger point therapy, strain-counterstrain, muscle energy technique, neuromuscular technique, myofascial release, and other therapeutic massage techniques. Paris[119] defined joint manipulation as "the skilled passive movement to a joint." Joint manipulation techniques are aimed at restoring motion at a joint and modulating pain. Joint manipulation techniques include nonthrust, thrust, and traction forces applied at various grades and directions.[119]

Soft-tissue manipulation is used to describe therapeutic massage and manual techniques for mobilizing soft tissue (e.g., muscles, connective tissue, fascia, tendons, ligaments)

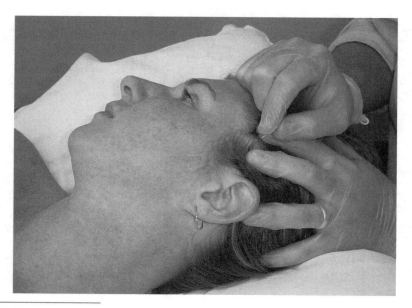

**Figure 9-10**   Trigger point dry needling temporalis muscle.

to improve the function of the muscular, circulatory, lymphatic, and nervous systems.[120] Some techniques are general for treating large areas using the palm of the hand and the forearm, for example, whereas other techniques are specific, such as deep stroking, transverse friction, and trigger point compression release using the thumb and fingertips. Postisometric relaxation (PIR) was a technique used for this patient with the goal of achieving muscle relaxation and elongation.[12,121] With the patient relaxed and the body supported, the therapist passively lengthened the muscle to its first barrier. The patient then performed a minimal isometric contraction of the muscle (10–25%) for 5 seconds during an inhalation while the therapist stabilized the muscle to be stretched. Then the patient relaxed completely and exhaled, while the therapist passively stretched the muscle to the new barrier. The technique was then repeated three to five times. This technique is very similar to contract/relax and hold/relax techniques. Specific muscles treated with this technique are indicated in Table 9-8 with the technique illustrated for the upper trapezius muscle in **Figure 9-11**. Subcranial inhibitive distraction (SID) is a myofascial technique described by Paris[60] that is aimed at releasing tension in suboccipital soft tissue and suboccipital musculature (**Figure 9-12**). The patient was lying supine with head supported. The therapist placed the three middle fingers just caudal to the nuchal line, lifted the fingertips upwards, resting the hands on the treatment table, and then applied a gentle cranial pull, causing a long axis extension. The procedure was performed with this patient for 2–5 minutes, as indicated in Table 9-8.

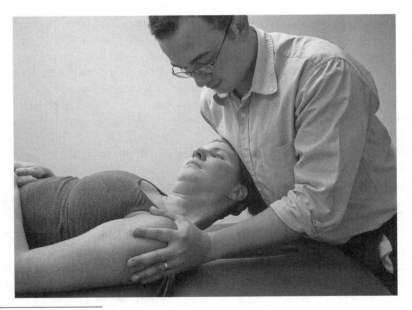

**Figure 9-11**   Post-isomedric relaxation upper trapezius muscle.

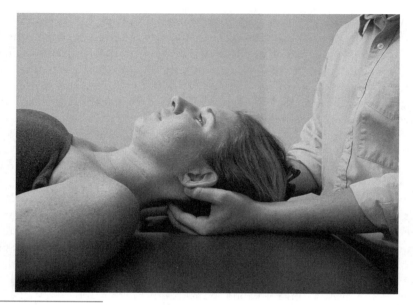

**Figure 9-12** Subcranial inhibitive distraction.

Mulligan[122,123] described reverse natural apophyseal glides as a mid- to end-range oscillatory mobilization indicated from the C7 vertebra down that were intended to aid in treatment of end-range loss of neck mobility, postural dysfunction (FHP with UT pain), and degenerative lower cervical or upper thoracic spine segments. The patient was seated and the therapist stood to the side and cradled the head to the body with forearm maintaining some neck flexion. Flexing the index finger IP joint and extending the MCP joints constituted the mobilizing handgrip. The thumb and index finger formed a V-shape that made contact with the articular pillars; then an anterior-cranial mobilization was applied gliding the inferior facet up on the superior one (**Figure 9-13**).

Rocabado[124] described long axis distraction of the upper cervical spine (C0–C2). The patient was lying supine with head in neutral. The therapist was sitting behind the patient and cradled the occiput with one hand while placing the same shoulder on the frontal bone to prevent head elevation. The opposite hand stabilized C2 with a pincer grip (**Figure 9-14**). Gentle cranial grade 3 distractions were applied six times with a 6-second duration.

Sustained natural apophyseal glides (SNAGS) involve concurrent accessory joint gliding and active physiological movement with overpressure at end-range.[122, 123] In this case, a C1–C2 SNAG to improve C1–C2 RR was performed with the patient sitting or standing and with the therapist behind the patient (**Figure 9-15**). The lateral border of the left thumb was placed on the lateral border of the left C1 transverse process and then

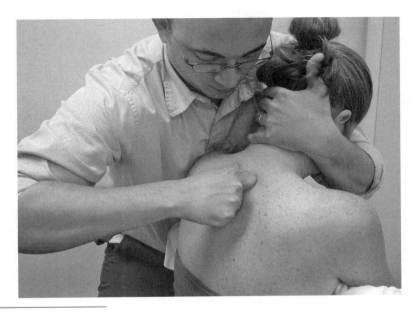

**Figure 9-13**   Reverse natural apophyseal glides.

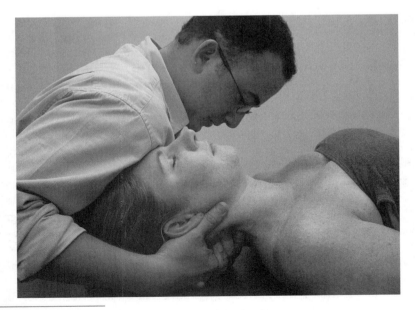

**Figure 9-14**   Long axis distraction upper cervical spine.

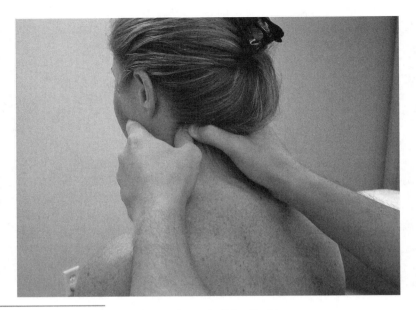

**Figure 9-15** Sustained natural apophyseal glide Cl–C2.

reinforced with the right thumb to give an anterior glide. The patient was asked to slowly turn her head to the right while the therapist maintained the anterior glide, also during return to starting position. The horizontal plane of the glide was maintained throughout the movement. If pain free, it was repeated five times.

Right lateral glide at C0–C1 was performed to improve C0–C1 SBL[124] (**Figure 9-16**). The patient was lying supine with head in neutral. The therapist was sitting behind the patient grasping the head by placing the medial side of the index finger on the mastoid process. A right lateral grade III glide was performed with the left hand using the nose as the center of rotation and this was repeated for three sets of 10 repetitions. The right hand simultaneously moved with the head to maintain stability.

Posterior-anterior (PA) glide progressive oscillations were performed to address restrictions of upper and mid-thoracic extension[60] (**Figure 9-17**). The patient was prone, and the therapist stood facing the patient. The therapist's cranial hand with elbow slightly bent was placed on the thoracic spine with the spinous process fitting in the hollow part of hand just distal to the pisiform bone. In time with the patient's breathing, at mid-exhalation, a series of four short progressive impulses were given in the PA direction ending at the patient's end-range (grade IV–IV++).

Traction manipulation as described by Kaltenborn et al[125] was performed for slight facet restrictions of upper and mid-thoracic extension (**Figure 9-18**). The patient lay supine with arms folded across the chest and hands on opposite shoulders. The therapist faced

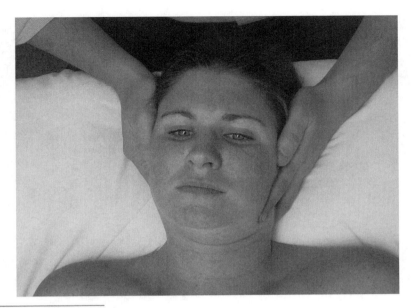

**Figure 9-16**  Right lateral glide C0–Cl.

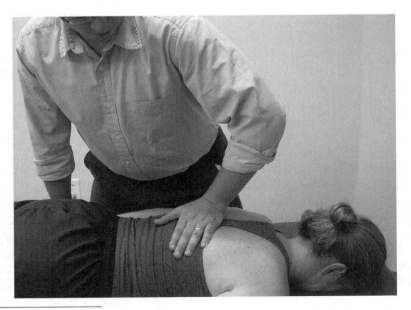

**Figure 9-17**  Postero-anterior glide progressive oscillation mid-thoracic spine.

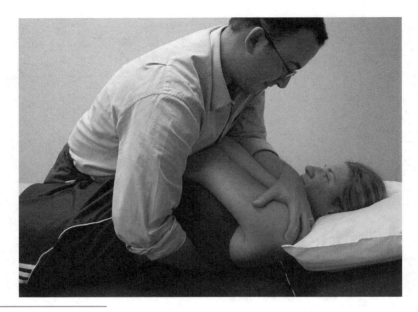

**Figure 9-18**    Traction manipulation upper and mid-thoracic spine.

the patient and eased her into a left sidelying position using his right hand. The therapist's left hand fixated the caudal vertebra of the segment with the thenar eminence on the right transverse process and the flexed third finger on the left transverse process. The therapist then rolled the patient back into a supine position with the right hand, maintaining the position of the left hand on the patient's back. The right hand and forearm were placed over the patient's crossed arms with the chest over the elbows. During an exhalation, a grade V linear mobilization was applied with the right arm and body moving the upper trunk in a posterior direction at right angle to the treatment plane through the facet joints.

TMJ long-axis distraction, medial glide, and lateral glide were performed to improve TMJ position, mobility, and stability, as described by Rocabado[124] (**Figures 9-19** through **9-21**). Bilateral TMJ manipulation was performed in this case; described here is an example of the procedure on the left. The patient was supine with the therapist sitting at the head of the table. The patient was asked to open her mouth minimally (10 mm). Using the right hand and wearing gloves, the therapist placed the palmar side of the thumb on cranial aspect of the bottom row of teeth on the lefthand side toward the molars while the index finger gently grasped the mandible. A gentle long-axis distraction was applied by performing an ulnar deviation of the wrist. To perform a medial glide or lateral distraction of the joint, the therapist changed the position of the hand to place the thumb on the inside aspect of the bottom row of teeth and grasped the lateral aspect of the

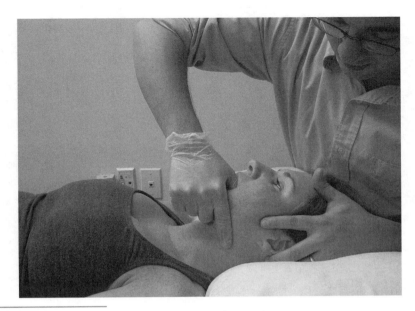

**Figure 9-19** Temporomandibular long axis distraction.

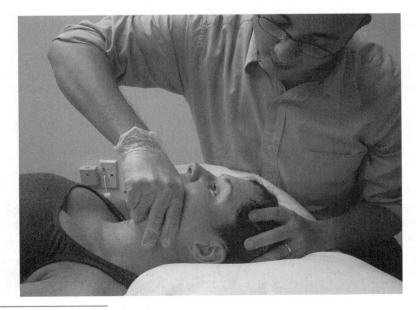

**Figure 9-20** Temporomandibular medial glide.

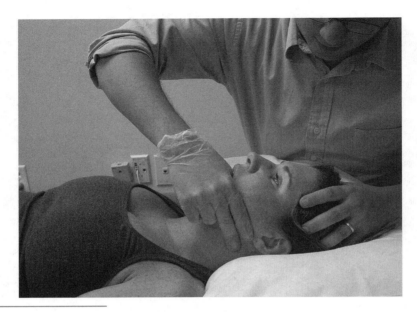

**Figure 9-21** Temporomandibular lateral glide.

mandible with the index finger. The therapist then performed an ulnar deviation of the wrist resulting in a medial glide. To do a lateral glide or medial distraction of the joint, the therapist kept the same hand position as the medial glide but the left hand was placed on the vertex of the head. The glide was performed by stabilizing the mandible with the right hand and performing a left head side-bend motion using the left hand resulting in a relative lateral glide of the joint. These TMJ manual interventions were performed as grade III mobilizations and repeated six times each. In between each direction, the hand was removed from the mouth and the patient was encouraged to swallow. Details on when these articular OMPT procedures were performed on this patient can be found in Table 9-8.

*Exercise Therapy*
Self-stretch exercises were provided for each muscle treated and were aimed at reducing muscle tension, decreasing pain, and improving flexibility. The general approach of performing the exercise was based on teaching the patient to stabilize one end of the muscle and then to passively stretch the other end to feel a gentle stretch. Directions were provided to hold the stretch for 20 seconds for three repetitions, two to three times per day. Slow, relaxed breathing was encouraged during the stretch. Neuromuscular re-education included verbal and manual cues that were used to provide proprioceptive feedback and to promote quality of movement. The neck clock exercise was used to induce relaxation,

decrease pain, and improve mobility and coordination of the head and neck complex.[120] This exercise involved the patient lying on her back with a towel roll to support the neck, knees bent, and feet flat. The patient was instructed to imagine the head against the face of a clock. Using the eyes or nose as a guide and the clock as a reference, she was asked to move the head into the 12:00 and 6:00 positions, then to repeat this for the 3:00 to 9:00 positions, doing this in both clockwise and counterclockwise directions. The patient was asked to repeat each direction 10 times. The shoulder clock exercise was aimed at inducing relaxation, reducing pain, and improving mobility and coordination for the neck and shoulder-girdle complex.[120] This exercise involved the patient lying on the side that was not targeted and imagining the shoulder against the face of a clock, where 12:00 is toward the head, 6:00 toward the hip, 3:00 toward the front, and 9:00 toward the back. The shoulder blade was moved between the different positions and directions, as it was for the neck clock exercise and, as for this exercise, this was repeated 10 times in each direction. AROM for anterior rotation of the head on the neck (also known as craniocervical flexion or axial extension) emphasized cervical muscular postural training and strengthening, craniocervical flexion mobility, and lengthening of the posterior craniocervical musculature often shortened in FHP, as noted in this patient.[120,124] The patient was again lying on her back with a towel roll to support the neck, knees bent, and feet flat. She was then instructed to perform a chin tuck and lift the back of the head upward off the floor holding this position for 6 seconds for six repetitions. Feedback was given to isolate the deep cervical flexors and to prevent an over-compensatory contraction of the SCM.

TMJ exercises were aimed at relieving joint irritation, promoting muscle relaxation, and reestablishing joint stability.[57,126] The patient performed AROM for 10 mm mouth opening (MO), 10 mm of right lateral excursion (LE), and 10 mm MO in LE for six repetitions each.[57,126] AROM for 10 mm MO was performed by applying gentle compression using thumb or fingertips through the bilateral shaft of the mandible, followed by a small excursion of mouth opening, equal to a small separation of the teeth, while keeping the tongue positioned against the palate at the roof of the mouth. AROM for 10 mm LE was performed to the opposite side of dysfunction or hypermobility, in this case to the right; 10 mm of LE is an approximate excursion equal to bringing the upper canine in line with the lower canine. The patient performed AROM of 10 mm MO in opposite LE by gently opening the mouth in the right lateral position. Throughout these exercises, the tongue was positioned at the roof of the mouth to maintain a minimal amount of stress to the TMJ. Manual guiding for these movements may initially be necessary to provide proprioceptive feedback and to encourage quality of motion.

The *Neck Program* is a patient education booklet that includes information on neck pathology, body mechanics with daily activities, and exercises. The exercises can be performed in a short period of time and they address four components of musculoskeletal neck care: (1) relaxation, (2) posture, (3) flexibility, and (4) strengthening. During the last visit, the patient was given the booklet, and the relaxation and posture sections were reviewed and performed. One additional visit was recommended to review and perform the flexibility and strengthening aspects, but the patient did not schedule another visit.

*Education*

Education for this patient included postural education, instruction on relaxation, self-application of a suboccipital release technique, and a TMJ self-care program. The therapist explained to the patient the role that posture played in relation to her complaints and musculoskeletal impairments, and what constituted good and bad postural alignment using the aid of a spine skeleton. Then functional tests were performed with the patient seated in front of a mirror to demonstrate the consequences of poor sitting posture. The patient was asked to assume her habitual posture. A vertical compression test was performed through the shoulders assessing alignment and stability. The patient was encouraged to see and feel any spinal instability as well as to note any pain. The posture was subsequently manually corrected and the test repeated so that the patient might note the positive changes in stability and discomfort. In her habitual posture, the patient was then directed to slowly turn her neck in each direction and then to raise her arms overhead noting ease of mobility and discomfort. After posture correction, the patient was directed to repeat the movements and note improvement in range and reduction in discomfort. The patient was taken through a series of postural adjustment steps that she could use to aid in correcting her posture. First, the concepts of base of support through the feet and chair adjustment were reviewed. The patient was then asked to roll her pelvis forward and backward noting the range of mobility, and then asked to overcorrect the lumbar lordosis, followed by slowly releasing the lordosis until she felt that her pelvis was in a comfortable, neutral position. The patient was encouraged to feel the pressure on the ischial tuberosities and the therapist explained how this was her neutral position. The patient was then shown the adjustment of the shoulder girdle into neutral while preventing the anterior ribs from elevating. The patient was instructed in the adjustment of the head position into neutral by performing a gentle chin tuck guided passively using the finger tips of the index finger and releasing the chin tuck at the point of a comfortable position. The patient was then shown strategies for maintaining the corrected sitting position using active sitting, lumbar or sacral roll, or broader lumbar supports. Finally, the patient was educated in body mechanics with proper dynamic posturing for home and work activities. These postural education concepts were based on the therapist's personal experience, the therapist's education, and teachings by Paris[60] and Johnson.[120]

Relaxation is addressed through teaching of relaxed positioning of the head, neck, and jaw incorporated with breathing techniques as described by Rocabado.[57] The positions of the head, jaw, and tongue have been shown to have potential adverse effects on TMJ compression, TMJ mobility, and periarticular muscle activity.[57] The patient was directed to lie in a supine position with towel support under the neck and pillow support under the head and then to note resting positions of her head, jaw, and tongue and to recognize her breathing pattern (e.g., through nose or mouth, with chest or abdomen). The patient was then directed to find the neutral position of the head, to position the tongue to the roof of the mouth with the tip behind the top two teeth, and to close the mouth but keep a small separation of the teeth. The patient was then directed to inhale through the nose allowing the breath to initiate from the abdomen by letting it naturally rise rather than via the chest and then to exhale slowly through the nose allowing the abdomen to naturally fall. This relaxation exercise was also instructed in a corrected sitting or standing posture and recommended as needed to relieve stress and tension. Conscious correcting of her posture and performing these relaxation exercises was encouraged once every hour for any duration.

A suboccipital release self-treatment technique was taught to address tension at the base of the head as well as for relieving headaches. The patient was educated on placing two tennis balls in a thin sock and then tying the sock to maintain stability of the balls. The technique was to be performed in a quiet dark room lying supine with the use of a neck roll to support the neck and a pillow to support the head with knees supported. The tennis balls were to be placed above the neck roll at the base of the head with additional support as needed under the head to prevent craniocervical extension. Lying in this position for 5 minutes while focusing on relaxation and breathing exercises, patients have described good success with the release of tension and pain as well as reducing or warding off headaches.

A TMJ self-care program was instructed for reducing pain, relaxing muscles, relieving intrajoint irritation, and maintaining gains achieved from therapeutic intervention.[57] Advice for self-care included a soft nonchewy diet, no wide opening of mouth (maximum of two fingers width), no biting, no gum chewing, prevention of direct pressure on mandible or sleeping on problematic side, yawning with tongue against the palate, tongue against the palate at rest, nasal breathing maintaining free airway space, and maintaining good posture.

## Outcomes

On the patient's last visit, she reported doing very well with no headache in the preceding month. The primary author recommended that the patient follow up for one additional visit to perform the flexibility and strengthening portions of the issued *Neck Program* and to review the entire program prior to discontinuation of therapy. However, the patient did not schedule another appointment for an unknown reason, so unfortunately objective data and outcome measures could not be reassessed.

Overall, the patient noted a significant decrease in headache frequency with progressive improvement since the start of therapy from more than once per week (daily) to one to four per month and finally to none in the month preceding her last therapy visit. Headache intensity also progressively improved since therapy onset from a reported *severe* to a *mild* intensity. Throughout the duration of PT treatment, the patient also reported cessation of tinnitus, less neck tenderness, and improved jaw and neck mobility and function. The patient reported improvement with the following activities of daily living: she was now able to do as much work as she wanted, able to drive longer distances with only slight neck pain, able to read as much as she wanted with only slight neck pain, and experienced some neck pain related only to a few recreational activities.

The last set of outcome measures completed by the patient was on the second-to-last visit. The results of the four HDI (**Table 9-10**) and NDI (**Table 9-11**) outcome measures completed throughout the treatment period are shown in **Figures 9-22** and **9-23**. The results of the HDI outcome measure showed a 31% improvement for the emotional score, a 42% improvement for the functional score, and a 36% improvement in the total score between the time of the initial evaluation and the second to last visit. During the same time period, the results of the NDI outcome measure showed an 18% improvement and—at one time—a 26% improvement for an earlier assessment date. Although specific subjective and objective signs of improvement were not assessed on the last visit date, which was approximately 1 month after the previous follow-up, there was noted significant improvement through the assessment of self-perceived outcome measures

**TABLE 9-10    HDI Outcome Measures**

|  | 10/18/04 | 11/11/04 | 1/13/05 | 3/31/05 |
|---|---|---|---|---|
| Frequency | >1/wk | >1/wk | 1–4/month | 1–4/month |
| Intensity | Severe | Moderate | Mild | Not completed |
| Emotional score (max 52) | 26 | 18 | 12 | 10 |
| Functional score (max 48) | 30 | 24 | 12 | 10 |
| Total score (max 100) | 56 | 42 | 24 | 20 |

**TABLE 9-11    NDI Outcome Measures**

|  | 10/18/04 | 11/11/04 | 1/13/04 | 3/31/05 |
|---|---|---|---|---|
| Total score (max 50) | 19 | 14 | 6 | 10 |
| Disability score | 38% | 28% | 12% | 20% |
| Disability | Moderate | Moderate | Mild | Mild |

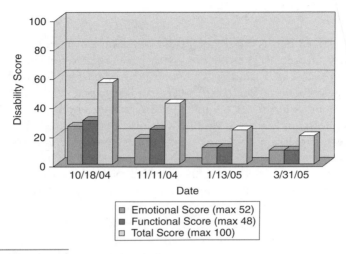

**Figure 9-22**    HDI outcome measures scores.

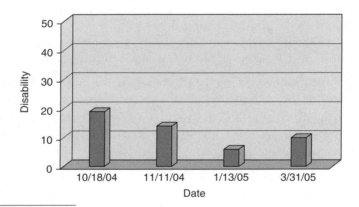

**Figure 9-23**    NDI outcome measure scores (total score).

used in this case. A 29% change in the HDI total score constitutes the $MDC_{95}$ for this measure.[39] A 7-point or 14% change in the NDI score constitutes the MCID for the NDI.[42] The change in the total score of the HDI outcome measure in this case was a decrease of 36%, which indicates that the MDC was exceeded and that a true change had indeed occurred in pain and disability due to the headache complaints. Similarly, the change in NDI score, which exceeded the established MCID for this measure, indicated that a true and meaningful change in neck-related disability had occurred during the course of treatment.

## Discussion

The patient described in this case report had a very complex presentation. Medical diagnoses included chronic TTH associated with pericranial tenderness, probable MH without aura, probable CGH, and TMD. Impairments identified during the PT examination included postural deviations (FHP), MTrPs and decreased length in the neck and jaw muscles, hypomobility in the C0–C2 and T1–T8 segments, and hypermobility of the left TMJ. Poor prognostic indicators, including the presence of possible central sensitization, emotional stress, depression, and the worsening nature of a chronic condition, further complicated the patient's presentation. Despite this complexity, the patient clearly improved over the course of treatment. She exceeded the MDC on the HDI indicating that a true improvement had occurred with regard to headache-related disability, while exceeding the MCID on the NDI implied that a true and clinically meaningful improvement also occurred for disability due to neck pain. In addition, the patient reported on the last visit after 1 month of no treatment that she had not experienced a single headache in the preceding month. This is especially significant considering that the patient initially described daily headaches. Although a case report does not allow us to infer a cause-and-effect relationship between intervention and outcome, true and meaningful changes in a previously worsening, chronic condition do imply that the PT management described was at least contributory to the positive changes noted.

At this point, we should mention and discuss two assumptions that are at the basis of the choices made in the PT diagnosis and management of this patient:

1. The impairments found during the PT examination as noted above can contribute to or even cause the medical headache diagnoses relevant to this patient.

2. By addressing these neuromusculoskeletal impairments, PT management can affect limitations in activities and restrictions in participation attributed to these medical headache diagnoses.

So what is the evidence linking the neuromusculoskeletal impairments noted in this patient to the medical diagnoses of chronic TTH associated with pericranial tenderness, probable MH without aura, probable CGH, and TMD?

Myofascial trigger points were among the main neuromusculoskeletal impairments identified and treated in this patient. Active MTrPs were diagnosed by way of subjective history, neck mobility tests, and manual palpation. The patient described her headache pain as a moderate to severe bandlike pain across her forehead; she reported her other head and neck pain as tenderness. Myofascial pain is often described as a dull, aching, tightening, or pressure-like pain of mild to moderate intensity.[12] The patient also complained of tinnitus in the left ear. Unilateral tinnitus may be associated with MTrPs in the deep masseter muscle. It is thought to be due to a referred sensory phenomenon or motor unit facilitation of the tensor tympani and/or stapedius muscles of the middle ear.[12] Various authors have claimed that head, neck, and shoulder girdle muscles are capable of referring pain into the head experienced as headaches.[12,20] Knowledge of myofascial referred pain patterns when interpreting the patient's pain diagram (Figure 9-1) indicated a possible involvement of the UT, SCM, SO, temporalis, and masseter muscles.[12] In addition, referred pain patterns for the masseter and temporalis were consistent with the reported facial pain; referral patterns for the upper, middle, and lower portions of the trapezius muscles were consistent with the patient's report of upper and lower neck pain.[12] Matching established referral patterns to a patient report of pain distribution then guided further examination: Referred pain recognized by the patient as part of her headache pain was elicited with compression of tender nodules within the left SCM and left UT. A trial of TrPDN on the first visit further confirmed the existence of active MTrPs by the elicitation of numerous LTRs with local and referred pain phenomena. In addition, the patient's cervical AROM test findings indicated myofascial tightness. Muscles with MTrPs are known to exhibit decreased flexibility and painful limitation to full stretch.

The primary author inferred in this case not only that MTrPs contributed to myofascial hypertonicity, myofascial tenderness, and referred pain into the head, neck, and face, but also that these trigger points played a major etiologic role in the chronic TTH diagnosed in this patient. Studies have shown that prolonged peripheral nociceptive input from pericranial myofascial tissue can sensitize the second-order neurons at the spinal and trigeminal level leading to impaired central nervous system (CNS) modulation of this nociceptive activity, thereby resulting in an increased general pain sensitivity.[7] In patients with chronic TTH with pericranial muscle tenderness, there appears to be just such a disruption of the balance between peripheral nociceptive input and CNS pain modulation.[7] The convergent afferent input in this scenario includes nociceptive input from muscles innervated by C1–C3, among which are the UT, SCM, and suboccipital muscles, and of those innervated by the trigeminal nerve, which includes the temporalis and the masseter muscles. In addition, we need to take into consideration the nociceptive input from possible segmental dysfunction of the upper cervical spine (C0–C3), thereby providing a potential explanation for the observed clinical link between and diagnostic confusion with regard to TTH and CGH. The resultant temporal and spatial summation is the CNS misinterpretation of the peripheral input leading to central sensitization.

The neuroanatomic explanation of how structures innervated by cervical nerve roots can refer pain into the head or face starts with the trigeminal nucleus caudalis. This nucleus descends as low as the C3 or C4 segments of the spinal cord. The trigeminocervical nucleus, a column of gray matter that is located adjoining to the trigeminal nucleus caudalis, exchanges sensory information from the upper cervical spinal nerve roots to the trigeminal nerve via interneurons, thereby explaining how cervical nociceptive input may be referred to the sensory receptive fields of the trigeminal nerve supplying the head and face, most commonly affecting the ophthalmic division, which in turn may lead to the perception of referred symptoms to the forehead, temple, or orbit. Because afferent sensory signals ascend or descend up to three spinal cord segments, nociceptive signals for spinal segments C6 or C7 may even interact with the trigeminocervical nucleus, and ultimately this may result in referral of pain into the head or face from structures as far distant as the lower neck region.[25]

Fernández-de-las-Peñas et al[13] provided clinical support for this proposed etiologic role for MTrPs in TTH. They found that there was a significant difference between a group of patients with chronic TTH and healthy controls with regard to the presence of active MTrPs ($P$ <0.001), but not for latent MTrPs ($P$ >0.05); they also noted that active MTrPs in the UT, SCM, and temporalis muscles were associated with chronic TTH.[13] In another study, Fernández-de-las-Peñas et al[127] also demonstrated significant ($P$ <0.001) between-group differences for active MTrPs in the SO muscles in patients with chronic TTH as compared to healthy controls; the between-group difference with regard to latent MTrPs was again not significant ($P$ >0.05). In addition, they found that chronic TTH subjects with active suboccipital MTrPs described greater headache intensity, duration, and frequency compared to those with latent MTrPs ($P$ <0.05). Furthermore, the characteristics of TTH noted in various studies[13,20] were very similarly described as pressure and/or tightness or increased tenderness of neck and shoulder muscles, and the similarity of this description with the documented nature of pain due to MTrPs further increases the plausibility of referred pain from MTrPs as contributory to TTH.

Assessing pericranial muscle tenderness and pressure pain thresholds are ways of evaluating diagnostic criteria with regard to the contribution of muscular disorders. Studies have shown that subjects with episodic and chronic TTH have increased muscle tenderness compared to subjects with MH and those without headaches.[128] In a random sample of 735 adults, 87% of those with chronic TTH and 66% of those with episodic TTH were found to also have signs of muscular disorders including increased tenderness recorded by either manual palpation or pressure algometry and/or increased EMG levels.[8] Relevant to the clinical examination of this patient, this same study also found that manual palpation for tenderness was more specific and sensitive than EMG and algometry.[8] This degree of pericranial muscle tenderness has also been shown to be strongly correlated to the frequency and intensity of TTH.[128]

Myofascial palpation revealed latent and active MTrPs using the recommended diagnostic criteria (Table 9-3). Although not specifically mentioned as a diagnostic criterion for MTrPs, in this patient myofascial hypertonicity was also noted during the palpatory examination of the muscles affected. Myofascial hypertonicity has been shown to be increased in patients with chronic TTH as compared to normal control subjects, irrespective of whether they had a headache that day.[129] Research[129] supports the clinical observation that hypertonic muscles are more tender than muscles with normal tone. In this patient, myofascial hypertonicity was indeed associated with tenderness.

Postural deviations as found in this patient have also been associated with TTH: Fernández-de-las-Peñas et al[130] demonstrated that subjects with chronic TTH had a higher prevalence of FHP compared to a healthy control group ($P$ <0.001). They also noted a significant negative correlation ($r = -0.5$; $P$ <0.04) between FHP and headache frequency, thereby linking a more pronounced FHP to a higher headache frequency. These same researchers again confirmed this significant negative correlation between FHP and headache frequency but also duration in a related study.[127] However, FHP is not limited to patients with TTH: Marcus et al[37] found spinal postural abnormalities in 90% of those with chronic headache of various types versus 46% of controls.[37]

Postural abnormalities of the cervical spine can theoretically also contribute to the activation of trigger points in head, neck, and shoulder musculature.[131] Shortening of the SO, semispinalis, splenii, UT, and SCM muscles is associated with FHP.[12] Fernández-de-las-Peñas et al[127] noted that patients with chronic TTH and active MTrPs had a greater FHP than patients with latent trigger points, although this difference was nonsignificant. The study also showed a positive correlation between the degree of FHP and the presence of active suboccipital MTrPs.[127]

Above we provided the neuroanatomic explanation for CGH; interconnections between the trigeminocervical nucleus and the trigeminal nucleus caudalis allow pain from cervical sources to be perceived as headache and facial pain. The postural deviation in this patient (i.e., FHP) is often a contributing factor to the onset and/or the maintenance of headaches, neck pain, and facial pain, because it may result in suboccipital compression with consequences on the trigeminocervical complex and vertebral artery, excessive compression of the facet joints and posterior surfaces of the vertebral bodies, alteration of cervical spine biomechanics, and altered proprioceptive input.[31] There has been notable study on the effects of poor activation, motor control, and endurance of the deep and postural tonic muscles of the neck and shoulder girdle as it relates to postural abnormalities, neck pain, and CGH.[91] A specific test has been used to test the tonic function of the deep cervical flexors,[91] but this test was not used in this case; rather, the primary author simply assumed that this impairment existed given the identified FHP resulting in a craniocervical extension position, suboccipital hypertonicity, and decreased craniocervical flexion mobility. In addition, the identification of C0–C2 segmental restrictions with—in our opinion—a sufficient degree of diagnostic confidence further strengthened the likelihood of a diagnosis of CGH.

Forward head posture has also been associated with TMD because it, too, leads to increased muscle tension of the muscles acting on the mandible, abnormal tongue position, tongue thrust and anterior open bite, and increased muscle activity of the muscles of mastication.[31]

The connection between MH and neuromusculoskeletal impairments as identified in this patient is less well supported in the research literature. Fernández-de-las-Peñas et al[132] reported a significantly ($P < 0.001$) greater number of active but not latent MTrPs in patients with MH as compared to healthy controls; trigger points were located mostly ipsilateral to the headache. Migraine subjects also had a significantly ($P < 0.001$) greater FHP than controls and more limited mobility in neck extension ($P = 0.02$) and flexion-extension combined ($P = 0.01$), leading those authors to hypothesize a contributory role for trigger points in the initiation or perpetuation of MH.

Our second assumption concerned the effect that PT management might have on limitations in activities and restrictions in participation related to headache complaints by addressing the identified neuromusculoskeletal impairments hypothesized to be related to the various headache diagnoses. Many headache sufferers seek numerous different treatment approaches, become dependent on medications to relieve their symptoms, and eventually accept their headaches as a fact of life. Treatment of chronic headache is varied and has included pharmacologic, nonpharmacologic, anesthetic, and surgical interventions. Pharmacologic treatment of headaches has included over-the-counter analgesics,[6,133] nonsteroidal anti-inflammatories,[6,14,17,25,29,133,134] tricyclic antidepressants,[6,14,17,25,133,134] anticonvulsants,[14,17,25,134] and muscle relaxants.[6,14,25] Nonpharmacologic treatment may include spinal manipulation,[24,25,29,38] so-called "conventional" PT,[6,14,16,24,25,29,38] transcutaneous electrical nerve stimulation (TENS),[6,25,29] biofeedback/relaxation therapy,[6,14,17,25,29,133] intraoral dental devices,[14,30] acupuncture,[135] wellness education,[6,14,16,38] and psychotherapy.[6,25,29,133] Anesthetic intervention for the treatment of headaches has included blocks of spinal roots, spinal nerves,[25,29] and zygapophyseal joints,[25] MTrP injections (using analgesics and botulinum toxin),[6,16,17,24,25] and neurolytic procedures (radiofrequency thermal neurolysis and cryoneurolysis).[24,25,29] Surgical interventions have included neurectomy, dorsal rhizotomy, microsurgical vascular and nerve decompression, and cervical spine fusion.[25,29] The PT plan of care for the patient described in this case report consisted of dry needling, myofascial and articular OMPT, exercise, and education, as discussed above.

The efficacy of TrPDN has been studied generally for the treatment of myofascial pain or trigger point inactivation[51,98,99,136–138] and specifically for use in patients with low back pain (LBP),[116,139–140] jaw pain,[141] hemiparetic shoulder pain,[142] and cervical radiculopathy.[118] A Cochrane review suggested that dry needling might be useful in combination with other therapies in the treatment of LBP.[139] A systematic review of 23 randomized controlled trials (RCT) of needling therapies in the treatment of myofascial pain found that direct trigger point needling was an effective treatment in decreasing symptoms, but efficacy compared to placebo could not be established.[51] A randomized controlled trial (RCT) that looked at the immediate effects of dry needling and acupuncture in the treatment of chronic neck pain found that dry needling was not effective in decreasing pain or improving mobility as compared to acupuncture.[143] However, this study did not take into account that dry needling often causes soreness immediately after treatment and pain relief is often reported 2–3 days later and may, therefore, have provided an inaccurate indication of the effectiveness of dry needling for chronic neck pain. Another RCT suggested that deep needling of MTrPs might be more effective than traditional acupuncture or superficial trigger point needling in the treatment of chronic LBP in the elderly.[140] However, only two studies have looked at the effect of TrPDN on various headache forms.[93,127] One RCT that compared dry needling of MTrPs in the neck and metoprolol in migraine prophylaxis for the treatment of MH found a significant reduction in headache frequency ($P <0.01$) for both groups and no between-group difference in frequency or duration.[136] The second RCT study—albeit one with a small sample size—looked at the effect of dry needling on TTH and found a significant improvement in headache indices, tenderness score, and neck mobility limitation.[93]

With regard to the research basis on the efficacy of OMPT, massage therapy has been deemed effective in the treatment of LBP due to MTrPs.[144] One study looked at the efficacy of ischemic compression technique and transverse friction massage for the treatment of active and latent MTrPs; both techniques produced significant improvement in pressure pain threshold and in visual analog pain scale scores without significant between-group differences.[145] Manual pressure release of latent MTrPs in the UT has shown a reduction in perceived pain and a significant increase in pressure tolerance ($P$ <0.001).[146] Lewit[121] treated 351 muscle groups in 244 patients with myofascial pain with the PIR technique and found immediate pain relief in 94%, lasting pain relief in 63%, and lasting relief of point tenderness in 23% of the sites treated.[147] Blanco et al[147] demonstrated the improvement of active mouth opening following a single treatment of PIR as used for the patient in this case report in subjects with latent MTrPs in the masseter muscle.

A systematic review of nine RCTs involving 683 patients into the efficacy of spinal manipulative therapy for chronic headaches that included TTH, MH, and CGH concluded that spinal manipulative therapy was more efficacious than massage for CGH and that it was of comparable efficacy to the use of prophylactic medication (amitriptyline) in the short-term treatment of tension-type and MH.[92] Another systematic review suggested that spinal manipulation has proven to be effective in CGH, but it has not been shown to be consistently effective in the treatment of TTH.[148] An RCT of 127 subjects with MH treated by chiropractic thrust manipulation for a maximum of 16 treatments over a 2-month period showed statistically significant improvement in favor of the treatment group with regard to headache frequency ($P$ <0.005) and duration ($P$ <0.01), headache-related disability ($P$ <0.05), and medication use ($P$ <0.001).[149] A systematic review of 20 RCTs that looked at efficacy of manual therapy for the treatment of mechanical neck disorders concluded that manual therapies combined with exercise therapy were more effective in improving pain and patient satisfaction in mechanical neck disorders with and without headaches than just manual therapy alone.[150] Although cervical SNAG techniques are widely used for the treatment of neck pain and mobility restrictions, little evidence has been provided on the biomechanical basis or on the efficacy of the technique.[151]

Jull et al[77] studied the effectiveness of various combinations of OMPT and an exercise program consisting of deep cervical flexor endurance training, scapular retraction exercises, postural education, and low-load cervical flexion and extension resistive exercises in 200 patients with cervicogenic headache. The three active treatments (OMPT, exercise therapy, and OMPT combined with exercise) reduced headache frequency and intensity more than the control therapy immediately post-intervention and after 12 months. The combined OMPT and exercise treatment showed clinically but not statistically relevant increased effect sizes over the other two treatment groups at 12 months.

A systematic review of studies that looked at the effectiveness of PT interventions for the treatment of TMD supported the effectiveness of the use of active and passive oral exercises and postural training exercises in reducing symptoms. However, most of the studies included only small sample sizes and were of poor methodology; only one study included OMPT treatments.[152]

We acknowledge that the case report described in this chapter has a number of limitations. As discussed earlier, the format of a case report does not allow us to infer a cause-and-effect relationship. Also, the lack of long-term follow-up and the lack of outcome data collected on the final visit negatively affect our careful assertion that there was a positive effect over the course of treatment. We also acknowledge that for many of the tests and measures and also with regard to the classification systems used to diagnose the headache (ICHD-II) and TMD (AAOFP diagnostic criteria), insufficient data are available on diagnostic accuracy to reach a diagnosis with research-based confidence. Despite plausible neuroanatomic explanations as provided above, the bulk of the clinical research linking the neuromusculoskeletal impairments theoretically amenable to PT management to the headache diagnoses relevant to this patient is correlational research; we need to remember that correlation does not imply causation. It is relevant to consider that neck pain accompanies 60–70% of all headache types.[153-155] In addition, recent research has established bidirectional interactions between afferents from the three upper cervical nerves and trigeminal afferents in the trigeminocervical nucleus.[156-158] In clinical terms, nociceptive afferent information originating in a structure innervated by the trigeminal nerve can therefore be perceived as neck pain. As also pointed out recently by Jull,[159] this bidirectional relationship might explain the high prevalence of neck pain (and perhaps of associated neuromusculoskeletal impairments in the cervical structures evident upon a physical examination as described in this chapter) as one possible symptom (and associated signs) of headache types where such cervical musculoskeletal impairments truly do not have an etiologic role. This chapter also has highlighted the fact that the research basis for the PT management of patients with headache—and specifically for the interventions used for this particular patient—is still too limited for confident research-supported designs of a plan of care for a patient as described in this case report. Instead, the plan of care remains based to a large extent on a pathophysiologic rather than a research-based rationale.

## Conclusion

This case provides a detailed account of the PT diagnosis and management of a patient with chronic headaches, facial pain, and neck pain. After ascertaining that there were no contraindications to PT examination, the therapist used the ICHD-II and AAOFP classification systems to classify the headache and TMJ complaints. Physical examination findings were evaluated based on a pathophysiologic and research-based rationale, and relevant impairments amenable to PT management were identified. The ICF disablement model was used to describe the patient's diagnosis, impairments, current functioning, and level of disability. The preferred practice patterns from the *Guide to Physical Therapist Practice*[85] were used as broad consensus-based guidelines for the development of a plan of care. Treatment incorporated TrPDN, OMPT, exercise therapy, and education. Over the course of treatment, true and meaningful changes were documented with regard to headache and neck pain-related disability. The patient also reported a noted decrease in headache frequency from daily to none over the month preceding the last visit. Despite the fact that a case report format as used in this chapter does not allow us to infer a cause-and-effect relationship between intervention and outcome, true and meaningful changes in a previously worsening, chronic condition do imply that the PT management described was at least contributory to the positive changes noted.

This case report has also shown a great many areas in need of further research. Data is lacking on the diagnostic accuracy of the clinical tests and measures and also on the diagnostic classification systems used for this patient. Research is also limited with regard to providing a causal or at least contributory link between the various headache types discussed in this case report and the neuromusculoskeletal impairments that might be amenable to PT management. Finally, research is lacking in the area of efficacy of the PT interventions used for patients with various headache types that might pose an indication for PT management (i.e., TTH, MH, CGH, TMD-related headaches, and occipital neuralgia). We hope that this chapter not only serves to make the clinical reasoning process related to PT diagnosis and management of patients with various headache types more transparent to the various health-care professionals involved in the care of such patients, but also that the identified areas in need of further study will lead to additional much needed research.

## References

1. Headache Fact Sheet. *Lifting The Burden*. Available at: http://www.l-t-b.org/pages/18/index.htm. Accessed May 20, 2006.
2. Boissonnault WG. Prevalence of comorbid conditions, surgeries, and medication use in a physical therapy outpatient population: A multi-centered study. *J Orthop Sports Phys Ther*1999;29: 506–519; discussion 520–525.
3. Olesen J. *The International Classification of Headache Disorders*. 2nd ed. Application to practice. *Funct Neurol* 2005;20(2):61–68.
4. Olesen J. *The International Classification of Headache Disorders*. 2nd ed. *Cephalalgia* 2004;24:1–150.
5. Schoenen J, MacGregor E, Holroyd K, et al. Tension-type headache. In: Olesen J, ed. *The International Classification of Headache Disorders*. 2nd ed. Oxford, UK: Blackwell; 2003.
6. Schulman EA. Overview of tension-type headache. *Curr Pain Headache Rep* 2001;5:454–462.
7. Jensen R, Bendtsen L, Olesen J. Muscular factors are of importance in tension-type headache. *Headache* 1998;38:10–17.
8. Jensen R, Rasmussen BK. Muscular disorders in tension-type headache. *Cephalalgia* 1996;16: 97–103.
9. Bendtsen L. Central sensitization in tension-type headache: Possible pathophysiological mechanisms. *Cephalalgia* 2000;20:486–508.
10. Meyer RA, Campbell JN, Raja SN. Peripheral neural mechanisms of nociception. In: Wall PD, Melzack R, eds. *Textbook of Pain*. 3rd ed. New York: Churchill Livingstone; 1994.
11. Dommerholt J. Persistent myalgia following whiplash. *Curr Pain Headache Rep* 2005;9:326–330.
12. Simons DG, Travell JG, Simons LS. *Travell & Simons' Myofascial Pain and Dysfunction: The Trigger Point Manual*. Vol. 1. Upper half of body. 2nd ed. Philadelphia, PA: Lippincott Williams & Wilkins; 1999.
13. Fernández-de-las-Peñas C, Alonso-Blanco C, Cuadrado ML, Gerwin RD, Pareja JA. Myofascial trigger points and their relationship to headache clinical parameters in chronic tension-type headache. *Headache* 2006;46:1264–1272.

14. Graff-Radford SB. Regional myofascial pain syndrome and headache: Principles of diagnosis and management. *Curr Pain Headache Rep* 2001;5:376–381.

15. Freund B, Schwartz M. Post-traumatic myofascial pain of the head and neck. *Curr Pain Headache Rep* 2002;6:361–369.

16. Davidoff RA. Trigger points and myofascial pain: Toward understanding how they affect headaches. *Cephalalgia* 1998;18:436–448.

17. Borg-Stein J. Cervical myofascial pain and headache. *Curr Pain Headache Rep* 2002;6:324–330.

18. Alvarez DJ, Rockwell PG. Trigger points: Diagnosis and management. *Am Fam Physician* 2002;65:653–660.

19. Han SC, Harrison P. Myofascial pain syndrome and trigger-point management. *Reg Anesth* 1997;22:89–101.

20. Fernández-de-las-Peñas C, Cuadrado ML, Gerwin RD, Pareja JA. Referred pain from the trochlear region in tension-type headache: A myofascial trigger point from the superior oblique muscle. *Headache* 2005;45:731–737.

21. Graff-Radford SB, Jaeger B, Reeves JL. Myofascial pain may present clinically as occipital neuralgia. *Neurosurg* 1986;19:610–613.

22. Borsook D, Burstein R, Moulton E, Becerra L. Functional imaging of the trigeminal system: Applications to migraine pathophysiology. *Headache* 2006;46(suppl):S32–S38.

23. Haldeman S, Dagenais S. Cervicogenic headaches: A critical review. *Spine J* 2001;1:31–46.

24. Jensen S. Neck related causes of headache. *Aust Fam Phys* 2005;34:635–639.

25. Biondi DM. Cervicogenic headache: Mechanisms, evaluation, and treatment strategies. *J Am Osteopath Assoc* 2000;100(suppl):S7–S14.

26. Alix ME, Bates DK. A proposed etiology of cervicogenic headache: The neurophysiologic basis and anatomic relationship between the dura mater and the rectus posterior capitis minor muscle. *J Manipulative Physiol Ther* 1999;22:534–539.

27. Martelletti P, van Suijlekom H. Cervicogenic headache: Practical approaches to therapy. *CNS Drugs* 2004;18:793–805.

28. Petersen SM. Articular and muscular impairments in cervicogenic headache: A case report. *J Orthop Sports Phys Ther* 2003;33:21–30; discussion 30–22.

29. Pollmann W, Keidel M, Pfaffenrath V. Headache and the cervical spine: A critical review. *Cephalalgia* 1997;17:801–816.

30. Benoliel R, Sharav Y. Craniofacial pain of myofascial origin: Temporomandibular pain and tension-type headache. *Compend Contin Educ Dent* 1998;19:701–704, 706, 708–710 passim; quiz 722.

31. Mannheimer JS, Rosenthal RM. Acute and chronic postural abnormalities as related to craniofacial pain and temporomandibular disorders. *Dent Clin North Am* 1991;35:185–208.

32. NHF Headache Fact Sheet. *National Headache Foundation.* Available at: http://www.headaches.org/consumer/presskit/NHAW04/Categories_of_Headache.pdf. Accessed May 20, 2006.

33. Leonardi M, Steiner TJ, Scher AT, Lipton RB. The global burden of migraine: Measuring disability in headache disorders with WHO's Classification of Functioning, Disability and Health (ICF). *J Headache Pain* 2005;6:429–440.

34. Stang PE, Crown WH, Bizier R, Chatterton ML, White R. The family impact and costs of migraine. *Am J Manag Care* 2004;10:313–320.

35. Schwartz B, Stewart W, Simon D, R. L. Epidemiology of tension-type headache. *JAMA* 1998;279:381–383.

36. Fishbain DA, Lewis J, Cole B, Cutler RB, Rosomoff RS, Rosomoff HL. Do the proposed cervicogenic headache diagnostic criteria demonstrate specificity in terms of separating cervicogenic headache from migraine? *Curr Pain Headache Rep* 2003;7:387–394.

37. Marcus DA, Scharff L, Mercer S, Turk DC. Musculoskeletal abnormalities in chronic headache: A controlled comparison of headache diagnostic groups. *Headache* 1999;39:21–27.
38. Mills Roth J. Physical therapy in the treatment of chronic headache. *Curr Pain Headache Rep* 2003;7:482–489.
39. Jacobson GP, Ramadan NM, Aggarwal SK, Newman CW. The Henry Ford Hospital Headache Disability Inventory (HDI). *Neurology* 1994;44:837–842.
40. Jacobson GP, Ramadan NM, Norris L, Newman CW. Headache disability inventory (HDI): Short-term test-retest reliability and spouse perceptions. *Headache* 1995;35:534–539.
41. Vernon H, Mior S. The Neck Disability Index: A study of reliability and validity. *J Manipulative Physiol Ther* 1991;14:409–415.
42. Cleland JA, Fritz JM, Whitman JM, Palmer JA. The reliability and construct validity of the Neck Disability Index and patient-specific functional scale in patients with cervical radiculopathy. *Spine* 2006;31:598–602.
43. Roy M. *Level I. Differential Diagnosis Part-A: Course Manual.* Fairfax, VA: North American Institute of Orthopaedic Manual Therapy, Inc.; 2002.
44. Gardner KL. Genetics of migraine: An update. *Headache* 2006;46(suppl):S19–S24.
45. Fedorak C, Ashworth N, Marshall J, Paull H. Reliability of the visual assessment of cervical and lumbar lordosis: How good are we? *Spine* 2003;28:1857–1859.
46. Youdas JW, Carey JR, Garrett TR. Reliability of measurements of cervical spine range of motion: Comparison of three methods. *Phys Ther* 1991;71:98–104; discussion 105–106.
47. Terwee CB, de Winter AF, Scholten RJ, et al. Interobserver reproducibility of the visual estimation of range of motion of the shoulder. *Arch Phys Med Rehabil* 2005;86:1356–1361.
48. Jepsen J, Laursen L, Larsen A, Hagert CG. Manual strength testing in 14 upper limb muscles: A study of inter-rater reliability. *Acta Orthop Scand* 2004;75:442–448.
49. Bertilson BC, Grunnesjo M, Strender LE. Reliability of clinical tests in the assessment of patients with neck/shoulder problems: Impact of history. *Spine* 2003;28:2222–2231.
50. Jepsen JR, Laursen LH, Hagert CG, Kreiner S, Larsen AI. Diagnostic accuracy of the neurological upper limb examination. I. Inter-rater reproducibility of selected findings and patterns. *BMC Neurol* 2006;6:8.
51. Cummings TM, White AR. Needling therapies in the management of myofascial trigger point pain: A systematic review. *Arch Phys Med Rehabil* 2001;82:986–992.
52. Gerwin RD, Shannon S, Hong CZ, Hubbard D, Gevirtz R. Interrater reliability in myofascial trigger point examination. *Pain* 1997;69(1–2):65–73.
53. Lew PC, Lewis J, Story I. Inter-therapist reliability in locating latent myofascial trigger points using palpation. *Man Ther* 1997;2:87–90.
54. Sciotti VM, Mittak VL, DiMarco L, et al. Clinical precision of myofascial trigger point location in the trapezius muscle. *Pain* 2001;93:259–266.
55. Schöps P, Pfingsten M, Siebert U. [Reliability of manual medical examination techniques of the cervical spine. Study of quality assurance in manual diagnosis.] (German) *Z Orthop* 2000;138:2–7.
56. Hong CZ, Kuan TS, Chen JT, Chen SM. Referred pain elicited by palpation and by needling of myofascial trigger points: A comparison. *Arch Phys Med Rehabil* 1997;78(9):957–960.
57. Rocabado M. *TMJ Evaluation and Treatment of the Craniomandibular System.* Course notes. St. Augustine, FL: University of St. Augustine; 2001.
58. Metcalfe S, Reese H, B S. The effect of high-velocity low-amplitude manipulation on cervical spine muscle strength: A randomized clinical trial. *J Manual Manipulative Ther* 2006;14:152–157.
59. Lewis J, Green A, Reichard Z, Wright C. Scapular position: The validity of skin surface palpation. *Man Ther* 2002;7:26–30.

60. Paris SV. *S1: Introduction to Spinal Evaluation and Manipulation*. Seminar manual. 3rd ed. St. Augustine, FL: Institute of Physical Therapy University of St. Augustine for Health Sciences; 1999.

61. Jull G, Zito G, Trott P, Potter H, Shirley D. Inter-examiner reliability to detect painful upper cervical joint dysfunction. *Aust J Physiother* 1997;43:125–129.

62. McGregor AH, Wragg P, Gedroyc WM. Can interventional MRI provide an insight into the mechanics of a posterior-anterior mobilisation? *Clin Biomech* 2001;16:926–929.

63. Pool JJ, Hoving JL, de Vet HC, van Mameren H, Bouter LM. The interexaminer reproducibility of physical examination of the cervical spine. *J Manipulative Physiol Ther* 2004;27:84–90.

64. Fjellner A, Bexander C, Faleij R, Strender LE. Interexaminer reliability in physical examination of the cervical spine. *J Manipulative Physiol Ther* 1999;22:511–516.

65. Huijbregts PA. Spinal motion palpation: A review of reliability studies. *J Manual Manipulative Ther* 2002;10:24–39.

66. Humphreys BK, Delahaye M, Peterson CK. An investigation into the validity of cervical spine motion palpation using subjects with congenital block vertebrae as a 'gold standard'. *BMC Musculoskelet Disord* 2004;5:19.

67. Jull G, Bogduk N, Marsland A. The accuracy of manual diagnosis for cervical zygapophysial joint pain syndromes. *Med J Aust* 1988;148:233–236.

68. Zito G, Jull G, Story I. Clinical tests of musculoskeletal dysfunction in the diagnosis of cervicogenic headache. *Man Ther* 2006;11:118–129.

69. Aprill C, Axinn MJ, Bogduk N. Occipital headaches stemming from the lateral atlanto-axial (C1-2) joint. *Cephalalgia* 2002;22:15–22.

70. Walker N, Bohannon RW, Cameron D. Discriminate validity of temporomandibular joint range of motion measurements obtained with a ruler. *J Orthop Sports Phys Ther* 2000;30:484–492.

71. Manfredini D, Tognini F, Zampa V, Bosco M. Predictive value of clinical findings for temporomandibular joint effusion. *Oral Surg Oral Med Oral Pathol Oral Radiol Endod* 2003;96:521–526.

72. Lobbezoo-Scholte AM, De Wijer A, Steenks MH, Bosman F. Interexaminer reliability of six orthopaedic tests in diagnostic subgroups of craniomandibular disorders. *J Oral Rehabil* 1994;21:273–285.

73. Israel HA, Diamond B, Saed-Nejad F, Ratcliffe A. Osteoarthritis and synovitis as major pathoses of the temporomandibular joint: Comparison of clinical diagnosis with arthroscopic morphology. *J Oral Maxillofac Surg* 1998;56:1023–1027; discussion 1028.

74. Holmlund AB, Axelsson S. Temporomandibular arthropathy: Correlation between clinical signs and symptoms and arthroscopic findings. *Int J Oral Maxillofac Surg* 1996;25:178–181.

75. Nilsson N, Bove G. Evidence that tension-type headache and cervicogenic headache are distinct disorders. *J Manipulative Physiol Ther* 2000;23:288–289.

76. Fernández-de-las-Peñas C, Alonso-Blanco C, San-Roman J, Miangolarra-Page JC. Methodological quality of randomized controlled trials of spinal manipulation and mobilization in tension-type headache, migraine, and cervicogenic headache. *J Orthop Sports Phys Ther* 2006;36:160–169.

77. Jull G, Trott P, Potter H, et al. A randomized controlled trial of exercise and manipulative therapy for cervicogenic headache. *Spine* 2002;27:1835–1843.

78. Moore MK. Upper crossed syndrome and its relationship to cervicogenic headache. *J Manipulative Physiol Ther* 2004;27:414–420.

79. Niere K, Robinson P. Determination of manipulative physiotherapy treatment outcome in headache patients. *Man Ther* 1997;2:199–205.

80. Griegel-Morris P, Larson K, Mueller-Klaus K, Oatis CA. Incidence of common postural abnormalities in the cervical, shoulder, and thoracic regions and their association with pain in two age groups of healthy subjects. *Phys Ther* 1992;72:425–431.

81. Agustsson H. *Evaluation and Treatment of the Craniomandibular System.* Course manual. St. Augustine, FL: University of St. Augustine; 2004.

82. Okeson JP. *Orofacial Pain: Guidelines for Assessment, Classification, and Management.* Hanover Park, IL: Quintessence Publishing; 1996.

83. The International Classification of Functioning, Disability, and Health. Available at: http://www.who.int/classifications/icf/en/. Accessed May 6, 2006.

84. Stucki G. International Classification of Functioning, Disability, and Health (ICF): A promising framework and classification for rehabilitation medicine. *Am J Phys Med Rehabil* 2005;84:733–740.

85. *Guide to Physical Therapist Practice.* 2nd ed. *Phys Ther* 2001;81:9–746.

86. Moog M, Quintner J, Hall T, Zusman M. The late whiplash syndrome: A psychophysical study. *Eur J Pain* 2002;6:283–294.

87. Choi YC, Kim WJ, Kim CH, Lee MS. A clinical study of chronic headaches: Clinical characteristics and depressive trends in migraine and tension-type headaches. *Yonsei Med J* 1995;36:508–514.

88. Holroyd KA, Stensland M, Lipchik GL, Hill KR, O'Donnell FS, Cordingley G. Psychosocial correlates and impact of chronic tension-type headaches. *Headache* 2000;40:3–16.

89. Leistad RB, Sand T, Westgaard RH, Nilsen KB, Stovner LJ. Stress-induced pain and muscle activity in patients with migraine and tension-type headache. *Cephalalgia* 2006;26:64–73.

90. Hanten WP, Olson SL, Lindsay WA, Lounsberry KA, Stewart JK. The effect of manual therapy and a home exercise program on cervicogenic headaches: A case report. *J Manual Manipulative Ther* 2005;13:35–43.

91. Jull G. Management of cervical headache. *Man Ther* 1997;2:182–190.

92. Bronfort G, Assendelft WJ, Evans R, Haas M, Bouter L. Efficacy of spinal manipulation for chronic headache: A systematic review. *J Manipulative Physiol Ther* 2001;24:457–466.

93. Karakurum B, Karaalin O, Coskun O, Dora B, Ucler S, Inan L. The 'dry-needle technique': Intramuscular stimulation in tension-type headache. *Cephalalgia* 2001;21:813–817.

94. Jull GA, Stanton WR. Predictors of responsiveness to physiotherapy management of cervicogenic headache. *Cephalalgia* 2005;25:101–108.

95. Tuttle N. Do changes within a manual therapy treatment session predict between-session changes for patients with cervical spine pain? *Aust J Physiother* 2005;51:43–48.

96. Gunn CC. *The Gunn Approach to the Treatment of Chronic Pain: Intramuscular Stimulation for Myofascial Pain of Radiculopathic Origin.* 2nd ed. New York, NY: Churchill Livingstone; 1996.

97. Travell J, Rinzler S, Herman M. Pain and disability of the shoulder and arm: Treatment by intramuscular infiltration with procaine hydrochloride. *JAMA* 1942;120:417–422.

98. Lewit K. The needle effect in the relief of myofascial pain. *Pain* 1979;6:83–90.

99. Hong CZ. Lidocaine injection versus dry needling to myofascial trigger point: The importance of the local twitch response. *Am J Phys Med Rehabil* 1994;73:256–263.

100. Chen JT, Chung KC, Hou CR, Kuan TS, Chen SM, Hong CZ. Inhibitory effect of dry needling on the spontaneous electrical activity recorded from myofascial trigger spots of rabbit skeletal muscle. *Am J Phys Med Rehabil* 2001;80:729–735.

101. Dommerholt J. Dry needling in orthopaedic physical therapy practice. *Orthop Phys Ther Pract* 2004;16(3):11–16.

102. Cummings M. Myofascial pain from pectoralis major following trans-axillary surgery. *Acupunct Med* 2003;21:105–107.

103. Cummings M. Referred knee pain treated with electroacupuncture to iliopsoas. *Acupunct Med.* 2003;21:32–35.

104. Ingber RS. Shoulder impingement in tennis/racquetball players treated with subscapularis myofascial treatments. *Arch Phys Med Rehabil* 2000;81:679–682.

105. Ingber RS. Iliopsoas myofascial dysfunction: A treatable cause of "failed" low back syndrome. *Arch Phys Med Rehabil* 1989;70:382–386.

106. Kaye MJ. Evaluation and treatment of a patient with upper quarter myofascial pain syndrome. *J Sports Chiro Rehabil* 2001;15(1):26–33.

107. Gozon B, Chu J, Schwartz I. Lumbosacral radiculopathic pain presenting as groin and scrotal pain: Pain management with twitch-obtaining intramuscular stimulation. A case report and review of literature. *Electromyogr Clin Neurophysiol* 2001;41:315–318.

108. Chu J, Takehara I, Li TC, Schwartz I. Electrical twitch obtaining intramuscular stimulation (ETOIMS) for myofascial pain syndrome in a football player. *Br J Sports Med* 2004;38:E25.

109. Gunn CC, Byrne D, Goldberger M, et al. Treating whiplash-associated disorders with intramuscular stimulation: A retrospective review of 43 patients with long-term follow-up. *J Musculoskel Pain* 2001;9:69–89.

110. Gerwin RD, Dommerholt J. *Trigger Point Needling.* Seminar manual. Bethesda, MD: Janet G. Travell, MD, Seminar Series; 2001.

111. Peuker E, Gronemeyer D. Rare but serious complications of acupuncture: Traumatic lesions. *Acupunct Med* 2001;19:103–108.

112. White A, Hayhoe S, Hart A, Ernst E. Survey of adverse events following acupuncture (SAFA): A prospective study of 32,000 consultations. *Acupunct Med* 2001;19:84–92.

113. MacPherson H, Thomas K, Walters S, Fitter M. A prospective survey of adverse events and treatment reactions following 34,000 consultations with professional acupuncturists. *Acupunct Med* 2001;19:93–102.

114. Walsh B. Control of infection in acupuncture. *Acupunct Med* 2001;19:109–111.

115. Chu J. The local mechanism of acupuncture. *Zhonghua Yi Xue Za Zhi* (*Taipei*). 2002;65:299–302.

116. Chu J, Yuen KF, Wang BH, Chan RC, Schwartz I, Neuhauser D. Electrical twitch-obtaining intramuscular stimulation in lower back pain: A pilot study. *Am J Phys Med Rehabil* 2004;83:104–111.

117. Chu J, Schwartz I. The muscle twitch in myofascial pain relief: Effects of acupuncture and other needling methods. *Electromyogr Clin Neurophysiol* 2002;42:307–311.

118. Chu J. Twitch-obtaining intramuscular stimulation (TOIMS): Long-term observations in the management of chronic partial cervical radiculopathy. *Electromyogr Clin Neurophysiol* 2000;40:503–510.

119. Paris SV, Loubert PV. *Foundations of Clinical Orthopaedics.* St. Augustine, FL: Institute Press; 1999.

120. Johnson GS, Johnson VS. *Functional Orthopedics I: Soft Tissue Mobilization, PNF and Joint Mobilization.* Course manual. Baltimore, MD: The Institute of Physical Art; 2001.

121. Lewit K, Simons DG. Myofascial pain: Relief by post-isometric relaxation. *Arch Phys Med Rehabil* 1984;65:452–456.

122. Mulligan B. *The Mulligan Concept: Spinal and Peripheral Manual Therapy Treatment Techniques.* Course manual. Baltimore, MD: Northeast Seminars; 2000.

123. Mulligan B. *Manual Therapy "NAGS", SNAGS", "MWMS" etc.* 4th ed. Wellington, New Zealand: Plane View Services; 1999.

124. Rocabado M. *CF3—Advanced Cranio-Facial.* Course notes. St. Augustine, FL: University of St. Augustine for Health Sciences; 2002.

125. Kaltenborn FM, Evjenth O, Kaltenborn TB, Morgan D, Vollowitz E, Kaltenborn F. *Manual Mobilization of the Joints: The Spine.* 4th ed. Minneapolis, MN: OPTP; 2003.

126. Rocabado M. *CF2—Intermediate Cranio-Facial.* Course notes. St. Augustine, FL: University of St. Augustine for Health Sciences; 2002.

127. Fernández-de-las-Peñas C, Alonso-Blanco C, Cuadrado ML, Gerwin RD, Pareja JA. Trigger points in the suboccipital muscles and forward head posture in tension-type headache. *Headache* 2006;46:454–460.

128. Jensen R, Rasmussen BK, Pedersen B, Olesen J. Muscle tenderness and pressure pain thresholds in headache: A population study. *Pain* 1993;52:193–199.

129. Ashina M, Bendtsen L, Jensen R, Sakai F, Olesen J. Muscle hardness in patients with chronic tension-type headache: Relation to actual headache state. *Pain* 1999;79(2–3):201–205.

130. Fernández-de-las-Peñas C, Alonso-Blanco C, Cuadrado ML, Pareja JA. Forward head posture and neck mobility in chronic tension-type headache: A blinded, controlled study. *Cephalalgia* 2006;26:314–319.

131. Gerwin RD, Dommerholt J. Treatment of myofascial pain syndromes. In: Weiner RS, Ed. *Pain Management: A Practical Guide for Clinicians,* 6th ed. Boca Raton, FL: CRC Press; 2002:235–249.

132. Fernández-de-las-Peñas C, Cuadrado ML, Pareja JA. Myofascial trigger points, neck mobility and forward head posture in unilateral migraine. *Cephalalgia* 2006;26(9):1061–1070.

133. Millea PJ, Brodie JJ. Tension-type headache. *Am Fam Physician* 2002;66:797–804.

134. Goadsby PJ, Boes C. Chronic daily headache. *J Neurol Neurosurg Psychiatry* 2002;72 (suppl 2):ii2–ii5.

135. Audette JF, Blinder RA. Acupuncture in the management of myofascial pain and headache. *Curr Pain Headache Rep* 2003;7:395–401.

136. Hesse J, Mogelvang B, Simonsen H. Acupuncture versus metoprolol in migraine prophylaxis: A randomized trial of trigger point inactivation. *J Intern Med* 1994;235:451–456.

137. Kamanli A, Kaya A, Ardicoglu O, Ozgocmen S, Zengin FO, Bayik Y. Comparison of lidocaine injection, botulinum toxin injection, and dry needling to trigger points in myofascial pain syndrome. *Rheumatol Int* 2005;25:604–611.

138. Ilbuldu E, Cakmak A, Disci R, Aydin R. Comparison of laser, dry needling, and placebo laser treatments in myofascial pain syndrome. *Photomed Laser Surg* 2004;22:306–311.

139. Furlan AD, van Tulder MW, Cherkin DC, et al. Acupuncture and dry-needling for low back pain. *Cochrane Database Syst Rev* 2005(1):CD001351.

140. Itoh K, Katsumi Y, Kitakoji H. Trigger point acupuncture treatment of chronic low back pain in elderly patients: A blinded RCT. *Acupunct Med* 2004;22:170–177.

141. McMillan AS, Nolan A, Kelly PJ. The efficacy of dry needling and procaine in the treatment of myofascial pain in the jaw muscles. *J Orofac Pain* 1997;11(4):307–314.

142. DiLorenzo L, Traballesi M, Morelli D, et al. Hemiparetic shoulder pain syndrome treated with deep dry needling during early rehabilitation: A prospective, open-label, randomized investigation. *J Musculoskel Pain* 2004;12(2):25–34.

143. Irnich D, Behrens N, Gleditsch JM, et al. Immediate effects of dry needling and acupuncture at distant points in chronic neck pain: Results of a randomized, double-blind, sham-controlled crossover trial. *Pain* 2002;99(1–2):83–89.

144. Chatchawan U, Thinkhamrop B, Kharmwan S, Knowles J, Eungpinichpong W. Effectiveness of traditional Thai massage versus Swedish massage among patients with back pain associated with myofascial trigger points. *J Bodywork Movement Ther* 2005;9:298–309.

145. Fernández-de-las-Peñas C, Blanco CA, Carnero JF, Page JCM. The immediate effect of ischemic compression technique and transverse friction massage on tenderness of active and latent myofascial trigger points: A pilot study. *J Bodywork Movement Ther* 2006;10:3–9.

146. Fryer G, Hodgson L. The effect of manual pressure release on myofascial trigger points in the upper trapezius muscle. *J Bodywork Movement Ther* 2005;9:248–255.

147. Blanco CR, Fernández-de-las-Peñas C, Xumet JEH, Algaba CP, Rabadan MF, Quintana MCLdl. Changes in active mouth opening following a single treatment of latent myofascial trigger points in the masseter muscle involving post-isometric relaxation or strain/counterstrain. *J Bodywork Movement Ther* 2006;10:197–205.
148. Fernández-de-las-Peñas C, Alonso-Blanco C, Cuadrado ML, Miangolarra JC, Barriga FJ, Pareja JA. Are manual therapies effective in reducing pain from tension-type headache? A systematic review. *Clin J Pain* 2006;22:278–285.
149. Tuchin PJ, Pollard H, Bonello R. A randomized controlled trial of chiropractic spinal manipulative therapy for migraine. *J Manipulative Physiol Ther* 2000;23(2):91–95.
150. Gross AR, Kay T, Hondras M, et al. Manual therapy for mechanical neck disorders: A systematic review. *Man Ther* 2002;7:131–149.
151. Hearn A, Rivett DA. Cervical SNAGs: A biomechanical analysis. *Man Ther* 2002;7:71–79.
152. McNeely ML, Armijo Olivo S, Magee DJ. A systematic review of the effectiveness of physical therapy interventions for temporomandibular disorders. *Phys Ther* 2006;86:710–725.
153. Fishbain DA, Cutler R, Cole B, Rosomoff HL, Rosomoff RS. International Headache Society headache diagnostic patterns in pain facility patients. *Clin J Pain* 2001;17:78–93.
154. Hagen K, Einarsen C, Zwart JA, Svebak S, Bovim G. The co-occurrence of headache and musculoskeletal symptoms amongst 51,050 adults in Norway. *Eur J Neurol* 2002;9(5):527–533.
155. Henry P, Dartigues J, Puymirat C, Peytour T, Lucas J. The association of cervicalgia-headaches: An epidemiologic study. *Cephalalgia* 1987;7:189–190.
156. Bartsch T, Goadsby PJ. Stimulation of the greater occipital nerve induces increased central excitability of dural afferent input. *Brain* 2002;125:1496–1509.
157. Bartsch T, Goadsby PJ. The trigeminocervical complex and migraine: Current concepts and synthesis. *Curr Pain Headache Rep* 2003;7:371–376.
158. Bartsch T, Goadsby PJ. Increased responses in trigeminocervical nociceptive neurons to cervical input after stimulation of the dura mater. *Brain* 2003;126:1801–1813.
159. Jull G. Diagnosis of cervicogenic headache. *J Manual Manipulative Ther* 2006;14:136–138.

Part 4

# Future Research Directions

Chapter 10

# Myofascial Pain Syndrome: Unresolved Issues and Future Directions

*Robert D. Gerwin, MD, FAAN*

## Introduction

Myofascial pain syndrome has progressed from the stage of classical clinical descriptions of local trigger point manifestations and referred pain symptoms to sophisticated descriptions of the biochemistry of the trigger point region by way of microdialysis techniques, the imaging of the trigger point taut band by special magnetic resonance imaging techniques, and explorations of the cerebral responses to trigger point activation. This chapter will explore areas of interest where studies are needed to provide critical information on the nature of the myofascial trigger point and its clinical presentations. It is hoped that the discussions in this chapter will help clinicians and researchers alike to formulate plans to study and address some of the issues that are raised. Whereas some of the studies considered in this chapter require sophisticated equipment, many require only an inquisitive mind and the willingness to organize clinical observations and to record them carefully. Of course, even clinical studies that record observations in an organized manner need to be well designed and approved by institutional review or ethical research boards.

## Etiology of Myofascial Trigger Points

### Generation of the Taut Band

The cause of trigger points is a matter of speculation. It appears evident from clinical inspection that a trigger point forms as a latent trigger point first and then becomes tender or not depending on the degree of activation. This sequence of events is assumed because latent trigger points exist without spontaneous pain. Pain is induced in muscle trigger points with physical activity. Trigger point tenderness does not occur except in regions of muscle hardness, but regions of muscle hardness occur without local or referred pain. It is concluded that muscle hardness or the taut band that occurs in the absence of pain is the first abnormality, and that the active trigger point is a more developed or secondary stage of the trigger point. However, this sequence of events, as simple as it is, has not been systematically studied and confirmed. *One study that needs to be done is the study of the relationship of the latent to active trigger point, or put another way, the study of the activation of trigger points.*

## Role of the Neuromuscular Junction in Trigger Point Formation

Trigger point pain does not occur in the absence of a taut band, as stated above. The mechanism of local and referred pain is well understood as a general phenomenon, based on the release of local neurotransmitters, hydrogen ions, potassium ions and cytokines peripherally, and the activation of nociceptive neurons in the dorsal horn centrally. The spread of nociceptive neuronal activation segmentally is also a well-described phenomenon, regardless of the tissue of pain origin. However, the underlying, initial change in muscle associated with the trigger point seems to be a motor phenomenon, the development of the taut band. How the taut band develops remains a matter of speculation and has not been proven. Simons' integrated hypothesis of the trigger point,[1] expanded on by Gerwin, Dommerholt, and Shah[2] and further elaborated on by Gerwin,[3] suggests that an excess of acetylcholine at the motor endplate, modulated by adrenergic facilitation or inhibition of neurotransmitter release, inhibition of acetylcholine esterase, and other modulating factors, such as adenosine concentration and feedback control of neurotransmitter release related to the frequency of endplate discharge, results in the development of localized muscle contraction. This is supported by the initial observations by Hubbard and Berkoff[4] of spontaneous low-amplitude electrical activity at the trigger point site, later called "endplate noise" by Simons. This activity is modulated by an α-adrenergic blocking agent[5] and by botulinum toxin,[6] indicating that it is related to acetylcholine release and is subject to sympathetic nervous system influences. Gerwin[3] has added the further consideration of a postsynaptic muscle dysfunction that increases intracellular calcium concentration through a leaky ryanodine receptor calcium channel on the sarcoplasmic reticulum membrane or through adrenergic-mediated second-messenger systems involving protein kinase C and cyclic-AMP, initiating actin–myosin interaction leading to muscle fibril contraction. McPartland and Simons[7] raised similar considerations in discussing possible molecular mechanisms of trigger point formation. Mense and Simons[8] have explored inhibition of acetylcholinesterase as a mechanism, but the results did not represent what is thought to occur at trigger points. *Thus, the biochemical mechanism for the establishment and maintenance of the persistent taut band or localized muscle hardness remains to be elucidated.*

## Peripheral Nerve Alterations in Myofascial Pain Syndrome

Peripheral nerve sensitization is well recognized in chronic pain syndromes. It has not been addressed in myofascial pain syndromes, where emphasis has been placed more on changes in muscle than in nerve. Nevertheless, it would seem reasonable that peripheral nerve sensitization would be a consequence of chronic myofascial pain just as it would in other chronic pain syndromes. Some manifestations of the myofascial trigger point are clearly related to a spinal reflex, such as the local twitch reflex.[9] Further studies have suggested that there is a central integration at the spinal cord level in animal trigger point models.[10] The role of the peripheral nerve at the neuromuscular junction and its relationship to anterior horn cell function, however, have been little studied.

A study of neuromuscular jitter by stimulated single fiber electromyography showed a significantly increased mean consecutive difference (jitter) in the trapezius and levator scapulae muscles in subjects with myofascial pain syndrome compared to controls.[11] This study demonstrated instability of peripheral endplate function that could be related to (1) peripheral motor nerve axonal degeneration and regeneration, or (2) motor neuron degeneration with development of collateral reinnervation. The implication is that the myofascial trigger point is a complex dysfunction with peripheral and/or central motor dysfunction as well as a sensory abnormality with peripheral and/or central hypersensitization. *Peripheral sensory nerve sensitization and peripheral motor nerve and anterior horn functional alterations in myofascial pain have not been widely studied. More research is needed on this aspect of myofascial trigger point generation, maintenance, and dysfunction.*

## Muscle Stress and Overuse

The general proposition is widely accepted that muscle overuse or biomechanical stress is the cause of the trigger point, resulting in the dysfunctional neuromuscular junction. This concept is central to Simons' integrated hypothesis of the trigger point and is expressed by Simons et al[1] as an energy crisis that they think is the primary cause of trigger point phenomena. Many studies show that supramaximal muscle contraction or overloaded eccentric contraction can damage muscle and lead to pain, including delayed-onset muscle soreness. Repetitive strain is considered a variant of muscle overload and is thought to have the same effect. Maintenance of fixed positions for long periods of time and sustained contraction of muscle as a result of emotional stress (anxiety, fear, depression) are also thought to produce muscle overuse. No studies, however, have shown that these phenomena actually lead to the development of the trigger point, although we have postulated that to be the case.[2] *Studies are needed, therefore, that investigate the kinds of muscle activity that lead to the development of the trigger point, particularly of the taut or contracted muscle band.*

Sustained low-level muscle contraction, in contrast to supramaximal contraction, has been implicated in the development of trigger points. The concept is that the earliest recruited and last deactivated motor units are overworked, particularly during prolonged tasks. This concept is supported by studies of ergonomic stress,[12,13] and well summarized by Dommerholt et al.[14]

Postural stresses are another form of mechanical muscle stress that has been related to myofascial trigger point formation and activation. Spondylosis with joint hypomobility results in a kind of postural dysfunction that is associated with neck, trunk, and low back pain. Myofascial trigger points are seen in these conditions, but there are few studies that specifically show such an association. The prevalence of myofascial trigger points in the upper trapezius, sternocleidomastoid (SCM), and levator scapular muscles in mid-cervical spine hypomobility was examined in a pilot study by Fernández-de-las-Peñas et al,[15] but the association of trigger point presence with hypomobility did not reach statistical significance. This study limited the trigger point evaluation to the region of the scapular insertion of the levator scapulae and to the vertical fibers of the trapezius muscle in the neck, in addition to the SCM. *A more expanded survey of cervical musculature looking at semispinalis and splenius capitis and cervicis, and suboccipital muscles, as well as the cervical fibers of the levator scapulae and the upper shoulder component of the trapezius muscle, might show such an association.* In fact, a previous study by the same primary investigator showed a statistically significant relationship between trigger points in the upper fibers of the trapezius muscle and C3–C4 hypomobility.[16] *Similar studies are relevant to mid-thoracic and lumbar spine regions as well, and indeed are relevant to joint hypomobility in general, including frozen shoulder and hip and knee osteoarthritis with hypomobility.*

## Weakness

Muscles harboring a trigger point are often weak, without atrophy.[1] The weakness is usually rapidly reversible immediately on inactivation of the trigger point. One postulated mechanism is the limiting of muscle contraction below the threshold that activates painful triggers. However, inhibition of effort or contractile force in one muscle is known to be the result of a trigger point in a different muscle, indicating some type of central inhibition of muscle activity. *Studies are needed to identify the central inhibitory and peripheral mechanisms that lead to trigger-point-induced, rapidly reversible weakness.*

## Hypoxia and Ischemia

The myofascial trigger zone or region is thought to be hypoxic, consistent with the concept that there is capillary compression and ischemia. Ischemia and hypoxia, in this construct, are inevitably connected. One study of tissue oxygen tension recorded temperatures in tender, tense indurations. There was a region of severe oxygen desaturation at the presumed core of induration, surrounded by a region of increased oxygenation, as if the core were ischemic and surrounded by a hyperemic zone.[17] Likewise, Travell[18] reported temperature studies of the trigger zone as early as 1954, showing an increase in temperature in the trigger point region. This would be consistent with a hyperemic area surrounding the trigger zone, but inconsistent with a hypoxic trigger zone core. Infrared studies of the skin overlying muscles affected by trigger points were done in the 1980s and 1990s, with varying results,[19,20] but address only the peri-trigger point tissue, and not the core of the trigger point itself. *Studies of the core of the trigger point of oxygen tension and of temperature would address the issue as to whether the trigger point is ischemic/hypoxic or not.*

## Biochemistry of the Trigger Point Region

Biochemical changes in the area of the trigger point have been identified by Shah et al[21,22] through studies of the trigger point region by microdialysis. Elevations of substance P, calcitonin gene-related peptide (CGRP), bradykinin, serotonin, and cytokines were found in active trigger point sites relative to the concentrations of these substances in latent trigger point regions and in normal muscle.[21] The pH of the trigger point region is low (between 4–5) compared to a pH of 7.4 seen normally. Further studies showed that the concentrations of these substances are also elevated at the active trigger point region compared to a distant muscle site, but that the concentrations of these substances are elevated at a distant site in subjects with active trigger points compared to subjects with latent or absent trigger points.[22] *This is a preliminary study that looked at only one distant site, but it raises the question about a possible systemic effect of chronic pain. Is the elevation of concentrations of these substances at sites distant to painful areas a general phenomenon or one unique to myofascial trigger points? Does this represent an acute or a chronic change? Do these changes reflect peripheral sensitization? There needs to be more work done by this ingenious technique looking at a wider selection of distant muscles and a variety of painful conditions.*

## Central Sensitization

So far the discussion has focused on the peripheral phenomena associated with the trigger point. The central connections of the trigger point are of interest because trigger point tenderness is most certainly associated with central sensitization and hypersensitivity, just as is the case with other tissues. The mechanisms of central sensitization and expansion of dorsal horn reference zones in acute muscle pain have been extensively studied by Mense.[23] One study of the central responses of trigger point pain did not show a difference in the numbers of neurons in the dorsal horn associated with trigger spots compared to controls.[10] Central sensitization has been extensively studied in fibromyalgia and other chronic pain states. It has been much less studied in myofascial pain syndromes. *The spread of central activity and signs of sensitization and development of hypersensitivity need to be examined in myofascial pain syndrome as it has been in other chronic pain states.* Another aspect of central responses to myofascial pain syndromes is the cerebral response to stimulation of myofascial trigger point. Painful stimulation of the trigger point results in activation of the cerebral cortex pain network in the primary and secondary somatosensory cortex, the inferior parietal lobe, and the link to the emotional (affective) cortex, the insula.[24,25]

## Referred Pain

Referred pain is a manifestation of central spread of pain perception via the spinal cord. Explanations for this include convergence of afferent nociceptive fibers on single sensory neurons and segmental spread of dorsal horn neuron activation through activation of ineffective synaptic connections centrally.[26] Referred pain patterns seen clinically continue to be identified and refined.[27, 28] New referred pain patterns have been described for headache.[29] *Further delineation of referral patterns from muscle continue to be made and are a helpful addition to our understanding of clinical pain syndromes. Areas of special interest include head referral patterns as related to headache and to trigeminal neuralgia, and to pelvic pain referral patterns that are insufficiently described. Careful clinical reports as well as experimental studies of pain referral patterns are both useful.*

# Epidemiology of Myofascial Pain

## Prevalence Studies

Studies on the epidemiology of myofascial pain syndrome are hampered by the lack of consensus about the criteria used to diagnosis the condition. This problem is addressed in the next section, "Diagnosis of Myofascial Pain Syndrome."

There are no prevalence studies of myofascial pain syndrome per se in the general population. One Canadian study showed 20% prevalence for musculoskeletal pain in a general population.[30] Pain complaints were found in 32% of a university primary care general internal medicine practice series of 172 patients, of which 30% were found to have myofascial pain (9% of the persons in the series).[31] Myofascial pain syndrome was diagnosed in 85% of persons evaluated in a pain rehabilitation referral center.[32] In a pain treatment referral program known for its interest in myofascial pain, within a larger neurological practice, 93% of persons with musculoskeletal pain had myofascial trigger points.[33]

Most other studies of the prevalence of myofascial pain syndrome have been confined to special populations. Myofascial pain syndrome (MPS) was detected in 61% of a series of 41 subjects with complex regional pain syndrome.[34] A study of 243 female sewing machine operators showed a prevalence of MPS of 15.2% in neck and shoulder muscles compared to 9.0% among 357 women serving as controls.[35] Single mothers, smokers, and those with perceived low support from colleagues and supervisors were at a higher risk for developing neck and shoulder pain.

## Gender Differences

Gender-related differences are known to exist in a variety of painful conditions, including migraine headache, fibromyalgia, interstitial cystitis, and irritable bowel syndrome. Differential responses based on gender are known to occur in musculoskeletal pain[36] and are represented in increased days of absence from work and greater expenditures for health care for women than men.[37] Occupational neck and shoulder pain is more common in women than in men.[38] Pressure pain thresholds are also lower for women. Injection of hypertonic saline in bilateral trapezius muscles, to simulate the real-life bilateral shoulder pain commonly experienced in certain work situations, resulted in greater pain inhibition in men than women 7.5 and 15 minutes after injection.[39] Baseline pain pressure threshold was lower in women, but the increase in pain pressure threshold (PPT) after a second injection of hypertonic saline was much greater in men than in women. The greater increase in PPT in men represents an increased hypoalgesia or increased nociceptive inhibition that is likely to be central. Glutamate-evoked muscle pain is also greater in women, whereas hypertonic saline-evoked pain is not, and glutamate-evoked afferent discharges are greater in female rats than males, suggesting that the effect is mediated peripherally.[40,41] One explanation is that there is an increased central sensitization in women, but another is that descending inhibition is weaker in females than in males. The exact mechanism(s) remains to be identified. A role for estrogen in the development of hypersensitization has been considered.[42] Nevertheless, one study of sex differences in recalled and experimentally induced muscle pain showed no difference between male and female subjects.[43] Estrogen facilitates the activation of the NMDA receptor in the rat,[44] offering one explanation of mechanism.

*Gender studies of myofascial pain are lacking, except by secondary inference. Direct evaluation of gender relationships to myofascial trigger point pain is needed. Mechanisms of gender differences in pain perception may then be evaluated in populations of males and females with myofascial pain syndrome.*

## Hypermobility

Hypermobility seems to be a relevant risk factor for the development of myofascial pain syndromes.[45] It has been considered to be a risk factor for the development of trigger points. The mechanism is thought to be the need for muscle to provide the support that ligaments ordinarily provide. Those persons with recurrent large joint dislocations or subluxation seem to be at an even higher risk for the development of trigger points.

*Studies of the prevalence of myofascial pain syndrome in the general population and as a comorbid condition associated with other conditions such as Lyme disease or hypermobility are needed. The role of female gender as a predisposing factor needs to be clarified and explained.*

## Diagnosis of Myofascial Pain Syndrome

The diagnosis of myofascial trigger points has long been controversial in the medical profession, because there had been no laboratory or imaging technique that was capable of confirming the clinical diagnosis. Diagnosis had been possible only by clinical history and examination, very similar to migraine and tension-type headache in that regard. Nevertheless, the literature was critical of the ability to make a diagnosis of myofascial trigger point pain until quite recently. Part of the problem was undoubtedly the failure to understand the nature of referred pain, an issue put to rest with the advances in the understanding of pain neurophysiology. Several attempts to demonstrate the clinical efficacy of physical examination failed to do so. It was only in 1997 that the first paper to establish interrater reliability in trigger point identification was published.[46] The most reliable findings in that study were localized tenderness, presence of a taut band, and pain recognition. Others have since confirmed the efficacy of physical examination in detecting myofascial trigger points. Interrater reliability to a precision of a square centimeter or so within a single muscle, indicating that examiners could independently identify the same taut band region, has been demonstrated.[47] Assessment of interrater reliability in the detection of trigger points continues to a topic of interest. A recent study looked at interrater reliability of palpation of myofascial trigger points in shoulder muscles.[48] They found that referred pain and the "jump sign" had the greatest degree of agreement among the blinded examiners. Identification of a nodule in a taut band and eliciting a twitch response had the two lowest degrees of agreement. Recognition of usual pain was not evaluated in that study. Degree of agreement among examiners varied with the muscle study, and even within different areas of a single muscle. The kappa coefficient (κ) for agreement on identifying a palpable nodule within a taut band varied from 0.11–0.75 (percentage of agreement varying from 45–90%). In clinical practice, feedback from patients allows assessment of reproducing clinically relevant pain elicited by palpation. Studies relating the presence of trigger points to treatment outcome (find a trigger point → inactivate the trigger point → measure the outcome) have not been done with the aim of delineating the criteria for trigger point identification or for reliability of the examination (e.g., multiple examiners identify a trigger point, it is treated, pain goes away) except in a preliminary report. Trigger points identified only by finding tenderness in a taut band showed a significantly greater increase in pain pressure threshold after treatment with either trigger point injection, dry needling, or manual compression than non-treated control sites.[49] *There continues to be a need to develop an objective, laboratory diagnostic procedure that would definitively identify the trigger point and relate the criteria to the elimination of trigger point pain. This would be highly useful for research studies, if not for day-to-day clinical practice.*

A review of the criteria used to diagnose trigger points concluded that there was limited consensus on case definition of trigger point syndrome.[50] Specifically, the authors noted that there has not been a consensus on the criteria for the definition of trigger point syndrome, despite the majority of authors citing Simons, Travell, and Simons[1] as the authoritative source for such criteria. For example, of 57 papers citing Simons, Travell, and Simons[1] as the source for the criteria defining MPS, the authors found that only 12 papers used the criteria correctly. The authors also noted that 30 papers that used algometry cited Fischer[51,52] as the authority for defining MTrP criteria, but that only one applied the criteria as described by Fischer. Over half of the studies used the criteria: (1) tender spot in a taut band of skeletal muscle and (2) recognition of usual pain or predicted pain referral pattern. The authors suggested that claims for effective interventions in treating myofascial pain syndrome should be viewed with caution until there are better validated criteria for case definition.

The development of criteria for the diagnosis of MPS was the object of an attempt initiated at the 1998 International Myopain Congress in Italy. A multicenter study was developed, but in the end only two centers completed the study. A merged data evaluation of the 80 subjects in the study showed that local tenderness, referred pain, and a palpable taut band were useful. However, agreement on diagnosis for both centers was weak (κ = 0.32).[53]

There has been no attempt to validate the clinical criteria with any objective criteria such as electromyographic evidence of endplate noise[54] or the biochemical changes identified with active myofascial trigger points, as reported by Shah et al.[21] *Validation of clinical diagnosis by palpation with these or other objective tests such as magnetic resonance elastography would help establish the reliability of the clinical examination, not as interrater reliability, but in terms of the reliability of the physical examination to identify those patients whose myofascial trigger point pain is verifiable by other means. Current laboratory studies that show abnormalities would have to be validated themselves by showing that they independently identify trigger points that can be treated resulting in pain relief and improved function.* Lucas et al[55] have done this with latent trigger points in the shoulder, by demonstrating that latent trigger points cause disordered sequencing of muscle recruitment for arm abduction, then showing the restoration of normal recruitment after treatment. *That kind of study can include identification of trigger points by a particular set of criteria, validate the identification by showing a specific impairment, and then restoring function by treating the identified trigger point.*

Skin resistance has been evaluated as a means of distinguishing myofascial trigger points in a superficial muscle from normal muscle tissue. Trigger points, whether active or latent, cause decreased skin resistance that can be used for identification, at least in a superficial muscle.[56] *The specificity of this skin resistance to myofascial trigger points needs to be established.*

Magnetic resonance elastography may emerge as an effective tool to identify the trigger point taut band. The technique involves the introduction of cyclic waves into the muscle and then using phase contrast imaging to identify tissue distortions. The speed of the waves is determined from the images. Shear waves travel more rapidly in stiffer tissues. The harder taut band can thus be distinguished from the surrounding normal muscle.[57,58]

*There remains a need to develop a consensus on the clinical features required to diagnose myofascial trigger points. There is also a need to develop objective laboratory criteria that can be used to standardize the diagnosis of MPS for research studies. These may also have clinical value if they can be used to confirm an examination made by physical examination. Elastography needs to be studied in a variety of trigger point pain syndromes.*

Another diagnostic issue has to do with the relative responsiveness of musculoskeletal tissues. Pain can arise from the junction of bone and tendon, from tendon alone, and from muscle, or from a combination of any of these components. Hypertonic saline and mechanical stimulation at all three sites showed greater pain to injection of the proximal tendon–bone junction and tendon than muscle, referred pain predominantly from tendon and bone–tendon junction stimulation, indicating that proximal bone–tendon junction and tendon are more sensitive and susceptible to sensitization by hypertonic saline,[59] although pain during eccentric loading was greater in the muscle belly.[60] These studies suggest that pain from tendon and bone–tendon junctions must be considered among the sources of musculoskeletal pain in addition to muscle. *Studies of myofascial pain and musculoskeletal pain in general should consider the possibility that local and referred pain can have a contribution from tendon and tendon–bone junction. Simons has alluded to enthesopathy as a source of pain, but this concept is often overlooked both in studies and in treatment.*

## Treatment Issues

Treatment of trigger point pain syndromes involves the relief of pain by inactivating the myofascial trigger point and then restoring normal biomechanics to the extent possible. Finally, those factors that initiated and maintained the pain syndrome need to be identified and corrected. There are unanswered questions associated with each of these stages of treatment. Trigger point inactivation can be accomplished by either noninvasive or invasive means (needling or injecting the trigger point). Prophylaxis or prevention of trigger point recurrence can also be accomplished by invasive and by noninvasive means.

## Manual Inactivation of Trigger Points

Manual inactivation of trigger points has been reviewed by Fernández-de-las-Peñas et al.[61] They found few randomized, controlled studies of the effectiveness of manual therapy in trigger point inactivation. The techniques used included trigger point compression, spray and stretch, strain/counterstrain, ultrasound, and various forms of muscle stretching. They noted that a limiting factor in assessing manual treatment techniques was the lack of uniform outcome measures. Most studies, but not all, used pressure pain threshold or an 11-point Likert numerical or visual pain scale. However, some studies used the McGill Short Form Pain Questionnaire or Quality of Life assessments. Range of motion has also been used as an outcome measurement of effectiveness of treatment. Moreover, some trials evaluate just one type of manual therapy and others evaluated a combination of manual therapies. The conclusion of these authors was that there was no rigorous evidence that the manual techniques studied have better outcome beyond placebo. The role of manual therapies was neither supported nor refuted by the results of their study. Rickards[62] looked at some manual interventions, but only two of the studies included in the review used typical manual treatments of trigger points used by trained physical therapists (ischemic compression). These two studies had short-term (immediate) benefit but no long-term follow-up. One of the two studies looked at a combination of heat, range-of-motion exercises, interferential current, and myofascial release. The other study looked at ischemic compression. *Clearly, more research is required on the efficacy of manual techniques in treatment of myofascial pain and some uniformity in selecting outcome measures would make cross-comparison of studies more feasible.*

The mechanism of pain reduction and softening of the taut band by manual therapy remains speculative. The effectiveness of a most commonly used manual technique of trigger point inactivation, trigger point compression, has been infrequently studied. A novel approach to evaluating the effectiveness of this approach utilized a digital algometer, demonstrating a benefit of manual compression with pain reduction and an increase in pain pressure threshold.[63] *Further controlled studies of the effectiveness of manual therapy techniques are warranted. Moreover, the mechanisms whereby the effects are mediated remain to be elucidated.*

## Noninvasive, Nonmanual Treatment Techniques

Treatments in this category include all forms of electrical stimulation, ultrasound, laser, and magnet therapies. One systematic review of the literature[62] reported that there is evidence to support the immediate benefit of transcutaneous electrical stimulation (TENS), but there is insufficient data to address long-term benefit. Conventional ultrasound was not more effective than placebo in neck and upper back pain based on the limited data available (one high-quality and two lower-quality studies). One recent study, nonblinded, showed a short-term improvement in pain pressure threshold with ultrasound.[64] In a follow-up study, Srbely et al[65] demonstrated that low-dose ultrasound can evoke short-term segmental antinociceptive effects on trigger points. Preliminary evidence supported the use of magnetic therapy, but data is very limited and studies were of only moderate quality.[62]

Another noninvasive approach to the inactivation of myofascial trigger points that has created much interest is the use of low-level laser. There have been mixed results in the studies that have been randomized, controlled, and blinded. Earlier studies have shown benefit,[66,67] but a more recent study showed no benefit.[68] *Consequently, this treatment modality, already increasing in use, needs to be further studied to determine its place in the treatment of myofascial pain syndromes.*

## Invasive Treatment of Myofascial Trigger Points

Invasive myofascial trigger point treatment is generally done by either dry needling or injection of substances. Deep dry needling was considered to be effective in some studies,[69] particularly in the management of myofascial pain syndromes. A recent Cochrane review concluded that dry needling might be an effective option in the treatment of persons with chronic low back pain.[70] One study showed that lidocaine diluted to 0.25% was the most effective concentration associated with the least postinjection soreness.[71] Substances other than lidocaine have been used for injection, most commonly some form of corticosteroid. Cummings and White[72] reviewed 23 papers and found the effect of needling was independent of the material injected. Moreover, there were no trials of sufficient quality or design to test the efficacy of any needling technique over placebo. Their conclusion was that direct needling of trigger points appears effective, that in three trials there was no difference between dry needling and injection, and that controlled trials are needed to determine if trigger point injections are more effective than placebo. An updated review found 15 randomized, controlled studies that met their inclusion criteria.[73] However, the small sample size, deficiencies in reporting, and heterogeneity of the studies precluded a definitive synthesis of the data. A review of acupuncture and trigger point dry needling came to much the same conclusion, that there is a paucity of studies that precludes making a definitive statement about the benefit of these techniques.[74] Trigger point injection (TPI) appeared to relieve symptoms when it was the sole treatment for whiplash syndrome, and for chronic neck, shoulder, and back pain. However, the authors concluded that there is no clear evidence that TPI is ineffective or beneficial, but that it is a safe procedure in experienced hands. No evidence supports or negates the use of any injectate over dry needling.

There is one study that compares TPI with lidocaine with intramuscular stimulation using acupuncture needles (dry needling).[75] Dry needling currently is most commonly done with acupuncture needles, so that this study is consistent with current clinical practice. The study demonstrated the effectiveness of both techniques in providing pain relief, better relief of depression with dry needling (!), and improvement in passive range of motion with both treatments. Post-treatment soreness was the same in both groups. Local twitch responses were elicited in 97.7% of subjects treated. An additional study by the same group evaluated peripheral dry needling without and with the addition of dry needling multifidi muscles (paraspinal dry needling) in the neck.[76] Although the addition of needling multifidi gave a small statistical advantage, both techniques were effective in relieving pain at 1 month. *Better studies are needed to settle the question of use of various injectates and of dry needling compared to trigger point injection, adequately powered, with common outcome measures, of both TPI and dry needling used as sole therapies and given in combination with other physical therapy approaches.* There is, however, a major difficulty in finding appropriate placebo or sham treatments in controlled studies. Many placebo treatments of myofascial trigger points are active, not inactive, placebos.

Acupuncture trigger point needling is a term used to describe inserting the acupuncture needle into a muscle trigger point. It has been used to treat myofascial trigger points in a manner identical to the dry needling technique described by physical therapists, physicians, and others. It has been shown to be effective in treating chronic neck pain[77] and chronic low back pain.[78,79] Blinding using sham needles was effective in these two studies. These studies further support the effectiveness of dry needling in treating myofascial pain syndromes. However, a recent systematic review of acupuncture and dry needling (deep needling techniques) concluded that there was only limited evidence from one study that deep dry needling was beneficial compared with standardized care.[74] Some studies were criticized because trigger points were not convincingly the sole cause of pain, although in clinical practice that is often the case. Treatment techniques (depth of insertion of the needle, location of needle placement, duration of needle insertion) varied, and cotreatment varied, all of which reduced the comparability of studies. *There is an additional need to develop a reliable way to assess needling technique effectiveness in myofascial trigger point pain syndromes. The clinical effectiveness of deep dry needling without injectate needs to be firmly established with additional credible studies, as well. Classical acupuncture needs to be better evaluated in trigger point treatment as well as deep dry needling.*

An interesting study looked at the effect of dry needling key trigger points on satellite trigger point activity.[80] In this single-blinded, randomized, controlled trial, inactivation of infraspinatus trigger points had a beneficial effect on trigger point manifestations (pain intensity and pressure pain threshold) in ipsilateral, proximal, and distal upper extremity muscles. This study suggests that there is a central modulating effect of dry needling inactivation of myofascial trigger points. *More studies of the peripheral and central effects of dry needling are needed to further elucidate the clinical effects and mechanism of action of this technique.*

The mechanism of action of trigger point needling has never been adequately elucidated. The results of dry needling seem to be about as effective as injection of local anesthetic, suggesting that local anesthetic is not absolutely necessary. Thus, it seems that it is the mechanical action of the needle itself that inactivates the trigger point. The mechanical stimulation of the trigger point by the needle causes a change in the substances that have been shown to be elevated in the trigger point region.[21] Some consideration has been given to disruption of the muscle cell wall by the needle, causing alterations of calcium influx into the cytoplasm. This mechanism does not seem credible, as disruption of the cell wall on a macroscopic basis would seem to result in major cellular functional disruption. A paper by Fine et al[81] in which well-documented trigger point inactivation associated with the injection of bupivicaine was significantly reversed with intravenous naloxone (10 mg) strongly suggests that endogenous opioids are involved in the needle-induced relief of pain and in the reversal of the physical manifestations of the trigger point. There have been no follow-up studies of this phenomenon. Moreover, there have been no studies of the effect of naloxone on the manual inactivation of the trigger point. *The mechanism of action of inactivation of trigger-point-related pain and taut band formation needs further investigation, including investigation of the role of endorphins in mediating the clinical response.*

Botulinum toxin has been used to inactivate trigger points. Theoretically, botulinum toxin should act like a long-lasting trigger point injection if it acts to prevent the development of the trigger point or inactivates it. One study showed that it reduced or blocked endplate noise at the trigger zone in the rabbit.[6] A number of randomized, controlled, double blind studies have been conducted, but many were small studies or did not utilize appropriate criteria for identification of trigger points. In addition, variable amounts of toxin have been used in the studies, lack of documentation of injecting precisely at the trigger zone, and lack of attention to treat the entire relevant functional muscle unit may have contributed to the inability to show efficacy.[82] *Studies of the effect of botulinum toxin inactivation of myofascial trigger points should meticulously use proper diagnostic criteria for identification of relevant active trigger points, take into consideration the effect of latent trigger points and treat them, and consider treatment of relevant trigger points in the entire functional muscle unit.*

Some new, interesting substances used for trigger point injection are presently being explored, such as bee venom and tropisetron.[83-85] Tropisetron is a 5HT3 antagonist that has been shown to alleviate pain in myofascial trigger point pain syndromes. It also has a more widespread analgesic effect. It may be the first specific injectate shown to have a positive benefit in the treatment of myofascial trigger point pain syndromes. *Tropisetron should be studied in more myofascial pain situations than low back pain, where it has been found to be effective.*

Baldry's technique of superficial dry needling has never been subjected to adequate study.[86] Baldry[86] proposed that this technique is effective and less invasive than inserting needles into muscle and avoids the potential complications of pneumothorax and other complications of deep needling. *Superficial dry needling as a treatment for myofascial trigger point pain needs to be properly studied for its underlying mechanisms and effectiveness, and compared to other treatment techniques.*

## Selected Specific Clinical Syndromes

### Headache

The role of myofascial trigger points in the generation of headache has recently been intensively studied.[87,88] The general concept put forth by these series of papers is that chronic tension-type headache is at least partly explained by referred pain emanating from trigger points in the head, neck, and shoulder muscles. Trigger points are considered to be responsible for the development of the central sensitization that initiates referred pain and headache. Trigger points in the trochlear region have been identified in unilateral migraine headache.[89] Forward-head postural dysfunction is associated with suboccipital muscle trigger points and chronic tension type headache.[90] Key to the concept that trigger points contribute to the development of headache is the finding that treatment of relevant trigger points results in reduction or elimination of headache. This has been shown in one elegant study by Giamberadino et al[91] in which inactivation of trigger points that referred pain to the headache areas resulted in reduction of headache frequency and intensity and a reduction in electrical pain thresholds. Another study, open labeled, showed that inactivation of trigger points in the head and neck by the injection of the long-acting local anesthetic ropivacaine decreased migraine headache frequency by more than 11% in more than 50% of subjects, and produced more than a 50% reduction in headache frequency in 17% subjects.[92] This study was problematic in that the authors talked about subcutaneous injection of trigger points and not intramuscular injections. Moreover, there was no mention of postinjection assessment of the treated trigger points to evaluate the effectiveness of the injections. *More studies are needed that study the inactivation of trigger points that refer pain to headache areas and/or cause scalp allodynia in a variety of headache types such as chronic tension-type headache, episodic tension-type headache, and chronic daily headache with either tension-type or migraine headache to see if such inactivation will reduce headache frequency and intensity and reduce associated scalp allodynia.*

## Fibromyalgia

There has long been a discussion about the relationship between myofascial pain and fibromyalgia, including whether myofascial pain evolves into fibromyalgia ("regional" pain evolving into "generalized" pain). Fibromyalgia is characterized by widespread musculoskeletal tenderness. Tender points theoretically are not associated with taut bands. However, myofascial trigger points are also tender, and many clinicians do not make a distinction between taut bands and trigger points. A preliminary report of 96 subjects evaluated for fibromyalgia and myofascial pain syndrome found 25 subjects who fulfilled the criteria for fibromyalgia.[33] Of these, 18 (72%) had trigger points as well as tender points. Central hypersensitization is considered to be the basis of fibromyalgia.[93] It is also likely to be implicated in the etiology of myofascial pain syndrome. There is interest, therefore, in whether persons with fibromyalgia have myofascial trigger points that account for the pain of fibromyalgia. *A study of fibromyalgia subjects for symptomatic myofascial trigger points would therefore be of interest.*

## Endometriosis and Other Pelvic Viscerosomatic Pain Syndromes

A serious pelvic pain problem is endometriosis, where recurrent abdominal pain is a common manifestation. Endometriosis is often treated by laparoscopic surgery when hormonal control is not effective to identify endometrial implants and remove them and to lyse adhesions. However, because abdominal pain usually recurs, laparoscopic surgical procedures tend to be repeated. Surgical excision of endometrial implants did not result in an improvement of 1-year outcome compared to sham surgery.[94] Jarrell and colleagues[94-96] explored the relationship of myofascial trigger points to visceral and pelvic pain syndromes, concluding that the cause of pain may not be the endometriosis itself, but rather abdominal wall trigger points that may represent pain referral from the affected viscera or even may reflect the development of trigger points from the surgical procedure itself. Jarrell[95] and Nazareno et al[97] found that treating abdominal trigger points alleviated the visceral pain syndromes. However, Nazareno et al did not define myofascial trigger points; it is not clear what criteria they used to direct the choice of injection site in the abdominal wall other than tenderness. They reported an 89% partial or complete relief of pain in both the short and long term, with no apparent greater benefit following the addition of corticosteroids to the injection mixture.

Another study examined the results of treatment of abdominal pain with point tenderness following surgery or diagnosis with abdominal adhesions, pelvic inflammatory disease, or nerve entrapment.[98] Treatment was by injection of local anesthetic and corticosteroids into trigger points. Again, this paper did not define how trigger points were defined or localized. The authors reported 95% of 140 treated patients were either pain free or had only mild pain after treatment, and that the benefit was sustained for 3 months: 86.5% retained the benefit.

Treatment of pelvic pain associated with interstitial cystitis responded to pelvic floor muscle trigger point treatment in a report of a small case series.[99] Pelvic floor pain syndromes and pelvic visceral pain syndromes such as noninfectious prostatitis, levator ani syndrome, irritable bowel syndrome, and interstitial cystitis commonly have pelvic floor and abdominal wall trigger points relevant to the complaint of pain, but are poorly understood.[100] *More needs to be done to define the myofascial contributions to viscerosomatic pain syndromes and to outline examination procedures and treatment protocols for these conditions.*

## Whiplash

Myofascial trigger points have been implicated in the mechanism of neck and shoulder pain in whiplash-associated disorders.[101] A review of manual treatment of following whiplash injury reported the common occurrence of trigger points in this condition, a finding also noted by others.[102] *Trigger point release techniques have been advocated as part of the treatment protocol in this condition, but the effectiveness of such treatment needs to be supported by careful clinical studies.*

## Radiculopathy

Myofascial trigger point pain may be the presenting symptom and the only sign of cervical or lumbar radiculopathy in some patients in this author's clinical practice. This phenomenon has not been well described in the literature, but certainly opens the question of the relationship of root compression and the development of trigger points and of the nature of at least a component of pain in radicular syndromes. A study of 191 subjects evaluated for suspected cervical radiculopathy were evaluated for myofascial pain syndrome as well as for other conditions.[103] Electrodiagnostic testing identified cervical radiculopathy in 52% of subjects and other neurological syndromes (plexopathy, peripheral nerve entrapments, or polyneuropathy) in 25%. Myofascial pain syndrome was found in 53% of persons with normal electrodiagnostic testing and also in 17% of patients with electrodiagnostic evidence of radiculopathy and 19% of those with other nerve diagnoses. Although diagnostic criteria for the identification of myofascial trigger point pain were not well defined in this study, the authors nevertheless highlight both the possibility that myofascial pain syndromes may mimic cervical radiculopathy and that it may be a symptomatic comorbidity of cervical radiculopathy. Moreover, this author has found that many patients with postlaminectomy pain syndromes have myofascial trigger point pain syndromes rather than recurrent disc herniation or scar formation. These findings have not been explored either in the literature. *The presence of myofascial pain syndrome as a presenting or complicating feature of radiculopathy, and the role of nerve root or peripheral nerve injury in the generation of myofascial trigger points, deserves greater attention and evaluation.*

## Conclusion

Research in myofascial pain has increased greatly since the basis for peripheral and central nervous system sensory sensitization became established. Much of the work on pain mechanisms in muscle and the effects of neural sensitization—such as the expansion of receptive fields—has been done by Mense and his associates. Hong and his group did many clinical studies both in the United States and in Taiwan. David Simons was often the catalyst if not the investigator in many studies that established the nature of the disorder in the trigger point dysfunction. The work of these individuals and others laid the groundwork for further studies that have been forthcoming now in ever-increasing numbers. The advent of more sophisticated imaging offers new ways to evaluate both the muscle harboring a trigger point as well as central responses to muscle trigger point pain. Nevertheless, there are many areas that need more detailed or innovative studies in order to expand our knowledge about the fundamental nature of the trigger point as well as to develop more effective ways of diagnosing and managing trigger-point-related pain. It is hoped that the comments in this chapter will direct attention to some of the areas that await further attention from those interested in the nature of muscle pain and in ways to alleviate it.

## References

1. Simons DG, Travell JG, Simons LS. *Myofascial Pain and Dysfunction: The Trigger Point Manual.* Vol. 1, 2nd ed. Baltimore, MD: Lippincott Williams & Wilkins; 1999.
2. Gerwin RD, Dommerholt J, Shah J. An expansion of Simons' integrated hypothesis of trigger point formation. *Curr Pain Headache Rep* 2004;8:468–475.

3. Gerwin RD. The taut band and other mysteries of the trigger point: An examination of the mechanisms relevant to the development and maintenance of the trigger point. *J Musculoskel Pain* 2008;15(suppl 13):115–121.

4. Hubbard DR, Berkoff GM. Myofascial trigger points show spontaneous needle EMG activity. *Spine* 1993;18:1803–1807.

5. Chen JT, Chen SM, Kuan TS, Chung KC, Hong CZ. Phentolamine effect on the spontaneous electrical activity of active loci in a myofascial trigger spot of rabbit skeletal muscle. *Arch Phys Med Rehabil* 1998;79:790–794.

6. Kuan TS, Chen JT, Chen SM, Chein CH, Hong CZ. Effect of botulinum toxin on endplate noise in myofascial trigger spots of rabbit skeletal muscle. *Am J Phys Med Rehabil* 2002;81;512–520.

7. McPartland JM, Simons DG. Myofascial trigger points: Translating molecular theory into manual therapy. *J Manual Manipulative Ther* 2006;232–239.

8. Mense S, Simons D. Lesions of rat skeletal muscle after local block of acetylcholinesterase ad neuromuscular stimulation. *J Appl Physiol* 2003;94:2494–2501.

9. Hong CZ. Persistence of local twitch response with loss of conduction to and from the spinal cord. *Arch Phys Med Rehabil* 1994;7:12–16.

10. Kuan TS, Hong CZ, Chen JT, Chen SM, Chien CH. The spinal cord connections of the myofascial trigger spots. *Eur J Pain* 2007;11:624–634.

11. Chang CW, Chen YR, Chang KF. Evidence of neuroaxonal degeneration in myofascial pain syndrome: A study of neuromuscular jitter by axonal microstimulation. *Eur J Pain* 2008;12:1026–1030.

12. Treaster D, Marras WS, Burr D, Sheedy JE, Hart D. Myofascial trigger point development from visual and postural stressors during computer work. *J Electromyogr Kinesiol* 2006;16:115–124.

13. Chen SM, Chen JT, Kuan TS, Hong J, Hong CZ. Decrease in pressure pain thresholds of latent myofascial trigger points in the middle finger extensors immediately after continuous piano practice. *J Musculoskel Pain* 2000;8(3):83–92.

14. Dommerholt J, Bron C, Franssen J. Myofascial trigger points: An evidence-informed review. *J Manual Manipulative Ther* 2006;14:203–221.

15. Fernández-de-las-Peñas C, Alonso-Blanco C, Alguacil-Diego IM, Miangolarra-Page JC. Myofascial trigger points and postero-anterior joint hypomobility in the mid-cervical spine in subjects presenting with mechanical neck pain: A pilot study. *J Manual Manipulative Ther* 2006;14:88–94.

16. Fernández-de-las-Peñas C, Fernández J, Miangolarra JC. Musculoskeletal disorders in mechanical neck pain: Myofascial trigger points versus cervical joint dysfunctions: A clinical study. *J Musculoskel Pain* 2005;13:27–35.

17. Brückle W, Suckfüll M, Fleckensteikng W, Weiss C, Müller W. Gewebe-pO2-Messung in der verspannten Rückenmuskulatur (m. erector spinae). *Z Rheumatol* 1990;49:208–216.

18. Travell J. Introductory comments. In: Foundation RCJMJ, ed. *Connective Tissues, Transactions of the Fifth Conference*. New York: Ragan C. Josiah Macy Jr. Foundation; 1954:12–22.

19. Pogrel MA, McNeill C, Kim JM. The assessment of trapezius muscle symptoms of patients with temporomandibular disorders by use of liquid crystal thermography. *Oral Surg Oral Med Oral Pathol Oral Radiol Endod* 1996;82:145–151.

20. Radhakrishna M, Burnham R. Infrared skin temperature measurement cannot be used to detect myofascial tender spots. *Arch Phys Med Rehabil* 2001;82:902–905.

21. Shah JP, Phillips TM, Danoff JV, Gerber LH. An in vitro micro-analytical technique for measuring the local biochemical milieu of human skeletal muscle. *J Appl Physiol* 2005;99:1977–1984.

22. Shah J, Danoff JV, Desai MJ, Parikh S, Nakamura LY, Phillips TM, Gerber LH. Biochemicals associated with pain and inflammation are elevated in sites near to and remote from active myofascial trigger points. *Arch Phys Med Rehabil* 2008;89:16–23.

23. Mense S. The pathogenesis of muscle pain. *Curr Pain Headache Rep* 2003;7:419–425.

24. Niddam DM, Chan RC, Lee SH, Yeh TC, Hsieh JC. Central modulation of pain evoked from myofascial trigger point. *Clin J Pain* 2007;23:440–448.

25. Niddan DM, Chan RC, Lee SH, Yeh TZ, Hsieh JC. Central representation of hyperalgesia from myofascial trigger point. *Neuroimage* 2008;39:1299–1306.

26. Mense S, Simons DG. *Muscle Pain: Understanding its Nature, Diagnosis, and Treatment.* Philadelphia, PA: Lippincott Williams & Wilkins; 2001.

27. Hwang M. Kang YK, Kim DH. Referred pain pattern of the pronator quadratus muscle. *Pain* 200;116:328–242.

28. Hwang M, Kang JK, Shin JY, Kim DH. Referred pain pattern of the abductor pollicis longus muscle. *Am J Phys Med Rehabil* 2005;84:593–597.

29. Fernández-de-las-Peñas C, Cuadrado RD, Gerwin RD, Pareja JA. Referred pain from the trochlear region in tension-type headache: A myofascial trigger point from the superior oblique muscle. *Headache* 2005;45:731–737.

30. Badley EM, Webster GK, Rasooly I. The impact of musculoskeletal disorders in the population: Are they just aches and pains? Findings from the 1990 Ontario Health Survey. *J Rheumatol* 1995;22:733–739.

31. Skootsky SA, Jaeger B, Oye RK. Prevalence of myofascial pain in general internal medicine practice. *West J Med* 1989;151:157–160.

32. Fishbain DA, Goldberg M, Meagher BR Steele R, Rosomoff H. Male and female chronic pain patients categorized by DSM-III psychiatric diagnostic criteria. *Pain* 1986;26:181–197.

33. Gerwin RD. A study of 96 subjects examined both for fibromyalgia and myofascial pain. *J Musculoskel Pain* 1995;3(suppl 1):121

34. Rashiq S, Galer BS. Proximal myofascial dysfunction in complex regional pain syndrome: A retrospective prevalence study. *Clin J Pain* 1999;15:151–153.

35. Kaergaard A, Andersen JH. Musculoskeletal disorders of the neck and shoulders in female sewing machine operators: Prevalence, incidence, and prognosis. *Occup Environ Med* 2000;57:528–534.

36. Treaster DE, Burr D. Gender differences in prevalence of upper extremity musculoskeletal disorders. *Ergonomics* 2004;15:495–526.

37. Rollman G, Lautenbacher S. Sex differences in musculoskeletal pain. *Clin J Pain* 2001;17:20–24.

38. Bergenudd H, Lindgärde F, Nilsson B, Petersson CJ. Shoulder pain in middle age. A study of prevalence and relation to occupational workload and psychosocial factors. *Clin Orthop* 1988;231:234–238.

39. Ge H-Y, Madeleine P, Cairns BE, Arendt-Nielsen L. Hypoalgesia in the referred pain areas after bilateral injections of hypertonic saline into the trapezius muscles of men and women: A potential experimental model of gender-specific differences. *Clin J Pain* 2006;22:37–44.

40. Cairns BE, Gambarota G, Svensson P, Arendt-Nielsen L, Berde CB. Glutamate-induced sensitization of rat muscle fibers. *Neuroscience* 2002;16:105–117.

41. Arendt-Nielsen L, Svensson P, Sessle BJ, Cairns BE, Wang K. Interactions between glutamate and capsaicin in inducing muscle pain and sensitization in humans. *Eur J Pain* 2008;661–670.

42. Isselee H, De Laat A, De Mot B, Lysens R. Pressure-pain threshold variation in temporomandibular disorder myalgia over the course of the menstrual cycle. *J Orofac Pain* 2002;16:105–117.

43. Dannecker EA, Knoll V, Robinson ME. Sex differences in muscle pain: Self-care behaviors and effects on daily activities. *J Pain* 2008;9:200–209.

44. Tang B, Ji Y, Traub RJ. Estrogen alters spinal NMDA receptor activity via a PKA signaling pathway in a visceral pain model in the rat. *Pain* 2008;137:540–549.

45. Nijs J. Generalized joint hypermobility: An issue in fibromyalgia and chronic fatigue syndrome. *J Bodywork Movement Ther* 2005;9:310–317.

46. Gerwin RD, Shannon S, Hong CZ, Hubbard, Gevirtz R. Interrater reliability in myofascial trigger point examination. *Pain* 1997;69:65–73.

47. Sciotti VM, Mittak VL, DiCarco L, Ford LM, Plezbert J, Santipadri E, Wigglesworth J, Ball K. Clinical precision of myofascial trigger point location in the trapezius muscle. *Pain* 2001;93:259–266.

48. Bron C, Franssen J, Wensing M, Oostendorp RAB. Interrater reliability of palpation of myofascial trigger points in three shoulder muscles. *J Manual Manipulative Ther* 2007;15: 203–215.

49. Gerwin R, Dommerholt J. Trigger point inactivation and the criteria for trigger point. *J Musculoskel Pain* 2004;12(suppl 9):24.

50. Tough EA, White AR, Richards S, Campbell J. Variability of criteria used to diagnosis myofascial trigger point pain syndrome: Evidence from a review of the literature. *Clin J Pain* 2007;23:278–286.

51. Fischer AA. Documentation of myofascial trigger points. *Arch Phys Med Rehabil* 1988;69:286–291.

52. Fischer AA. New developments in diagnosis of myofascial pain and fibromyalgia. *Phys Med Rehabil Clin North Am* 1997;8:1–21.

53. Staffel K, del Mayoral del Moral, Lacomba MT, Jung I, Russell IJ. Factors that influence the reliability of clinical assessment for the classification of the myofascial pain syndrome. *J Musculoskel Pain* 2007;15(suppl 13):36.

54. Simons DG, Hong C-Z, Simons LS. Endplate potentials are common to mid-fiber myofascial trigger points. *Am J Phys Med Rehabil* 2002;81:212–222.

55. Lucas KR, Polus BI, Rich PS. Latent myofascial trigger points: Their effect on muscle activation and movement efficiency. *J Bodywork Movement Ther* 2004;8:160–166.

56. Shultz SP, Driban JB, Swanik CB. The evaluation of electrodermal properties in the identification of myofascial trigger points. *Arch Phys Med Rehabil* 2007;88:780–784.

57. Chen Q, Bensamoun S, Basford J, Thompson JM, An K-N. Identification and quantification of myofascial taut bands with magnetic resonance elastography. *Arch Phys Med Rehabil* 2007;88:1658–1661.

58. Chen Q, Basford J, An K-N. Ability of magnetic resonance elastography to assess taut bands. *Clin Biomech* 2008;23:623–629.

59. Gibson W, Arendt-Nielsen L, Graven-Nielsen T. Referred pain and hyperalgesia in human tendon and muscle belly tissue. *Pain* 2006;120:113–123.

60. Gibson W, Arendt-Nielsen L, Graven-Nielsen T. Delayed onset muscle soreness at tendon-bone junction and muscle tissue is associated with facilitated referred pain. *Exp Brain Res* 2006;174:351–360.

61. Fernández-de-las-Peñas C, Sohrbeck-Campo M, Fernández-Carnero J, Miangolarra JC Manual therapies in myofascial trigger point treatment: A systematic review. *J Bodywork Movement Ther* 2005;9:27–34.

62. Rickards LD. The effectiveness of non-invasive treatments for active myofascial trigger point pain: A systematic review of the literature. *Int J Osteopathic Med* 2006;9:120–136.

63. Fryer G, Hodgson L. The effect of manual pressure release on myofascial trigger points in the upper trapezius muscle. *J Bodywork Movement Ther* 2005; 9:248–255.

64. Srbely JZ, Dickey JP. Randomized controlled study of the antinociceptive effect of ultrasound on trigger point sensitivity: Novel applications in myofascial therapy. *Clin Rehabil* 2007;21:411–417.

65. Srbely JZ, Dickey JP, Lowerison M, Edwards AM, Nolet PS, Wong LL. Stimulation of myofascial trigger points with ultrasound induces segmental anti-nociceptive effects: A randomized controlled study. *Pain* 2008;139:260–266.

66. Ilbuldu E, Cakmak A, Disci R, Aydin R. Comparison of laser, dry needling and placebo laser treatments in myofascial pain syndrome. *Photomed Laser Surg* 2004;22:306–311.

67. Gur A, Sarac AJ, Cevik R, Altindag O, Sarac S. Efficacy of 904 nm gallium arsenide low level laser therapy in the management of chronic myofascial pain in the neck: A double-blind and randomized-controlled trial. *Lasers Surg Med* 2004;35:229–235.

68. Dundar U, Evcik D, Samli F, Pusak H, Kavuncu V. The effect of gallium arsenide aluminum laser therapy in the management of cervical myofascial pain syndrome: A double blind, placebo-controlled study. *Clin Rheumatol* 2007;26:930–934.

69. Dommerholt J, Mayoral del Moral O, Gröbli C. Trigger point dry needling. *J Manual Manipulative Ther* 2006;14:E70–E87.

70. Furlan A, Tulder M, Cherkin D, et al. Acupuncture and dry-needling for low back pain: An updated systematic review within the framework of the Cochrane Collaboration. *Spine* 2005;30:944–963.

71. Iwama H, Ohmori S, Kaneko T, Watanabe K. Water-diluted local anesthetic for trigger-point injection in chronic myofascial pain syndrome: Evaluation of types of local anesthetic and concentrations in water. *Reg Anesth Pain Med* 2001;26:333–336.

72. Cummings TM, White AR. Needling therapies in the management of myofascial trigger point pain: A systematic review. *Arch Phys Med Rehabil* 2001;82:986–992.

73. Scott NA, Guo B, Barton PM, Gerwin RD. Trigger point injections for chronic non-malignant musculoskeletal pain: A systematic review. *Pain Med* (in press).

74. Tough EA, White AR, Cummings TM, Richards SH, Campbell JL. Acupuncture and dry needling in the management of myofascial trigger point pain: A systematic review and meta-analysis of randomized controlled trials. *Eur J Pain* 2009;13:3–10.

75. Ga H, Ko HJ, Choi JH, Kim CH. Intramuscular and nerve root stimulation versus lidocaine injection of trigger points in myofascial pain syndrome. *J Rehabil Med* 2007;39:374–378.

76. Ga H, Choi JH, Yoon HY. Dry needling of trigger points with and without paraspinal needling in myofascial pain syndromes in elderly patients. *J Altern Compl Med* 2007;13:617–623.

77. Itoh K, Katsumi Y, Hirota S, Kitakoji H. Randomized trial of trigger point acupuncture compared with other acupuncture for treatment of chronic neck pain. *Compl Ther Med* 2007;15:172–179.

78. Itoh K, Katsumi Y, Kitakoji H. Trigger point acupuncture treatment of chronic low back pain in elderly patients; A blinded RCT. *Acupunct Med* 2004;22:170–177.

79. Itoh K, Katsumi Y, Hirota S, Kitakoji H. Effects of trigger point acupuncture on chronic low back pain in elderly patients: A sham-controlled randomized trial. *Acupunct Med* 2006;24:5–12.

80. Hsieh YL, Kao MJ, Kuan TS, Chen SM, Shen JT, Hong CZ. Dry needling to a key myofascial trigger point may reduce the irritability of satellite MTrPs. *Am J Phys Med Rehabil* 2007;86:397–403.

81. Fine PG, Milano R, Hare BD. The effects of myofascial trigger point injections are naloxone reversible. *Pain* 1988;32:15–20.

82. Ho K-Y, Tan K-H. Botulinum toxin A for myofascial trigger point injection: A qualitative systematic review. *Eur J Pain* 2007;11:519–527.
83. Statz T, Müller W. Treatment of chronic low back pain with tropisetron. *Scand J Rheumatol* 2004;119(suppl):76–78.
84. Müller W, Fiebich BL, Stratz T. New treatment options using 5-HT3 receptor antagonists in rheumatic diseases. *Curr Top Med Chem* 2006;6:2035–2042.
85. Dommerholt J, Gerwin RD. Neurophysiological effects of trigger point needling therapies. In: Fernández-de-las-Peñas C, Arendt-Nielsen L, Gerwin RD, eds. *Diagnosis and Management of Tension-Type and Cervicogenic Headache*. Sudbury, MA: Jones & Bartlett; 2010:247–260.
86. Baldry P. Management of myofascial trigger point pain. *Acupunct Med* 2002;20:2–10.
87. Fernández-de-las-Peñas C, Arendt-Nielsen L, Simons DG. Contributions of myofascial trigger points to chronic tension type headache. *J Manual Manipulative Ther* 2006;14:222–231.
88. Fernández-de-las-Peñas C, Cuadrado ML, Arendt-Nielsen L, Simons DG, Pareja JA. Myofascial trigger points and sensitization: An updated pain model for tension-type headache. *Cephalalgia* 2007;27:383–393.
89. Fernández-de-las-Peñas C, Cuadrado ML, Gerwin RD, Pareja JA. Myofascial disorders in the troclear region in unilateral migraine. *Clin J Pain* 2006;22:548–553.
90. Fernández-de-las-Peñas C, Alonso-Blanco C, Cuadrado ML, Gerwin RD, Paruza JA. Trigger points in the subocciptial muscles and forward head posture in tension-type headache. *Headache* 2006;46:454–460.
91. Giamberadino MA, Tafuri E, Savini A, Fabrizio A, Affaitati G, Lerza R, Di Ianni L, Lapenna D, Mezzetti A. Contribution of myofascial trigger points to migraine symptoms. *J Pain* 2007;8:869–878.
92. Garcia-Leiva JM, Hildago J, Rico-Villademoros F, Moreno V, Calandre EP. Effectiveness of Ropivacaine trigger points inactivation in the prophylactic management of patients with severe migraine. *Pain Med* 2007;8:65–70.
93. Mense S. Neurobiological concepts of fibromyalgia—the possible role of descending spinal tracts. *Scand J Rheumatol* 2000;113(suppl):24–29.
94. Jarrell J. Myofascial dysfunction in the pelvis. *Curr Pain Headache Rep* 2004;8:452–456.
95. Jarrell J, Robert M. Myofascial dysfunction and pelvic pain. *Can J CME* 2003;Feb:107–116.
96. Jarrell J. Gynecological pain, endometriosis, visceral disease, and the viscero-somatic connection. *J Musculoskel Pain* 2008;16(1–2):21–27.
97. Nazareno J, Ponich T, Gregor J. Long-term follow-up of trigger point injections for abdominal wall pain. *Can J Gastroenterology* 2005;19:561–565.
98. Kuan LC, Li YT, Chen FM, Tseng CJ, Wu SF, Duo TC. Efficacy of treating abdominal wall pain by local injection. *Taiwanese J Obstet Gynecol* 2006;45:239–243.
99. Doggweiler-Wiygul R, Wiygul JP. Interstitial cystitis, pelvic pain, and the relationship to myofascial pain and dysfunction: A report on four patients. *World J Urol* 2002;20:310–314.
100. Srivivasan AK, Kaye JD, Moldwin R. Myofascial dysfunction associated with chronic pelvic floor pain: Management strategies. *Curr Pain Headache Rep* 2007;11:359–364.
101. Fernández-de-las-Peñas C, Palonecque del Cerro L, Fernandez Carnero J. Manual treatment of post-whiplash injury. *J Bodywork Movement Ther* 2005;9:109–119.
102. Gerwin RD, Dommerholt J. Myofascial trigger points in chronic cervical whiplash syndrome. *J Musculoskel Pain* 1998;6(suppl 2):28.
103. Cannon DE, Dillingham TR, Miao H, Andary MT, Pezzin LE. Musculoskeletal disorders in referral for suspected cervical radiculopathy. *Arch Phys Med Rehabil* 2007;88:1256–1259.

# Index